YOU NEED TO KNOW . . .

- Just because it says "salad" doesn't mean it's low calorie. Some fast-food salads can push 900 calories and contain nearly 50 grams of fat.
- Ultra-popular blended coffee drinks are ruinously high in calories. You could be consuming 750 calories, 20 grams of fat, and 121 grams of carbs for a drink.
- That "healthy" bran muffin could easily be pushing 500 calories.

. . . THAT THERE ARE ALTERNATIVES

- A company that makes muffins—in 9 delicious flavors, including chocolate and peanut butter chip—that weigh in at about 200 calories.
- Soy chips—available in flavors such as creamy ranch and white cheddar—can make a delicious alternative to potato chips, and have only 70 calories and 1.5 grams of fat in a serving.
- While one tablespoon of tartar sauce packs in 74 calories and 7.5 grams of fat, one tablespoon of cocktail sauce has only 15 calories and is nearly fat-free—a hands-down winner.

THE DIET DETECTIVE'S
Calorie
BARGAIN BIBLE

More than 1,000 Calorie Bargains®
in Supermarkets, Kitchens, Offices, Restaurants,
at the Movies, for Special Occasions, and More

CHARLES STUART PLATKIN

POCKET BOOKS
NEW YORK   LONDON   TORONTO   SYDNEY

Pocket Books
A Division of Simon & Schuster, Inc.
1230 Avenue of the Americas
New York, NY 10020

First Pocket Books paperback edition May 2008

POCKET and colophon are registered trademarks of Simon & Schuster, Inc.

For information about special discounts for bulk purchases, please contact Simon & Schuster Special Sales at 1-800-456-6798 or business@simonandschuster.com.

Cover design by Cheung Tai, cover photos © Getty Images

Manufactured in the United States of America

10   9   8   7   6   5   4   3

ISBN-13: 978-1-4165-6660-1
ISBN-10:   1-4165-6660-0

This book is dedicated to my daughter,
Parker South, a constant inspiration;
to my parents, Linda and Norton, who have
always and continue to be a driving force in my life;
and to my wife, a patient, considerate,
and caring friend, Shannon.

Contents

THE DIET DETECTIVE'S
Calorie
BARGAIN BIBLE

Introduction

This book is about living well, eating well by choosing well, and losing weight. I will take you by the hand, teach you how to seek out Calorie Bargains—foods that are as satisfying as snacks like chips and candy but with fewer calories—and lead you through the confusing food maze that characterizes eating in America today.

Want to know how to find tasty, satisfying compromises that will not leave you feeling deprived? Look no further, because here are the answers. Dying for Domino's Pizza? Switch from stuffed crust to thin crust and forget the extra cheese, and you'll save 200 calories. Fainting for chocolate ice cream? Try Weight Watchers Smart Ones chocolate mousse bars at only 40 calories each. Want whipped cream? Did you know that Reddi-wip has only 15 calories in a two-tablespoon serving? With *The Diet Detective's Calorie Bargain Bible* in hand, you will be able to eat your way through any occasion, including ball games, barbecues, birthday parties, business meetings, and holiday celebrations, without gaining weight.

The Diet Detective has done the legwork for you—separating truth from myth, dispelling misconceptions, and letting you know which are the best choices for meals and snacks at every time of day, every day of the week, throughout the year. No food has escaped the scrutiny of the Diet Detective.

As the satisfied readers of my popular column know only

too well, I don't beat around the bush, and I don't leave anything to chance. I name names—brands, fast-food chains, family and casual dining restaurants—so that wherever you go, you'll know what to eat. Leaving no food source undetected, I take you from restaurants to supermarkets and into the kitchen, even letting you know what choices to make on special occasions like Thanksgiving and Super Bowl Sunday.

In short, *The Diet Detective's Calorie Bargain Bible* takes you back to what experts have always known to be the simple, basic truth: Successful weight loss depends on finding a variety of filling foods that you enjoy eating, getting the most food for the fewest calories (which includes eating fewer carbs and/or fats), and burning more energy than you consume. This book is not about a diet I created for you to follow. More than six years in the making, it is the only guide that solves the mystery of how to eat more of the foods you like, wherever you are—and weigh less.

Part One

FIND YOUR CALORIE BARGAINS

This is a book about bargains. We look for bargains in clothing, electronics, food, and travel—to name just a few. We go to discount price clubs, cut coupons, and wait until things go on sale so that we can get more for less. We want to spend wisely and know that we're getting the most for our money.

What if we were as cost conscious about our calorie consumption as we are about our spending?

Unfortunately, we have a finite number of calories in our bodies' budget, just as we have limited funds in our pocketbooks. So how can we be sure that we're making good use of the foods we consume? The answer: Look for Calorie Bar-

Using *The Diet Detective's Calorie Bargain Bible*:

1. Figure out your daily calorie needs.
2. Learn about Calorie Bargains.
3. Take the Three-Day Food Challenge.
4. Keep *The Diet Detective's Calorie Bargain Bible* handy to find out which foods are Calorie Bargains® and Calorie Rip-offs™ while eating out, eating at home, or eating anywhere.
5. Figure out *your* Calorie Bargains and Calorie Rip-offs. (You can use *The Diet Detective's Count Down,* which lists more than 7,500 foods, with their exercise equivalents, to help you keep on track.) Or you can go to the Diet Detective website at www.dietDetective.com and use the free food search tool.
6. Stay on the lookout for Calorie Bargains and Calorie Rip-offs.

gains. These are foods that are relatively low in calories and high in nutrients, but still taste great and satisfy your strongest temptations. You use these "cheaper" foods to replace others you eat regularly that are more calorically "expensive." But remember, if it doesn't satiate you, a Calorie Bargain can easily turn into a Calorie Rip-off, because you'll end up eating more of it, consuming more calories, and gaining more weight.

> A Calorie Bargain is not just something that is lower in calories, it should be healthier—in fact, the ultimate Calorie Bargains are fruits and vegetables.

You can find your own Calorie Bargains using these three easy steps:

STEP 1: Think of a food that you typically eat each day. It might be a guilty pleasure or simply a high-calorie food you think might be worth replacing—if you had a good substitute.

Example: The food I eat now that I'm willing to change: Lay's regular potato chips, 150 calories per serving.

The serving size I would eat in a typical sitting (be honest!): three servings, about four handfuls.

Total calories: $150 \times 3 = 450$ calories.

STEP 2: Now try to think of a substitute for that food. It's got to be something you think you might like, and it's got to have fewer calories.

Example: My potential Calorie Bargain: air-popped popcorn, 25 calories per serving. Serving size I would eat in a typical sitting (be honest!): three servings, about four handfuls.

Total calories: $25 \times 3 = 75$ calories.

You just saved a whopping 375 calories. So if you normally eat chips three times a week, and you replace them with popcorn, you could lose as much as 15 pounds in a year!

Learn to Get Good Value

You have to learn to know a good thing when you see it. Understanding value in food is important, and it's important to think before you eat. Again, *remember*, Calorie Bargains are only to be used to *replace* something that you are already eating on a regular basis. A Calorie Bargain should *never* be added to your existing diet; it is only a replacement for higher fat and higher calorie foods. And if it doesn't satiate you, you'll end up eating more food, consuming more calories, gaining more weight, and losing that Calorie Bargain. So be careful. Experiment, negotiate, and keep track of your failures and successes.

Your initial goal should be to reduce your calorie intake by 100 to 200 calories a day for maintenance, and about 250 to 400 calories per day for weight loss. This means you should substitute at least 20 percent of your current diet with Calorie Bargains for weight loss and 10 percent of your current diet for weight maintenance. As you become a skilled detective, however, you'll be able to find even bigger bargains.

Bargain Hunting

The food I eat now that I'm willing to substitute: _____

_____

Serving size I would eat in a typical sitting: _____

Total calories: _____

My potential Calorie Bargain: _____

_____

Serving size I would probably eat in a typical setting: _____

_____

Total calories: _____

How many calories I saved by making the switch: _____

Rate It: Is this a good choice? Why do I think it will or won't last? _____

_____

_____

STEP 3: Make sure you can live with the food choice you just made, and that you will not overindulge to make up for the fact that you're eating a food that is lower in calories and higher in nutrient density. If you consume more of the Calorie Bargain than you did of the substituted food, you will defeat the purpose.

Here's one of mine. I used to eat chips, cookies, and ice cream, averaging about 600 calories in an evening. Now I substitute pan popcorn. I don't love air-popped corn, so I started experimenting and found a way to use regular kernels, a skillet, and cooking spray. Put the kernels in a deep pot lightly coated with vegetable cooking spray, cover, and turn on the heat. Make sure to open the lid slightly from time to time to release the steam. Shake the pot during cooking. After a number of burned batches, I was finally able to get it right: 5 cups (popped) equals 150 calories. Calorie savings: about 450.

Celebrity Calorie Bargains

I've spent years finding Calorie Bargains for myself and getting tips on others from readers, so I began to wonder what health "celebrities" do to create the Calorie Bargains that help them stay fit. Here are a few notables:

Mike Huckabee, governor of Arkansas, lost more than 100 pounds and made healthy living a priority for his administration. Used to eat premium ice cream: 2 cups, 550 calories.

 Calorie Bargain: Yarnell's Guilt Free "CarbAware" ice cream made with Splenda. "You can't tell the difference between this and regular premium ice cream, which it has replaced in my diet. Yarnell's is amazingly good, and it's what we serve at the governor's mansion. Guests are shocked to find out it's a sugar-free, low-fat, low-carb product." Breakdown: 2 cups, 250 calories.

 Calorie savings: 300.

Bobby Flay, chef/restaurateur, cookbook author, and television personality. Used to eat: "When I was younger, I loved eating breakfast sandwiches consisting of fried eggs, bacon, and cheese every morning on my way to work." Breakdown: 440 calories.

 Calorie Bargain: "Now I prepare healthy smoothies for breakfast or yogurt with fresh fruit." Breakdown: 16-ounce low-calorie smoothie (no sugar), about 150 calories; low-fat yogurt with fruit, 220 calories.

 Calorie savings: about 250.

Denise Austin, fitness expert, author, fitness DVD personality (star of more than forty exercise videos and DVDs). Used to eat: baked potato (100 calories) with 2 tablespoons of sour cream (about 120 calories) and 1 tablespoon butter (60 calories) for a total of 280 calories. Frappuccino and whipped cream at Starbucks, 390 calories.

 Calorie Bargain: "I've replaced the sour cream and butter with two tablespoons of salsa for thirty calories. And you can make your own coffee treat with a lot less calories. Use ice cubes, a half cup of skim milk (about fifty calories), and a half cup of decaf coffee. Froth it up and blend it."

 Calorie savings: 150 for the potato extras; 340 for the coffee drink.

What's a Calorie Anyway?

Calories have a bad rap. When you hear the word, it conjures up images of eating cakes, candies, and other sin foods. *The Diet Detective's Calorie Bargain Bible* is here to help you appreciate calories rather than seeing them as something that ends up ruining your day. Calories should be viewed as energy that keeps you going. The only problem is that if you get too many of them, you end up stockpiling unused energy, and that's what turns into fat.

Ok. What exactly *is* a calorie? It's a measure of energy: the capacity to do work. Science defines a calorie as the amount of energy required to raise the temperature of 1 gram of water by 1 degree Celsius. But in our everyday struggle to eat well and exercise, it is easy to forget the simple functional purpose of calories: to fuel our body's day-to-day activities.

Calories at Rest

If you want to start keeping track of your calories in order to lose weight, the first thing you need to know is how many calories you *should* eat each day. Sounds simple, right? You thought carbs and fat were controversial? Well, even calories have their issues.

How many calories should you try to cut from your diet?

The first step is to figure out how many calories you need in a day. To do this, you must determine your resting metabolic rate (RMR). That's the number of calories you need to support the unconscious work of your body, such as your heartbeat and breathing.

There are a variety of methods for estimating caloric needs, including a complex formula called the Harris Benedict equation (HBE), considered the "gold standard." It takes into account your height, weight, gender, and age. However, two people with the same height, weight, gender, and age can have entirely different RMRs. In fact, one of the biggest determinants of RMR is body composition; specifically, your ratio of muscle to fat. The more muscle you have, the more calories you burn at rest.

Once you've determined your RMR, you probably think that all you have to do to lose weight is cut down on the number of calories you consume. But that's not the whole story. Your metabolic rate basically tells you how many calories your body needs to operate when you do *nothing*—that's all. If you simply cut calories from your RMR, you will lose weight, but the wrong kind of weight: mostly lean muscle tissue.

> **Q. Will I still lose weight if my RMR is not 100 percent accurate?**
>
> A. Yes. Figuring out your caloric needs should be used as a guideline, sort of a starting point. That's why it's acceptable that these measurements are not 100 percent accurate. But you should also weigh yourself at least every thirty days, because the scale doesn't lie. Then adjust your eating accordingly.

What about Activity?

Your resting metabolic rate is only a part of the equation for determining your daily caloric needs. After you figure that out, you need to factor in your activity level, and this is where the problems begin. To determine how many calories you're burning from activity, you would typically choose from a pre-determined scale ranging from "sedentary" all the way to "extreme activity." Sedentary activities include sitting, driving, lying down, or standing in one place for most of the day, and not doing any type of exercise, which would mean tacking on about 20 percent more calories to your RMR. (Keep in mind, your RMR doesn't change, it's your activity level that can influence calories burned.) Extreme activities include heavy manual labor, army and marine recruit training, or competitive athletics, and would allow you to eat more than double the calories required simply to maintain your body weight when you're at rest.

Trying to estimate someone's activity level is no easy task, and standards can easily be misapplied. What is moderate activity for an elite athlete is quite different from what's moderate for the average Jane. For instance, according to the guidelines, a competitive athlete might burn 2,400 calories per day at rest. Double that, according to the guidelines, and the same person's caloric needs would be 4,800 per day. But someone training for the Tour de France cycling competition, for example, might actually burn 10,000 calories per day—so the formula can be significantly inaccurate.

That said, the following is the most widely accepted method of determining your calorie needs (Harris Benedict equation):

STEP 1: Calculate Your Resting or Resting Metabolic Rate (RMR)

> **Female:** 655.1 + (4.35 × weight in pounds) + (4.699 × height in inches) − (4.676 × age)

Male: $66.5 + (6.25 \times$ weight in pounds$) + (12.71 \times$ height in inches$) - (6.775 \times$ age$)$

STEP 2: Calculate Your Caloric Needs

Now that you've determined your RMR, multiply it by your activity factor:

- **Sedentary:** 1.2 (you sit, drive, lie down, or stand in one place for most of the day and don't do any type of exercise).
- **Light activity:** 1.3 to 1.4 (you're sedentary for most of the day and do light activity, such as walking, for no more than two hours daily).
- **Moderate activity:** 1.5 (you're on your feet most of the workday, with light lifting only, and do no structured exercise).
- **Very active:** 1.6 to 1.7 (your typical workday includes several hours of physical labor, such as light industry and construction-type jobs).

Diet Detective's What You Need to Know

Daily Caloric Budget—the Simple Way: You can determine a rough estimate of your own caloric budget by first assigning 10 calories per pound for a female and 11 calories per pound for a male. Then multiply that number by your activity level: 1.2 if you're sedentary and up to 1.8 if you are very active. For example, a 130-pound female who is somewhat active would have a budget of 1,300 calories multiplied by 1.5, or 1,950 calories per day. If you want to lose weight, you'll need to eat fewer calories than you have in your budget. If you eat more than your budget, you'll gain. For a more exact calculation (or if you're not a math student), you can go to: www.DietDetective.com for a free calculator that uses a more exact formula for determining your daily caloric budget. You plug in height, weight, age, and gender, and it will give you your RMR along with your daily caloric budget.

- **Extreme activity:** 2 to 2.4 (you do heavy manual labor, army or marine recruit training, or are a competitive athlete).

Your RMR multiplied by your activity factor is your total daily calorie allowance for weight maintenance.

To lose weight, you will need to increase your level of activity and/or decrease your caloric intake until you are burning more calories than you consume.

What's a Cup of Coffee?

Just putting milk and/or sugar in your tea or coffee can add up to quite a few calories.

- Half-and-half (⅛ cup, or 2 tablespoons): 39 calories.
- Whole milk (⅛ cup, or 2 tablespoons): 19 calories.
- Skim milk (⅛ cup, or 2 tablespoons): 11 calories.
- Sugar: 16 calories per teaspoon.

Just 3 cups of coffee with 2 tablespoons of half-and-half and 2 teaspoons of sugar could add up to 213 calories a day, or 22 pounds in a year.

Try using Splenda instead of sugar. Is Splenda healthy? While I'm sure it's healthier to eat natural foods, the evidence seems to indicate that Splenda is not unhealthy or harmful. Also try skim milk instead of half and half.

Take the Three-Day Food Challenge

I know what some of you are thinking: Another food-diary recommendation—not again! Yes, it can be a pain to keep a food diary if you've never done it before, or if you're not the journal type. All I'm saying is to try it for a few days. It's a challenge to take a good, hard look at what you eat for three straight days. But if you do it accurately, you can learn a lot about your eating habits in a very short time. You can discover clues that will help you develop a diet plan that's going to work for you. But to figure out how to make changes in the way you eat, you've got to pin down *how you eat already*. You need to figure out your comfort zone. Here's a visual of what I mean:

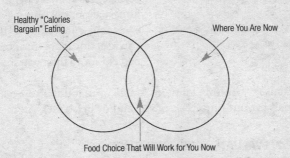

For your diet to work, it's got to be comfortable. It's got to be somewhere between the circle on the left and the circle on the right. It has to be in *the middle zone*—where you're comfortable and satisfied with what you eat, but also at the weight you want to be.

Fit Tip: Can't keep a food diary? Use your camera phone or a digital camera to snap photos of every food you eat. Then at the end of each night, put your photos on your computer or simply review them on your phone, write them down, and tally them up. Do this for at least three days.

The Advantages of Keeping a Three-Day Food Diary

- It creates a tangible, in-your-face look at your everyday eating habits.
- Being able to see what you're eating at all times can help you realize what you shouldn't be eating.
- You can pinpoint which times of the day are your Unconscious Eating Times and your Eating Alarm Times.

STEP 1: KEEP A FOOD DIARY

Keep It Real: Record every single thing that goes into your mouth, including beverages, bites off someone else's plate, or samples at the grocery store.

Portion Distortion: Learn to be honest about portion size. As a general rule, assume that you're eating 30 percent to 40 percent more than you think.

No Excuses: Use this guide to track your food! Keep blank journals in your office, car, purse, and/or briefcase!

STEP 2: EVALUATE YOUR FOOD DIARY

At the end of three days, your diary should provide you with a clear picture of what, how, when, and why you eat what you do. Here's what you should look for:

Triggers: A trigger is anything that makes it difficult for you to stick to your weight-loss goal. It could be a mood, an event—

Create Your Own Food Diary

Here's a rundown of exactly what you should be recording:

Meal, Time, and Place

Record the approximate time you sit down to eat. This will help you find the eating schedule that works best for you. Also, record which meal it is (breakfast, midmorning, and so on) and where you eat it—whether it is on the run, at your desk, at a restaurant, and so forth.

Hunger Level

Record your level of hunger on a scale of 1 to 5, with 1 being the least hungry and 5 being the most hungry. Aim to be between 3 and 4 when you're eating. You never want to let yourself get too hungry, and you certainly don't want to eat when you're not hungry at all.

Dining Companions

Write down who you ate with and what you talked about. This information could offer clues to unconscious eating or stress eating.

Feelings and Mood

Record how you feel before, during, and/or after you eat. Before is probably the most important because it can have the greatest effect on how and what you eat. Try to keep track of whether you have general feelings like being happy or sad, or specific ones like "stressed at work," "angry at spouse," or "having a great day." You will see that this really helps you to pinpoint which emotions affect your eating habits the most.

Food and Drink

Record all the individual foods you eat and beverages you drink, including accurate portion sizes and even brand names (nutrient content can vary by brand). Anything that goes in your mouth should be in your food diary—including little nibbles from the refrigerator and bites from other people's plates!

Nutrient Information

Use the free food search information on DietDetective.com to determine and record the calories (and/or carbs) for each food/meal you eat. You can also download a version of DietDetective.com Food Diary Form to print and use to write down the information mentioned above. Total your calories at the end of the day to make sure you are staying within your goal. You can do this while relaxing at home each evening.

even a certain food. Look for patterns of emotions, foods, or times of day that contribute to excessive calorie consumption.

Meal Patterns: Skipping meals or waiting too long to eat can lead to overeating later in the day. If your meals are more than four hours apart, try scheduling a snack in between.

Unconscious Eating: It's easy to consume massive amounts of high-calorie and high-fat foods while sitting in front of the TV or at the computer. Keeping a food diary helps you keep this unconscious eating in check.

Failure to Plan: If high-calorie and high-fat fast foods or vending machine snacks appear frequently in your food diary, it may be a sign of poor planning. A food diary allows you to see your weak spots and plan for them.

Unbalanced Meals: Are some of your meals heavy on the carbs? Or maybe a protein overdose? Not choosing balanced meals can lead to excessive hunger, which in turn can result in overeating.

Fruits and Veggies: These are your weight-loss allies. Your ultimate goal is to eat at least five servings of fruits and veggies a day. (By the way, that's a minimum recommendation of five total, not five of each.) If you're not having any now, work your way up slowly.

STEP 3: REVIEW YOUR DIARY

Your diary will show you which foods you eat most often. This is where *The Diet Detective's Calorie Bargain Bible* comes in. Read this book to discover which Calorie Bargains are most appealing to you and use them as substitutes or replacements for those foods that are higher in calories. This book will also teach you to spot Calorie Rip-offs—those foods not worth the splurge. Check out the free food search database on Diet Detective .com for calorie information on all your favorite foods.

Q: Do fats, carbohydrates, protein, and alcohol all have the same number of calories per gram?

A: No. Fat is the most expensive calorically, with 9 calories per gram; then alcohol with 7 calories per gram. Carbohydrates and protein both have 4 calories per gram. Total calories are nothing more than a combination of the fats, carbohydrates, and protein in a particular food. So if a food has 1 gram of fat (9 calories), 2 grams of carbohydrate (8 calories), and 1 gram of protein (4 calories), it would have a total of about 21 calories.

Calorie Bargain Spotlight

Make a Better Burger

If you make your burger using lean ground beef instead of regular ground beef (or get even better results by using ground turkey), you'll have the same size burger, but you'll be getting more calories from protein and fewer from fat, and the total number of calories will be lower even though the burger is the same size. Or you could mix regular ground beef with mushrooms, peppers, and onion before forming the burger. Again, you'll have the same size burger, but it will be much lower in calories—and you'll be getting the health benefits of all those vegetables as well.

The Power of One

When I talk to people who are trying to lose weight, I often come across the dieter's paradox: They "hardly eat anything," but still they don't lose weight. This seems to be one of our biggest problems; we never believe we're eating anything.

It's been reported in the *New England Journal of Medicine* that people attempting to lose weight tend to underestimate the amount they eat by as much as 47 percent and to overestimate their physical activity by as much as 51 percent. When scientists at the U.S. Department of Agriculture's (USDA) Beltsville Human Nutrition Research Center in Maryland asked ninety-eight men and women how much they ate in a twenty-four-hour period, they found that 6 out of 7 women underreported by an average of 621 calories, and 6 out of 10 men underreported by an average of 581 calories.

When the American Institute for Cancer Research did a study asking Americans to determine the portion sizes of eight specific foods, only 1 percent got them all right. Sixty-one percent couldn't get more than four correct.

That's why taking the Three-day Food Challenge and keeping an accurate record of *everything* you consume—including a single grape or a stick of gum—is so important. Think about it: Just 25 extra calories per day means an additional 2½ pounds per year. Multiply that by ten years, and you've just put on 25 pounds. That's how it happens. Below are the calorie counts for "just one" of a few different foods. The point of presenting the calorie "costs" of these foods isn't to get you to stop eating them but to get you to think about your food before you eat it. And remember that you would have to walk for one minute to burn off every 4 calories that you eat in excess of your daily calorie budget (an average of 2,000).

One Pringles Potato Chip vs. One McDonald's French Fry

Believe it or not, one french fry has only 5 calories, while a single Pringle is double at 10 calories.

One Stick of Wrigley's Juicy Fruit Chewing Gum vs. One Piece of Bazooka Bubblegum

Who would think that chewing two or three pieces of gum a day adds up to 4½ pounds per year? The winner here is Juicy Fruit at 10 calories, compared to Bazooka's 15.

One M&M Chocolate Candy vs. One Jelly Belly vs. One Peppermint Altoid

M&M's can be a pretty good deal at times, especially if you're comparing them to a regular candy bar (one bite of a Hershey's bar with almonds has 37 calories)—which always seems to disappear so fast. Also, if you're sharing M&M's, they split up nicely because you can pass the bag back and forth. However, they have 4.3 calories per piece, which add up fast as you're popping them into your mouth.

As far as jelly beans go, I hear a lot about them being low in fat, but they're still 4 calories per bean. If you're satisfied with a few, that's great, but watch out for unconscious consumption. Altoids and other mints are another story. They supposedly serve a function—to freshen your breath—so the calories don't matter, right? Sorry, but all calories count, and please spare me the argument that it takes work to suck on the mint. One Altoid has almost 3½ calories.

One Bite-size Cube of Cheddar Cheese vs. One Famous Amos Chocolate Chip Cookie

Clearly the cheese is the better choice nutritionally, but cheese is not a health food you can consume without guilt: One bite-size (½ inch) cube has 55 calories, whereas the cookie has only 37.5. Whenever possible, go with low-fat cheese. A great one is Cabot Cheese 50% Reduced Fat Cheddar—35 calories per ½-inch cube.

One Fritos Original Corn Chip vs. One Cashew Nut

Here again, the cashew has health benefits that far outweigh those of the nutritionally bland corn chip; however, cashews have 8.5 calories per nut, whereas Fritos have 5 per chip. So just because nuts are healthful doesn't give you carte blanche to overindulge; you're supposed to eat nuts in place of something else in your diet that's high in calories and nutritionally inferior, not simply add them.

What Makes It Difficult for You to Eat Healthfully?

Eating healthfully isn't easy, so recently DietDetective.com asked more than three hundred people what makes it difficult for them to eat better. Here are the obstacles mentioned most often and how to overcome them.

Too Many Tempting Foods

Survey results: 27.7 Percent.

Facts: This is by far the most common complaint and excuse for not being able to eat healthfully. Everywhere you go, there's fast food, cupcakes, doughnuts, fried chicken—the list is endless. In fact, many public health advocates call this an "obese-friendly environment." So, yes, it's tough to eat healthfully.

Solution: Planning is really the only way to overcome the problem. Don't think simple willpower is going to get you past indulging in all those tempting foods. Plan ahead. Think about where you're going and what healthy foods will be available. Try to mentally rehearse making healthier choices in the most tempting situations.

For instance, find the healthier choices on fast-food menus before you get there; most fast-food restaurants have information on their websites. When traveling or in stressful situations, keep healthy food (including ready-to-eat foods such as low-cal soups, frozen dinners, cereals, and fruit) readily available. Keep junk foods out of your house—they're too tempting. The research shows that if you have those foods around, you're likely to eat them. Do a housecleaning and dump all the junk food you find. And don't be a diet hero: Avoid cues that tempt you. If you drive by Dunkin' Donuts on the way to work, and you can't resist stopping for a box of doughnuts, change your route. Also, don't head to the supermarket when you're starving—eat a snack beforehand. (For more information on this, check out http://www.dietdetective.com/content/view/3/156/.)

Lack of Time

Survey Results: 16.9 Percent.

Facts: For Americans who are rushing to get a healthy meal on the table between work, soccer, ballet class, and sleep, time is often the missing ingredient. This lack of time leads many people to rely on unhealthy versions of takeout, fast food, and easy-to-fix convenience foods.

Solution: The truth is that it's not easy to eat healthfully when you're busy, particularly when it's not a priority in your life. But even if you have no time to buy healthy food and cook at home, you still have options. You can make convenience and fast foods work for you. For instance, find out what healthy offerings you might enjoy at your favorite restaurant (try getting menus in advance). Go to the supermarket and buy a selection of tasty low-calorie frozen dinners; some of them are delicious. Try batch cooking: Pick one day of the week to prepare an entire week's worth of healthy meals.

High Price of Eating Healthfully

Survey Results: 14.2 Percent.

Facts: It may seem cheaper and simpler to eat unhealthy foods. And in many cases it is. However, according to analysis from the USDA Economic Research Service, more than half of the sixty-nine forms of fruit and eighty-five forms of vegetables included in the analysis were estimated to cost twenty-five cents or less per serving, and 86 percent of all vegetables and 78 percent of all fruits cost less than fifty cents a serving.

Solution: Plan your meals and shopping lists in advance. Search out coupons and specials on supermarket websites. To cut shopping time and avoid impulse purchases, write the list according to the grocery aisles and sections where foods are kept. You probably know the store you shop in pretty well; if you map out your route, you will be more likely to stick to the plan. Bring your lunch to work or school. Don't wait until you're starving to eat. Also, keep in mind that sin foods are often more expensive than healthier choices. For instance, one apple pie generally costs three times more than five apples. (For more information, check out: http://www.dietdetective .com/content/view/69/158/.)

No Motivation

Survey Results: 9.8 Percent.

Facts: Healthy food can seem boring and bland. Plus, it takes more work to eat healthfully. However, eating healthy foods can be exciting and tasty if you put forth some effort.

Solution: Take a few minutes to write down all the reasons you want to eat healthier. For instance, "I've been diagnosed with heart disease and need to start eating better." Or "I just feel better about myself when I eat properly." Try to come up with as many reasons as possible. Anytime you have doubts and need motivation, you can refer back to your list. That's why you need to make sure it is meaningful. Make eating healthfully more exciting and enjoyable by learning healthy recipes and finding tasty, healthy restaurants.

Eat Out Frequently

Survey Results: 8.6 Percent.

Facts: Up to 50 percent of our food budget is spent eating out, and foods purchased outside the home are generally higher in calories and saturated fat and lower in fiber and nutrients such as calcium than home-prepared foods.

Solution: There are lots of ways to eat out, have a good time stuffing your face, and still eat healthfully. Start by picking places that offer healthy choices. Also, follow a few of these tips:

- Limit mayo, tartar sauce, creamy dressings, and extra cheese.
- Ask for dressing, sauces, butter, or sour cream on the side.

- Use mustard, ketchup, salt, pepper, or vinegar as fat-free ways to season your food.
- Watch nuts, croutons, and other salad add-ons.
- Chicken and fish are good choices only if they're grilled or broiled, *not* breaded or deep fried.
- Avoid large portions. Split your entrée with a family member or ask for a half portion.
- Read the menu. Avoid any of the following words: à la mode (with ice cream on top), au gratin (covered with cheese), battered, bisque, breaded, buttered, cheese sauce, creamy or rich, crispy, deep fried, deluxe, fried, hollandaise (sauce made with butter and egg yolks), jumbo, nuts, scalloped, sautéed (unless you make a special request for it to be prepared in a small amount of oil), and tempura (deep fried).
- Don't be afraid to ask questions or make special requests.

Unsupportive Family Members

Survey Results: 4.6 Percent.

Facts: Family members can really put a damper on your diet. Also, family can influence your behavior; if your spouse doesn't eat healthfully, it can make it difficult for you to eat right.

Solution: Don't let your family throw you off track. Set boundaries for yourself when dining out or eating at home; make sure that you keep track of your "difficult" family eating situations and think in advance about how you're going to overcome them. Give yourself permission not to eat the same foods they're eating, so that you can remain on track. Also, remember to talk with your family and let them know you want their help—not to police your eating but to support your healthy eating choices.

Diet Detective's What You Need to Know

Let Your Fingers Do the Walking: Search for your Calorie Bargains right in your home—on your computer. FreshDirect is a supermarket delivery service in New York City, but you can take advantage of its fabulous website (www.freshdirect.com) no matter where you live. The site offers an impressive amount of nutrition information, arranged in whatever order you choose, for almost every single food in the supermarket. Look for details of every ingredient, as well as the Nutrition Facts panel, at no charge. Just be sure to input a valid New York City zip code when prompted (try 10011).

Unhealthy Food at Work

Survey Results: 4.3 Percent.

Facts: What with all the birthdays, parties, coworkers bringing in unhealthy foods, and the stress of the workplace, the office can be a minefield for anyone trying to stay healthy.

Solution

Be Social: Team up with a coworker who is also determined to lose weight. An office diet buddy can provide you with emotional support and reminders.

Plan: Gather menus from all local restaurants as well as convenient takeout and fast-food eateries. Then scan them for healthy foods. Narrow your choices and highlight them. Pack a healthy lunch: Bring your own low-cal sandwiches or buy healthy microwave meals (see if you can keep food in an area of the fridge or freezer).

Set rules: Many offices are breeding grounds for nibbling just because snack foods are available. Decide in advance what you will and will not eat.

Vending Machines: These are filled mostly with unhealthy choices. Bring your own healthy snacks.

Diet Detective's What You Need to Know

Diet Cheat Sheet

Food and Diet

- Calorie Bargains: Find three or four lower-calorie versions of what you typically eat three to four times a week and make substitutions you can live with forever. Make sure you don't overindulge in the newly found Calorie Bargain—that defeats the purpose.
- Plan ahead: Come up with a list of preapproved foods you know are low in calories so you can avoid making too many on-the-spot decisions when you're traveling or eating out.
- Fast Food Is OK: There are low-calorie options available. Learn them before arriving at the restaurant.
- Singles Only: Buy single-serving snack foods; never buy in bulk.
- Read it: Check food labels and never eat anything that contains more than 15 calories without thinking about it. That includes cookies, crackers, and chips (each chip can have as many as 15 calories).
- Buy frozen and ready-to-eat: Most of us are pressed for time. Go to the supermarket and stock up on healthy low-calorie frozen foods (such as Lean Cuisine, Healthy Choice, and Kashi); also pick up cereals (under 120 calories per cup) and low-cal soups. When you're too tired or too busy to cook, use these tasty, lean alternatives to eating out.
- Switch: from whole milk to skim, from eggs to egg whites, and from soda to water or no-calorie iced tea.

- Eat more fiber: It helps keep you full longer. Foods that are high in fiber include fruits, vegetables, nuts, cereals, legumes (i.e., beans and lentils), and whole-grain breads and pastas.

Nutrition

- Calories: Calories are made up of carbs, fats, and protein. Fats are the most "expensive," with 9 calories per gram. Carbs and protein have 4 calories per gram. Also, know your calorie "budget."
- As a quickie guide, figure 10 calories per pound for women and 11 calories per pound for men. Then multiply that by your activity level (sedentary = 1.2, lightly active = 1.35, moderately active = 1.5, very active = 1.65, extremely active = 2.0). Reduce your calorie budget to lose weight. Know the cost of a calorie and shop wisely, because every 40 calories over your calorie budget will require ten minutes of walking to burn off.
- Carbs: Learn the good carbs from the bad ones. Good: whole grains, vegetables, and fruit. Bad: starchy foods such as white pasta and white rice, candy, cakes, and sugary drinks. To lose weight, eliminate or limit bad carbs. Low-carb diets are not all bad. If you can live on a low-carb diet, and it works for you, go for it, but avoid low-carb products that are high in calories.
- Fat: It's not all bad. You need some fat to make you feel full and stay healthy. Limit unhealthy saturated fats and trans fats. Stick to monounsaturated and polyunsaturated fats such as olive oil and canola oil.
- Protein: It can help you lose weight by keeping you full. Just make sure to limit protein sources that are bundled with saturated fat (for example, fatty meats, cheeses, whole dairy products, and others— see Sources of Protein on page 213).
- Lose it: Find out exactly how much weight you need to lose by determining your body mass index (BMI) and using that as a guide. For more information on BMI, check out http://www.dietdetective.com/content/view/1148/156/.

Food and Behavior

- Avoid willpower: Don't think all you need is a good dose of willpower to go against your nature, which is to want sugary and fatty foods. To avoid unhealthy foods that entice you, keep junk foods out of your house. Don't go to the supermarket when you're ravenous—eat something first. Over time, the healthy stuff tastes great.

- Use forward thinking: Plan ahead for weak "diet" moments. For instance, if you know that Friday is "muffin day" in your office, come up with a healthier alternative that helps prevent you from becoming weak in the knees.
- Review: Check out all menus from restaurants you frequent beforehand. Come up with three or four preselected healthy choices. Call ahead to find out how various dishes are prepared.
- Form patterns: Make your new eating behaviors automatic by doing them over and over again. You shouldn't need to take breaks from your diet. If you have to take a break, you made too many compromises in the first place, and your diet will not last. New eating behaviors need to be comfortable and not too restrictive.
- Make it excuse proof: Don't let your family give you an excuse to overeat. Make sure they're aware of your diet and don't bring unhealthy foods into your home.
- Find a reason why: It helps to know why you actually want to get in shape. For health reasons? Vanity? Think you already know? Make sure. Write it down.
- Create a goal: How long do you expect it will take to lose the weight you want? A healthy goal is about ½ to 1 pound per week. Take it slow; no need to rush.

Activity and Diet

- Combine it: Research shows that you need to combine diet with activity to lose and maintain your weight.
- Make it necessary. Incorporate increased physical activity into your daily life. It should be like brushing your teeth. You do it every day, seven days per week, and most of the time without thinking. Having trouble? Try making the activity useful—in other words, something you need to do anyway—such as actually walking the dog instead of just letting him or her out in the backyard.

- Get motivated: Come up with an activity you will enjoy, so that it doesn't seem as if it's a burden.
- Take a walk: Walking is the number one form of activity to control weight. Locate all available parks, recreation centers, and bike and hiking paths in your area, and use them.

A Final Word about Using *The Diet Detective's Calorie Bargain Bible*

The Diet Detective's Calorie Bargain Bible is meant to be a guide that you can keep in your desk at work, in the glove compartment of your car, your pocketbook or purse, in the kitchen—wherever you can have easy access to it when you're around food or are making food decisions. It's divided into categories that will make it easier to find the particular foods or food situations in which you're most likely to find yourself. Browse through the fast-food section to see which restaurants offer healthier breakfasts. Or find out how to stay healthy the next time you go to the movies—it's all here for you to browse, read, learn, and be entertained.

Free Weight Loss Program for Book Purchasers

The purchaser of this book will receive free access to the Diet Detective's Weight Loss Program (no credit card required). Simply email us your proof of purchase, which can include a receipt from any bookstore or bookseller, and you will be emailed a free access code. Send proof of purchase emails to freediet@DietDetective.com, and you will receive free access to the Diet Detective's sophisticated weight-loss program at no cost.

Calorie Bargain Spotlight

Calorie Bargain: Vitalicious VitaMuffins and VitaTops

The Why: Have you gone to Dunkin' Donuts and ordered a "healthy" honey bran raisin muffin? If so, you may be surprised to learn that one muffin has 480 calories. Even fat-free muffins can be diet disasters. They're typically only a few calories lower than the regular versions, plus the taste is often disappointing.

The Health Bonus: Vitalicious, a New York City–based company, has come up with a great all-natural product that has fewer than half the calories of a regular muffin yet is packed with fiber and tastes great.

What We Liked Best: They come in a variety of flavors, but of all the ones we tasted, we loved the MultiBran and the Deep Chocolate versions best. The muffins weigh 4 ounces, which is perfect for portion control. And because they're so filling (because of the fiber), you really can't eat too many, so you can avoid any serious diet damage. The company even sells muffin tops that weigh only 2 ounces and fit perfectly into a toaster. Not only that, but if you happen to miss your daily multivitamin, you're covered, because these muffins are jam-packed with vitamins. Vitalicious even makes great baking mixes—you can make your own VitaMuffins and VitaBrownies.

What We Liked Least: Orders from the website are processed only on certain days.

The Price: $18 per dozen muffins; $17 per dozen muffin tops.

Offerings: Deep Chocolate, AppleBerryBran, BlueBran, CranBran, MultiBran, Banana Nut, Dark Chocolate Pomegranate, Double Chocolate Dream, Fudgy Peanut Butter Chip.

Website: www.vitalicious.com.

Where to Buy: They are available online or by phone at 877-VITA-877.

Ingredients:

MultiBran Muffin

Water, organic evaporated cane juice, wheat flour, egg whites, wheat bran, molasses, raisins, soy bran, oat bran, modified food starch, wheat gluten, sea salt, sodium acid pyrophosphate, natural flavors, baking soda, corn starch, cinnamon, xanthan gum, monocalcium phosphate, distilled monoglycerides, vitamin C, vitamin E, iron, biotin, vitamin A, zinc, vitamin B_{12}, vitamin D_3, folic acid, vitamin B_5, vitamin B_6.

Deep Chocolate VitaTop

Water, whole wheat flour, organic evaporated cane juice, egg whites, chocolate chips (sugar, chocolate liquor, cocoa butter, butterfat, soy lecithin added as an emulsifier, vanilla), cocoa (processed with alkali), soy fiber, inulin, dried honey, wheat gluten, leavening (sodium acid pyrophosphate, sodium bicarbonate), natural flavors, lecithin, sea salt, xanthan gum, vitamin C, vitamin E, iron, biotin, vitamin A, zinc, vitamin B_{12}, vitamin D_3, folic acid, vitamin B_5, vitamin B_6.

Nutritional Analysis per Serving

4-ounce MultiBran Muffin	2-ounce Deep Chocolate VitaTop
200 calories	100 calories
0 g fat	1.5 g fat
6 g protein	
24 g carbs	25 g carbs
8 g fiber	6 g fiber
720 mg sodium	230 mg sodium

Compare these to some other muffins:

- Au Bon Pain Raisin Bran Muffin (5¾ ounces): 410 calories, 9 g fat, 74 g carbs, 9 g fiber.
- Au Bon Pain Low-fat Chocolate Cake Muffin (4.15 ounces): 320 calories, 2 g fat, 74 g carbs, 4 g fiber.
- Dunkin' Donuts Reduced-fat Blueberry Muffin (5 ounces): 400 calories, 5 g fat, 7 g carbs, 3 g fiber.

Part Two

WHAT TO EAT WHEN YOU'RE EATING OUT

The Basics

Eating out is a huge part of our lives. In fact, the National Restaurant Association estimates that we eat almost six meals per week outside the home (about 290 times per year)—which means it's important to know how to eat and still stay trim.

The problem is that when we go out to eat, we don't want to spoil our fun by eating "healthy." Here are a few tips to help you stay on track. And remember, you don't have to apply every tip to make things work. Just pick the few that work and fit into your life.

Plan Ahead: If you do nothing else, this alone will help you stick to a healthy eating lifestyle.

A Complete Overhaul of Your Diet Is Not Required

Just a few small changes in the way you order can make a big difference. Even cutting a mere 100 calories every time you eat out can result in losing more than eight pounds in a year (290 × 100 calories = 29,000 calories, and 3,500 calories = 1 pound). Something as simple as not putting sour cream on your baked potato or skipping that extra piece of bread can go a long way. Don't think it doesn't matter—it does. Get into a pattern and stick to it every time.

- Call the restaurant ahead of time to find out what healthy options are available, and/or check out the website. You can probably even place a special order in advance.
- If no healthy options are available, nearly every restaurant will let you order plain grilled chicken, fish, or lean meat with some type of vegetable or salad.
- Dine at an earlier or later time; special instructions don't take as long if you eat during off-peak dining hours.
- Be aware that it's harder to make the right choices when dining out with a group of friends—don't give in to peer pressure.

Eat Consciously: Don't eat just to eat. For many of us, dipping into the bread basket is something to keep us busy until the real meal comes. To avoid being tempted, ask the waitperson not to bring bread to the table. Or, if you must have a slice of bread, at least don't smother it with butter or dip it in olive oil.

- French bread (4 slices): 384 calories, 4 g fat, 72 g carbs.
- Garlic bread (4 slices): 545 calories, 21 g fat, 75 g carbs.
- Butter (2 pats): 72 calories, 8 g fat, 0 g carbs.
- Olive oil (2 tablespoons): 240 calories, 27 g fat, 0 g carbs.

Snacking on peanuts or other bar treats to pass the time while waiting for your dining companions just adds additional calories.

- Peanuts (¼ cup): 212 calories, 18 g fat, 7 g carbs.
- Tortilla chips (1 cup): 130 calories, 7 g fat, 16 g carbs.
- Pretzels (1 cup): 171 calories, 2 g fat, 36 g carbs.

Eat Before: Avoid going out to eat when you're starving. Have a high-fiber snack like an apple or even a bowl of cereal before heading off to the restaurant. Don't skip meals before eating out in order to save calories; the hungrier you are, the more you will eat. Try drinking water before your meal—it will fill up your stomach a little.

Avoid Large Portions: If you're making the decision about where to eat, choose wisely. Steer clear of buffets and all-you-can-eat restaurants. Avoid fixed-price menus; they encourage you to overeat high-calorie foods. If you know that the restaurant serves huge portions, don't try to be a "diet hero" by assuming that you won't eat everything on your plate. Ask the server to wrap up half your portion in a takeout box before you even start.

Skip the Fries and Extra Pasta: If you think you're going to have "just one" or "a couple of bites" and leave the rest, well, you're mistaken. Just say no to the side of fries or pasta. Replace it with a healthy portion of broccoli steamed with garlic or another type of vegetable or salad.

- French fries (1 medium order): 450 calories, 22 g fat, 57 g carbs.
- Pasta with meat sauce (1 cup): 301 calories, 10 g fat, 33 g carbs.

Don't Be Afraid to Ask: Don't be embarrassed to ask your waitperson questions or make special requests. If you don't ask, you'll be the only one to suffer. I often tell the server that I'm allergic to certain foods or even go so far as saying I have a medical condition (just to make it simpler). Remember, restaurants want you to be satisfied, because your business is important to them, so don't be shy. Ask how your dish is prepared even if it's called "light" on the menu. Also, make sure to ask:

- "Is this dish fried?"
- "Can you make this dish without frying?"
- "Can you steam the vegetables or fish?"
- "What is the sauce made with?"
- "Can you prepare this without the cheese/sauce?"
- "Can you serve the sauce on the side?"
- "How large is the serving?"
- "How many ounces is the beef/chicken/fish?"
- "Can you make this dish without soy sauce or MSG?"

On the Side: Ask for dressing, sauces, butter, or sour cream on the side, instead of on the dish itself.

- Sour cream (2 tablespoons): 62 calories, 6 g fat, 1 g carbs.
- Thousand Island dressing (2 tablespoons): 118 calories, 11 g fat, 5 g carbs.
- Caesar dressing (2 tablespoons): 155 calories, 17 g fat, 1 g carbs.

Liquid Donuts: Don't go overboard on the alcohol; it adds excess calories and stimulates your appetite. If you want a drink, have it with your meal rather than before. Remember, nonalcoholic drinks (soda, juice, sweetened iced tea) add up too. Just two or three sodas have about 400 calories!

- Dry table wine (8 ounces): 165 calories, 0 g fat, 3 g carbs.
- Beer (12 ounces): 148 calories, 0 g fat, 13 g carbs.
- Margarita in a pint glass: 676 calories, 0 g fat, 43 g carbs.

Go Out, Eat Skinny

*At-a-Glance List of Lower-cal Options at Your
Favorite Restaurants*

Caribbean and African
Look for: poached, steamed, or grilled dishes; stews, curries (without coconut or coconut milk).
Look out for: fried foods; coconut, peanuts, cream, puddings, fritters.
Best bet: broiled fillet red snapper, or jerk chicken without sauce.

Chinese
Look for: stir-fried, simmered, steamed, or roasted foods; bean curd (not fried), lobster sauce, tomato sauce, light sauce, oyster sauce, brown rice.
Look out for: fried, crispy, or breaded foods; eggs, peanuts or cashews, hoisin sauce, fruit, sweet-and-sour sauce, soy or teriyaki sauce (high in sodium).
Best bet: steamed chicken, fish, or tofu with vegetables, sauce on the side.

Indian, Thai, or Vietnamese
Look for: stir-fried, steamed, or simmered foods; soup (without coconut milk), kebabs, biryani (without nuts), curried vegetables.
Look out for: crispy or fried items; coconut, cream.
Best bet: tandoori or tikka (grilled, skewered Indian dish), or any steamed fish with vegetables.

Italian
Look for: marinara, primavera, or arrabiata sauces; roasted, grilled, or steamed foods; thin-crust pizza, pasta, tomatoes.
Look out for: foods that are fried, stuffed, or prepared parmigiana style; Alfredo, white, or carbonara sauces; cheese.
Best bet: pasta with tomato-based sauce; chicken or fish prepared without oil.

Japanese

Look for: broiled, grilled, or steamed items; sushi, sashimi, soup, hijiki, oshitashi.

Look out for: fried or battered foods; soy, teriyaki, or tamari sauces (high in sodium); tempura, duck, cream cheese, or mayo (in sushi), eel, fish roe.

Best bets: vegetable or fish sushi rolls (not fried) or tuna nigiri.

Mexican

Look for: grilled items (like fajitas); simmered, shredded, or minced items; soft tortillas/soft tacos, beans, enchilada sauce, salsa.

Look out for: deep-fried foods; tacos, taco salad, cheese, chips, guacamole, nachos, huevos rancheros, sour cream, bunuelos.

Best bet: char-grilled chicken burrito or fajita (dry; no oil) with salsa, no cheese.

Steak House

Look for: grilled or baked foods or meats prepared au jus; sirloin, filet, chicken, shrimp.

Look out for: battered or fried foods; béarnaise or hollandaise sauce; New York strip, T-bone, porterhouse, or rib-eye steak; prime rib; onion rings.

Best bet: filet mignon prepared without oil with small baked potato and salad on the side.

Restaurant Shockers

So now you have the basics, but you're still not fully armed. Most people believe that if you want to eat healthy at a restaurant, all you have to do is know the "right" way to order your food. However, I've learned secrets from several restaurant insiders that will shock even the savviest restaurant aficionados.

You've Been Grilled

That's right, even the grill is not sacred. I don't know how many times I've recommended that people order their food grilled. But according to food-safety expert Jeff Nelken, "Oftentimes breakfast cooks save the bacon fat and use it on the grill to make lunch and dinner foods." Also, the grill itself may not be what you think it is. When we order foods grilled, most of us assume they'll be cooked on an open flame, but many times it's a flat-top grill, where some type of grease or oil is necessary to create an even cooking surface, increase the cooking speed, and prevent the food from sticking. Also, even though foods are called "flame grilled" on the menu, they or the grill may have been brushed with oil to prevent sticking. Even "grilled" fish/seafood is always brushed with some type of oil.

Fit Tip: Ask if the restaurant uses a flat-top or flame grill. If it's flat-top, request that your food be grilled in a pan with cooking spray instead of oil. Nelken suggests telling the server that you just returned from the hospital and need the food prepared according to your doctor's instructions. Another option would be to frequent restaurants where you can see the food being cooked in an open kitchen.

Oil Slick

There is oil in almost every restaurant dish, and while oils such as canola and olive are healthier than others, they all have approximately 120 calories per tablespoon. So even if you go to the trouble of ordering an egg-white omelet, believing that you're making a healthy choice, it could be doused in oil. Or you might order grilled or steamed vegetables, but they may have been marinating in oil for hours, if not all day. It's difficult to get grilled or steamed veggies without oil, because they must be made to order—which takes a lot of time in a busy kitchen. And certain vegetables are worse than others. Eggplant, for example, absorbs a lot of oil—just look on your plate; you can see it.

There's oil in other healthy foods as well. Because fat and oil help preserve cooked food, busy restaurants usually partially cook poultry and fish, then coat them in butter or oil until they're ready to be finished, says Billy Strynkowski, executive chef of *Cooking Light* magazine. "Even if you order your chicken 'dry' with the sauce on the side, poultry is always pan-fried in oil or clarified butter." Pasta, potatoes, and rice, again, are often partially cooked and filmed with some type of fat so they stay fresh and don't clump together, adds Juventino Avila, chef and instructor at the Institute of Culinary Education in New York City. Oh, and if you think that having simple rice and beans at your favorite Mexican restaurant is healthy, think again: The rice is fried, then steamed.

Fit Tip: Be aware of where you're eating. Restaurants typically want to please their patrons; however, most of the time, unless the restaurant promotes itself as healthy, it just doesn't have the equipment, materials, time, or utensils to do it right, according to Avila. Almost all the chefs agree: If you want your food cooked a certain way, make sure to tell your server that you have an allergy (to butter or whatever it is you want eliminated). This usually encourages the chef to make up a new batch of veggies, chicken, and so on without those added calories. Avila also recommends calling the restaurant in advance and making sure it can provide the food exactly the way you want it prepared.

Butter Me Up

Even if something is not doused in oil, you still may not be calorie safe, because it can have added butter or cream. Toasted buns are often covered in butter; even steaks have butter drizzled on them before they're sent out. "And restaurants always finish sauces with butter or cream, even if the words *butter* or *cream* are not in the sauce's name," says Cooking Light's Strynkowski. "For example, a white wine sauce is always finished with butter."

Fit Tip: Be suspicious, be inquisitive, and make sure to get a straight answer from the server (who should ask the chef). Always invoke the "allergic reaction" or "medical condition" excuse to be on the safe side.

Puree Fantasy

Pureed soups, potatoes, and vegetables are often full of cream and/or butter to make them smooth and tasty. Also, anything that looks creamy and velvety probably has butter or cream. Some restaurants do make thick, creamy soups without butter or cream, but if that's the case, your server will almost always make a point of telling you. Restaurants know that many customers are concerned about cutting the fat in their diets, and they want to let you know when they've done something they think you'll appreciate.

Fit Tip: Ask your server about the ingredients and the preparation method. Ask specifically if the dish has any cream, and, if not, what was used instead. Natural, healthy, low-calorie thickening agents include pureed potato, roasted garlic, and arrowroot. If there is no thickening agent, well, they probably used butter or cream.

Sodium Surprise

Calories are not all you get when dining out: Many restaurants go heavy on the seasoning, including sodium. Most places put salt on almost everything they make, especially the marinades. Some chicken producers even inject chickens with a sodium solution to add flavor.

Fit Tip: Ask for no salt or sodium. In addition, ask if your dish has been marinated, and if so, in what.

Allergies

Almost eleven million Americans have allergies to foods such as peanuts, fish, milk, and wheat. Even if your food is not made with the offending ingredient, it still may not be allergen free. Cooks, food handlers, utensils—almost anything can infect an allergic individual, warns Nelken. A server comes out with four or five plates, and if one has a peanut sauce or fish oil, the odds are that the server has it on his or her hands and can transfer it to your dish.

Fit Tip: Call ahead and don't take risks. If you believe something contains or has been contaminated with an allergen, avoid it.

Salad Surprise

According to many chefs, any pretossed salad (particularly those made in large batches) could have up to a quarter cup of dressing, when a tablespoon usually suffices.

Fit Tip: Order a simple vinaigrette dressing made with vinegar, olive oil, and an acid such as lemon juice or grapefruit juice, and always ask for it on the side.

Whole-grain Mystery

When we see wheat-crust pizza, whole-wheat pasta, or wheat buns on a menu, most of us automatically think *healthy*. But according to Marjorie K. Livingston MS, RD, an assistant professor at the Culinary Institute of America in New York, there's no real way to be sure that you're really getting a whole-grain product. In fact, most of the time you're getting products that just have brown coloring, maybe with some whole-grain flour. "There really is no definition of whole grain for restaurants. Even something like a bran muffin often has very little bran in it; you're mostly getting a muffin with coloring," says Livingston.

Fit Tip: Ask the manager to find out if what you're ordering is truly a 100 percent whole-grain product. If he or she is not 100 percent sure, it's probably not.

It Must Be True

Even though there is no law requiring restaurants to provide nutrition information, they are required to do so if they make a nutritional claim (low sodium, low fat, low cholesterol, healthy, light, and so forth) or a health claim about the relationship between a nutrient or food and a disease or health condition ("heart healthy").

The following are sample nutritional claims on menus:

- **Light:** Means the item has fewer calories and less fat than the food to which it's being compared. Restaurants may, however, use the term *light* for reasons other than as a nutrient-content claim. For example, "lighter fare" may mean smaller portions. But the intended meaning must be clarified on the menu.
- **Healthy:** Means the item is low in fat and saturated fat, has limited amounts of cholesterol and sodium, and provides significant amounts of one or more of the key nutrients vitamins A and C, iron, calcium, protein, or fiber.

Calorie Bargain Spotlight

Calorie Bargain: Metromint

The Why: I'd take an iced tea or diet soda over a glass of water any day, so I wasn't terribly optimistic about the newest addition to the world of lightly flavored waters. But Metromint exceeded all my expectations.

The Health Bonus: The concept is simply adding mint to water, which not only tastes great but also has been said to calm nerves, freshen breath, and reduce congestion.

What We Liked Best: I can really imagine giving up a lifelong commitment to iced tea for one of these refreshing spearmint- or peppermint-infused beverages.

What We Liked Least: the cost.

The Price: $1.39 to $2 per bottle, $6.99 to $7.49 for 6-pack, $38 for 24-pack.

Offerings: spearmint, peppermint, lemonmint, orangemint.

Website: www.metromint.com.

Where to Buy: Safeway, Wild Oats Marketplace, company website.

Ingredients: water, mint.

Nutritional Analysis per Serving: 500 Milliliters
0 calories
0 g fat
0 g carbs
0 g protein
0 g fiber
0 g sodium

Fit Tip: Keep in mind that restaurants are not required to have their food analyzed, as are food manufacturers. They may make their claims based on any "reasonable" information, such as databases, cookbooks, or other secondhand sources, so the information they provide is probably not 100 percent accurate.

Restaurant Calorie Rip-offs

Sometimes when you walk into a fast-food restaurant, even if you're looking for healthy choices, it's a matter of choosing the least of all evils on the menu. To make your choices a bit easier, I've sleuthed some of the worst of America's dining-out disasters. Remember, to maintain current weight, the average person should consume about 2,000 calories per day.

Burger King (www.bk.com/#menu=3,-1,-1)

- Triple Whopper with Cheese: 1,230 calories, 82 g fat, 52 g carbs, 71 g protein.
- Chocolate Shake (king size): 1,260 calories, 38 g fat, 204 g carbs, 21 g protein.
- Enormous Omelet Sandwich: 730 calories, 45 g fat, 44 g carbs, 37 g protein.
- Double Croissan'wich with sausage, egg, and cheese: 680 calories, 51 g fat, 26 g carbs, 29 g protein.
- Tendercrisp Chicken Sandwich: 780 calories, 44 g fat, 73 g carbs, 26 g protein.

When it comes to fast food, there's really nothing more over-the-top than the Triple Whopper. Do you really need three slabs of meat to fill you up? And if your daily budget is

2,000 calories, you probably don't want to start your day by spending 700 of them on the Omelet Sandwich or the Double Croissan'wich.

Hardee's (www.hardees.com/content/downloads/nutrition.pdf)

- Monster Thickburger: 1,420 calories, 108 g fat, 46 g carbs, 60 g protein.
- Loaded Breakfast Burrito: 780 calories, 51 g fat, 38 g carbs, 40 g protein.
- Loaded Biscuit 'N' Gravy Breakfast Bowl: 770 calories, 54 g fat, 49 g carbs, 20 g protein.
- Big Country Breakfast Platters:
  - Ham: 970 calories, 53 g fat, 90 g carbs, 33 g protein.
  - Breaded Pork Chop: 1,220 calories, 68 g fat, 102 g carbs, 48 g protein.
  - Chicken: 1,140 calories, 61 g fat, 105 g carbs, 44 g protein.

At 1,410 calories, the infamous Monster Thickburger takes first place in the unhealthiest-fast-food category. But the greatest numbers of disastrous options are actually on the breakfast menu. Unless you plan on crawling into a cave and hibernating after your meal, there's really no need to consume so many calories at once—especially for breakfast.

McDonald's
(www.mcdonalds.com/usa/eat/nutrition_info/nutrition_lists.html)

- Double Quarter Pounder with Cheese: 740 calories, 42 g fat, 40 g carbs, 48 g protein.

- Deluxe Breakfast with Large Biscuit: 1,380 calories, 67 g fat, 159 g carbs, 36 g protein.
- Hotcakes and Sausage: 780 calories, 33 g fat, 106 g carbs, 15 g protein.
- Chocolate Triple Thick Shake (32 ounces): 1,160 calories, 27 g fat, 203 g carbs, 27 g protein.
- Chicken Selects Premium Breast Strips (10 pieces): 1,260 calories, 66 g fat, 92 g carbs, 78 g protein.

I was surprised that the Deluxe Breakfast, the Hotcakes and Sausage, and the Chicken Selects all pack more calories than the Double Quarter Pounder. But the worst choice of all is probably the Chocolate Triple Thick Shake, because it isn't even a meal.

Wendy's (www.wendys.com/food/pdf/us/nutrition.pdf)

- Large French Fries: 540 calories, 24 g fat, 69 g carbs, 7 g protein.
- Chicken Club Sandwich: 610 calories, 31 g fat, 49 g carbs, 39 g protein.
- Chicken BLT Salad with Homestyle Garlic Croutons and Honey Mustard Dressing: 650 calories, 43.5 g fat, 29 g carbs, 36 g protein.
- Southwest Taco Salad with Reduced-fat Sour Cream, Seasoned Tortilla Strips, and Ancho Chipotle Ranch Dressing: 680 calories, 39 g fat, 48 g carbs, 34 g protein.

Wow, bet you thought salad was a healthy choice. Not so fast. Also, at 650 calories, the Chicken Club Sandwich is not a great choice.

Subway (www.subway.com/subwayroot/MenuNutrition/Nutrition/pdf/NutritionValues.pdf)

- Double Meat Meatball Marinara (6-inch): 860 calories, 42 g fat, 82 g carbs, 2,480 mg sodium, 37 g protein.
- Double Meat Italian BMT (6-inch): 630 calories, 35 g fat, 49 g carbs, 2,850 mg sodium, 34 g protein.

Although many Subway offerings are very good, there are exceptions. Case in point: the Double Meat Meatball Marinara Sandwich, which has more calories than a Double Quarter Pounder with Cheese from McDonald's. Oh, and watch out for the sodium.

Kentucky Fried Chicken (www.yum.com/nutrition/menu.asp)

- Crispy Twister sandwich: 600 calories, 33 g fat, 49 g carbs, 26 g protein.
- Famous Bowls—Rice with Gravy: 620 calories, 28 g fat, 67 g carbs, 2,130 mg sodium, 26 g protein.
- Famous Bowls—Mashed Potato with Gravy: 740 calories, 35 g fat, 80 g carbs, 2,330 mg sodium, 27 g protein.
- Chicken Pot Pie: 770 calories, 40 g fat, 70 g carbs, 33 g protein.

While the Pot Pie and the Crispy Twister—a sandwich of deep-fried chicken smothered in mayonnaise—certainly are not great ideas for the diet conscious, you need to be especially cautious about the sides. Both the rice and gravy and the potatoes and gravy will send your total calorie count soaring.

Starbucks (www.starbucks.com/retail/nutrition_info.asp)

- White Chocolate Frappuccino Blended Crème with whipped cream (24 ounces): 760 calories, 21 g fat, 121 g carbs, 20 g protein.
- Strawberries & Crème Frappuccino Blended Crème with whipped cream (24 ounces): 750 calories, 15 g fat, 135 g carbs, 16 g protein.

Seven hundred calories is steep any way you cut it, but in this case you're not even getting anything to eat for all those calories. You can save more than 100 calories by skipping the whipped cream, but even so, you're still consuming a meal's worth of calories with no real food to show for it. You need to remember that these drinks are not substitutes for coffee—they're substitutes for banana splits and ice cream sundaes.

Dunkin' Donuts
(www.dunkindonuts.com/aboutus/nutrition/nutrition.pdf)

- Sausage Egg Cheese Croissant Sandwich: 690 calories, 51 g fat, 40 g carbs, 22 g protein.
- Chocolate Chip Muffin: 630 calories, 26 g fat, 89 g carbs, 10 g protein.
- Jelly Stick: 530 calories, 29 g fat, 61 g carbs, 4 g protein.

"Sticks" have even more calories than "fancy" doughnuts, and check out that breakfast sandwich.

P. F. Chang's China Bistro
(www.pfchangs.com/cuisine/menu_main.aspx)

- Chang's Spare Ribs: 1,280 calories, 79 g fat, 47 g carbs, 92 g protein.
- Anything named kung pao; for example, kung pao chicken: 1,240 calories, 80 g fat, 58 g carbs, 74 g protein.
- Tam's Noodles with Savory Beef and Shrimp, 1,700 calories, 94 g fat, 144 g carbs, 58 g protein.
- Great Wall of Chocolate: 2,240 calories, 89 g fat, 376 g carbs, 20 g protein.

Chinese food is almost never a great bet for dieters, but if you're going to indulge, at least steer clear of calorie disasters like the spare ribs, which are actually just an appetizer. What is there to say about the Great Wall of Chocolate other than buyer beware?

Ruby Tuesday (www.rubytuesday.com/files/nutrition.pdf)

Note: Protein info not specifically listed for Ruby Tuesday.
- Colossal Burger: 1,943 calories, 141 g fat, 74 g carbs.
- Spinach Artichoke Dip: 1,328 calories, 80 g fat, 108 g carbs.
- Fresh Chicken & Broccoli Pasta: 2,061 calories, 128 g fat, 109 g carbs.
- Carolina Chicken Salad: 1,025 calories, 72 g fat, 38 g carbs.

Kudos to Ruby Tuesday for providing nutrition information, but all I can say is: Wow! All these options are not only high in calories but also sneaky little diet disasters. Don't be fooled by words like *spinach, broccoli*, and especially *salad*—in this case, they are all Calorie Rip-offs. The chicken and broccoli pasta and the burger each has about a day's worth of calories.

Pizza Hut (www.yum.com/nutrition/documents/ph_nutrition.pdf)

- Stuffed Crust Meat Lover's Pizza (1 slice, 14-inch pie): 520 calories, 29 g fat, 38 g carbs, 26 g protein.
- 6-inch Personal Meat Lover's Pan Pizza: 890 calories, 49 g fat, 70 g carbs, 41 g protein.

The Stuffed Crust Meat Lover's Pizza might just be the worst pizza option out there for a dieter. Only two pieces, and you're looking at more than 1,000 calories—and if you kick off your meal with breadsticks and wash it down with a soda, you'd better prepare yourself to get off the couch the next morning and run a marathon to undo all the damage.

Chili's (www.chilis.com/menu/)

- Awesome Blossom w/Seasoned Rice: 2,710 calories, 203 g fat, 194 g carbs, 24 g protein.
- Fajita Steak Quesadilla with Guacamole: 1,890 calories, 100 g fat, 154 g carbs, 86 g protein.
- Black Bean Burger (without bun or toppings): 650 calories, 12 g fat, 96 g carbs, 38 g protein.
- New England Clam Chowder (bowl): 940 calories, 65 g fat, 54 g carbs, 34 g protein.

The Awesome Blossom is about the worst appetizer on any menu. And at more than 1,700 calories, none of the quesadillas is a safe bet.

Denny's (www.dennys.com/en/page.asp?PID=1&ID=23)

- Mini Burgers (six) with Onion Rings: 2,220 calories, 136 g fat, 179 g carbs, 3,834 mg sodium, 76 g protein.
- Grand Slam Slugger with Hash Browns: 1,040 calories, 55 g fat, 97 g carbs, 38 g protein.

The Italian Chicken Melt is a poor option, but the calories and sodium in those Mini Burgers are off the charts. In terms of breakfast choices, the Sausage Bowl and the Grand Slam Slugger are just two examples of many calorie-packed items.

Bob Evans (www.bobevans.com)

- Sunshine Skillet: 948 calories, 72 g fat, 36 g carbs, 37 g protein.
- Country Biscuit Breakfast: 659 calories, 45 g fat, 40 g carbs, 24 g protein.
- Border Scramble Omelet: 855 calories, 70 g fat, 15 g carbs, 41 g protein.
- Farmer's Market Omelet: 911 calories, 74 g fat, 15 g carbs, 42 g protein.

Who knew you could cram so many calories into an egg-based dish, when the eggs themselves have only 75 calories apiece?

Fast Food

Researchers reported in the British medical journal *The Lancet* that people who ate fast food twice a week gained 10 pounds more over fifteen years than those who did so less than once a week. And the Cleveland Clinic has made attempts to remove McDonald's and other fast-food concessions from its hospital campus.

OK, so fast food is unhealthy and can make you fat—but almost any food you eat too much of can make you fat. And, yes, it can be difficult to eat healthfully at a fast-food restaurant, but it can be done. Here are a few tips, as well as some foods you can actually eat.

Go to the Net

Don't just walk in; look at the menu board and start picking. Almost every fast-food restaurant has nutrition information available online, so check the internet and have your order already planned before you get to the register. Also, mentally prepare yourself for suggestions by the counter person—get ready to say, "No thanks."

Watch the Weight

Just because a food is low in calories doesn't mean it's a bargain. Check the serving size and look at the grams to compare the weight with that of other foods you normally eat. Look to see how much of the food you have to eat in order to feel satisfied. And make sure that you don't deprive yourself; eat a real meal, which is about 350 to 600 calories for lunch or dinner, depending on your gender, height, and weight.

> ### Diet Detective's What You Need to Know
> **Fast Food Basics:**
>
> - As always, say no to mayo, tartar sauce, creamy dressings, and extra cheese. Don't be shy—ask questions about preparation.
> - Use mustard, ketchup, salt, pepper, or vinegar as fat-free ways to season your food.
> - For salads, watch the nuts, croutons, and other add-ons.
> - Chicken and fish can be good choices—but *only* if they are grilled or broiled, *not* breaded or deep fried.
> - Instead of cheese, opt for lettuce, tomato, and onion. Removing just one slice of cheese can save you about 100 calories.
> - Order a salad or broth-based soup to enjoy before your main meal.

Don't Take Their Word

Even if an item is labeled "low carb" or "healthy," don't take the restaurant's word for it. Review the information and ask yourself: Is this lower in calories than what I would normally choose to eat? And don't be fooled by menu items you'd think would be healthy but aren't, like the Taco Bell Fiesta Salad, which packs 870 calories and 47 grams of fat.

Make Better Choices

Look below for some of the better choices available at your favorite fast-food restaurants.

McDonald's
(www.mcdonalds.com/app_controller.nutrition.index1.html)

- Premium Grilled Chicken Classic Sandwich (without mayonnaise): 370 calories, 4.5 g fat, 50 g carbs, 32 g protein.
- Bacon Ranch Salad with Grilled Chicken (before dressing): 260 calories, 9 g fat, 12 g carbs, 33 g protein.
- Caesar Salad with Grilled Chicken (before dressing): 220 calories, 6 g fat, 12 g carbs, 30 g protein.

Fit Tip: Always choose grilled rather than crispy chicken, and hold the mayo. Newman's Own Low Fat Balsamic Vinaigrette is the best dressing at 40 calories for 2 ounces, while Newman's Own Ranch dressing has a whopping 170 calories and Newman's Own Caesar dressing has 190.

Calorie Bargain Spotlight

Calorie Bargain: McDonald's Southwest Salad with Grilled Chicken

The Why: It's fast, good, and low in calories. The salad, ordered with the grilled (not crispy) chicken, has a nice mix of lettuce, a few black beans, pieces of corn, and a few pieces of crispy tortilla. It makes for a satisfying lunch or dinner, even without any fries.

Note that this calorie count doesn't include dressing or croutons. So skip the Butter Garlic Croutons, which are 60 calories, and ask for

Newman's Own Low-fat Balsamic Vinaigrette or Newman's Own Low-fat Family Recipe Italian Dressing, which have about half the calories of the creamy dressing the salad usually comes with.

The Health Bonus: The salad has 7 grams of fiber. Wow.

What We Liked Best: a lean, healthy, and filling salad, from the drive-through, for about five bucks.

What We Liked Least: It's one of the most expensive items on the menu. Also, it's very high in sodium.

The Price: approximately $5.15 (with tax).

Offerings: available with grilled or crispy chicken. You gotta go for the grilled, or it'll cost you an extra 7 grams of fat and 80 calories.

Website: www.mcdonalds.com.

Where to Buy: At a McDonald's near you (www.mcdonalds.com/usa/rest_locator.html).

Ingredients: salad mix, grilled chicken breast filet, Southwest vegetable blend, cilantro lime glaze, shredded cheddar/Jack cheese, limes, chili lime tortilla strips, liquid margarine.

Nutritional Analysis per Serving
320 calories
9 g fat
30 g carbs
30 g protein
7 g fiber
970 mg sodium

Wendy's (www.wendys.com/food/pdf/us/nutrition.pdf)

- Ultimate Chicken Grill Sandwich: 370 calories, 8 g fat, 44 g carbs, 33 g protein.
- Plain 10-ounce baked potato with Buttery Best Spread and a side salad with fat-free French dressing: 440 calories, 6 g fat, 88 g carbs, 9 g protein.
- Two quarter-pound Classic Singles without buns and nothing on them except ketchup: 430 calories, 28 g fat, 4 g carbs, 38 g protein.
- Mandarin Chicken Salad with almonds (no noodles) and fat-free French dressing instead of the sesame dressing: 380 calories, 13 g fat, 41 g carbs, 28 g protein. You can also ask for the salad without the almonds and save another 130 calories.

Fit Tip: Get two Ultimate Chicken Grill Fillets without bread for a total of only 260 calories. If you add ketchup, it's another 15. Eight slices (about 6 ounces) of Roasted Turkey Breast is only 160 calories.

Burger King (www.bk.com/Nutrition/PDFs/brochure.pdf)

- Tendergrill Chicken Sandwich (without sauce): 400 calories, 7 g fat, 49 g carbs, 36 g protein. With the sauce, it's 450 calories, 10 g fat, 53 g carbs, 37 g protein. If you get the Tendergrill without any bread or sauce, just plain chicken, it's only 150 calories—not bad.
- BK Veggie Burger (without mayonnaise): 340 calories, 8 g fat, 46 g carbs, 23 g protein. (Add another 110 calories if you want the mayo.)

- Angus Steak Burger—low carb: 260 calories, 18 g fat, 2 g carbs, 24 g protein.
- Tendergrill Chicken Garden Salad (without dressing): 240 calories, 9 g fat, 8 g carbs, 33 g protein. If you want the dressing, it's 300 calories, 9 g fat, 24 g carbs, 33 g protein.
- Side Garden Salad (15 calories) with Ken's Light Italian Dressing (120 calories) and garlic croutons (60 calories): 195 calories, 13 g fat, 15 g carbs, 2 g protein. Or go with Ken's Fat-free Ranch Dressing, which is only 60 calories for 2 ounces.

Fit Tip: Anything low carb that comes without mayo, ketchup, or a bun will save you a bundle of calories. For a list of carb counts go to (www.bk.com/Nutrition/PDFs/Low%20Carb%20handout%204-3-06.pdf). Even a Whopper with just the patty, pickles, onions, tomatoes, lettuce, and ketchup is only 255 calories. Burger King's website is very helpful for finding nutritional information.

Subway (www.subway.com/subwayroot/MenuNutrition/Nutrition/pdf/NutritionValues.pdf)

- 6-inch Veggie Delite sandwich: 230 calories, 3 g fat, 44 g carbs, 9 g protein.
- 6-inch Turkey Breast sandwich: 280 calories, 4.5 g fat, 46 g carbs, 18 g protein.
- 6-inch Double Ham Sub: 350 calories, 7 g fat, 49 g carbs, 28 g protein.
- Minestrone soup (10-ounce bowl): 90 calories, 0.5 g fat, 17 g carbs, 4 g protein.
- Roasted Chicken Noodle Soup (1 cup): 80 calories, 2 g fat, 11 g carbs, 6 g protein.

Fit Tip: Order your sandwich without mayo or other special sauces. Opt for vinegar or mustard instead. If you want a bag of chips, choose Baked Lay's. And if you're really hungry, ask for a double-meat 6-inch sub with roast beef (360 calories), turkey (340 calories), or ham (350 calories). The soups are also very low in calories. For instance, a 10-ounce bowl of Tomato Garden Vegetable with Rotini is only 90 calories. Subway has a great program called FreshFit: Pick one of its sandwiches with less than 6 grams of fat and get a choice of baked chips, apple slices, or raisins, and, for a beverage, 1 percent low-fat milk, water, or diet soda.

Chick-fil-A (www.chickfila.com/MenuTable.asp)

- Chick-fil-A Southwest Chargrilled Salad with one packet Fat-free Honey Mustard Dressing: 300 calories, 6 g fat, 37 g carbs, 22 g protein.
- Chick-fil-A Chargrilled Chicken Garden Salad: 180 calories, 6 g fat, 9 g carbs, 22 g protein.
- Reduced-fat Raspberry Vinaigrette Dressing: 80 calories, 2 g fat, 15 g carbs, 0 g protein.
- Spicy Chicken Cool Wrap: 410 calories, 12 g fat, 44 g carbs, 35 g protein.

Fit Tip: If you order the chicken sandwich, ask for it without butter. You can also get a Chargrilled Chicken "sandwich" without the bun and pickles for only 100 calories. And try the Diet Lemonade—it has only 30 calories for 12 ounces (medium) and is very tasty.

Taco Bell (www.yum.com/nutrition/documents/tb_nutrition.pdf)

- Two Fresco Style Chicken Ranchero Tacos: 330 calories, 8 g fat, 41 g carbs, 25 g protein.

- Fresco Style Burrito Supreme (Chicken): 350 calories, 8 g fat, 50 g carbs, 19 g protein.
- Fresco Style Grilled Steak Soft Taco with Fresco Style Mexican Rice: 320 calories, 9 g fat, 47 g carbs, 13 g protein.

Fit Tip: Order everything "Fresco Style"—with salsa and without cheese or sauce. All the Fresco Style Burrito Supremes and Enchiritos are pretty good and come in decent-size portions. The regular Gordita and Chalupa are not too high in calories either, but the portions are smaller.

Jack in the Box
(www.jackinthebox.com/ourfood/index.php?section=7)

- Asian Chicken Salad (no wonton strips) with almonds and Low-fat Balsamic Dressing: 290 calories, 12 g fat, 25 g carbs, 19 g protein.
- Chicken Fajita Pita with salsa: 305 calories, 10 g fat, 32 g carbs, 23 g protein.
- Chicken Sandwich (without the mayo-onion sauce), a Side Salad (hold the croutons), and Low-fat Balsamic Dressing: 410 calories, 16 g fat, 48 g carbs, 18 g protein.

Fit Tip: The plain hamburger is 300 calories, which is not bad, but the specialty burgers range from 900 to more than 1,000.

Arby's (www.arbys.com/nutrition/printable.php?type=nutrition)

- Regular Roast Beef Sandwich: 320 calories, 14 g fat, 34 g carbs, 20 g protein.
- Martha's Vineyard Salad with Light Buttermilk Ranch Dressing: 276 calories, 8 g fat, 24 g carbs, 26 g protein.

- Medium Roast Beef Sandwich, 415 calories, 21 g fat, 34 g carbs, 31 g protein. (This has a generous amount of meat; drop the bun, and it's only 239 calories.)

Fit Tip: The bun is what costs you the most calories in any sandwich, so you might want to use only half and save about 100 calories.

Kentucky Fried Chicken
(www.yum.com/nutrition/documents/kfc_nutrition.pdf)

- Tender Roast Sandwich without sauce: 300 calories, 4.5 g fat, 28 g carbs, 37 g protein.
- Roasted Caesar Salad without dressing and croutons: 220 calories, 8 g fat, 6 g carbs, 30 g protein.
- Roasted BLT Salad (without dressing): 200 calories, 6 g fat, 8 g carbs, 29 g protein.

Fit Tip: If you take the skin and breading off the Original Recipe chicken breast, you'll save a whopping 190 calories and 13.5 grams of fat! And if you want a side, choose green beans (50 calories) or a large corn on the cob (150 calories). For salad dressing, use the Hidden Valley Original Ranch Fat-free Dressing—it's only 35 calories—or the Hidden Valley Golden Italian Light Dressing, which is 45 calories.

Long John Silver's
(www.ljsilvers.com/nutrition/res/pdf/brochure.pdf)

- Baked Cod with two Corn Cobettes: 310 calories, 10 g fat, 27 g carbs, 27 g protein
- Shrimp and Seafood Salad with Lite Italian Dressing: 350 calories, 17 g fat, 33 g carbs, 19 g protein.

Fit Tip: Fish and seafood can be healthy—as long as they're not battered and fried. Avoid the tartar sauce; it's 100 calories per ounce. The cocktail sauce is only 25 calories per ounce.

Blimpie (www.blimpie.com/na/nutritional_facts.php)

- Grilled Chicken Salad: 350 calories, 27 g fat, 9 g carbs, 18 g protein.
- Garden Vegetable Soup: 80 calories, 0.5 g fat, 14 g carbs, 5 g protein.
- Hot Grilled Chicken Sub: 370 calories, 9 g fat, 50 g carbs, 25 g protein.

Fit Tip: If you want potato salad, go with the mustard version rather than the regular to save 110 calories. Also, if you're a low-carb person, Blimpie has a carb-counter menu at www.blimpie.com/bcc/BCC_Menu.pdf.

Carl's Jr. (http://www.carlsjr.com/nutrition)

- Charbroiled BBQ Chicken Sandwich: 360 calories, 4 g fat, 48 g carbs, 34 g protein.
- Charbroiled Chicken Salad: 260 calories, 7 g fat, 16 g carbs, 34 g protein.
- The Low Carb Six Dollar Burger (served without a bun): 490 calories, 37 g fat, 6 g carbs, 33 g protein.

Fit Tip: Use Low-fat Balsamic Dressing on the salads; it's only 35 calories per serving. Watch out for some of the fancier hamburgers, such as the Super Star with Cheese, at 930 calories; the Double Western Bacon Cheeseburger, at 970 calories; and especially the Six Dollar burgers, ranging from 1,010 to 1,520 calories.

Diet Detective's What You Need to Know

Nutrient Density: There is no one accepted definition of "nutrient density," says Joanne R. Lupton, PhD, a professor of nutrition at Texas A&M University. That said, the overall concept is how much nutrient value you get for each calorie consumed. "Nutrient-dense foods provide high amounts of nutrients at a low-calorie cost." For a food to be considered nutrient dense, it must provide substantial amounts of vitamins and minerals and relatively fewer calories.

As Dr. Katz, associate professor of public health and director of the Prevention Research Center, at Yale University School of Medicine, explains that the opposite of *nutrient dense* is *calorie dense*, or *nutrient dilute*—foods that mainly supply calories, with relatively few nutrients. These are often referred to as "empty calories": calories that provide few or no health benefits.

Foods that are nutrient dense should provide 50 percent more in nutrients than they cost in calories. Take sunflower seeds, for example. A ¼ cup packs about 200 calories, which doesn't seem like a Calorie Bargain when you consider that a can of Sprite has only 140 calories and a Hershey's Kiss has only 25. But that ¼ cup of seeds also provides more than 20 percent of the daily value for folate and vitamin B_5 and over 25 percent for phosphorous, tryptophan, copper, magnesium, and manganese. Meanwhile, the 200 calories are only about 11 percent of daily calorie needs. So you're getting twice as many nutrients as calories.

Some foods are almost always nutrient dense: whole grains and whole-grain products, fruits, vegetables, and legumes. Remember that a food doesn't have to be extremely low in fat or calories to be nutrient dense—it just has to counterbalance the calorie count with an exceptional level of nutritional value.

Casual Dining

Many of our restaurant meals are eaten at "casual dining" restaurants such as T.G.I. Friday's, Chili's, Applebee's, Olive Garden, Outback Steakhouse, Denny's, Red Lobster, Ruby Tuesday, and P F. Chang's China Bistro. Believe it or not, dining at these restaurants can cost you more calories than eating fast food. It's important to know how to eat out and not take in an entire day's worth of calories (1,800 to 2,500) at one sitting. Here are a few healthier choices and tips to keep in mind when you decide to go casual:

T.G.I Friday's (www.tgifridays.com)

The following are all 500 calories or less and 10 grams or less of fat per serving:

- Dragonfire Chicken: marinated chicken breast with stir-fried brown rice and Cilantro Lime seasoned broccoli.
- Zen Chicken Pot Stickers: fire-grilled dumplings stuffed with minced chicken and vegetables.
- Santa Fe Chicken Salad: Get the Chipotle Ranch dressing on the side.
- Lo-Phat Chicken Salad: chilled sautéed chicken with low-fat Cilantro Lime dressing.

Fit Tip: Just because the menu says "Right Portion, Right Price" doesn't mean it's a healthier choice. Watch out for the appetizers (often loaded with fat), salads (may have more than 700 calories with dressing), steak and ribs (T.G.I. Friday's is known for these particularly fattening foods), and everything on the Atkins-approved menu.

Outback Steakhouse (www.outbacksteakhouse.com)

- Shrimp and Veggie Griller, Chicken and Veggie Griller, or Steak and Veggie Griller: Request no butter or glaze and skip the pineapple. Get a baked potato with ketchup or salsa (no butter or sour cream) instead of rice; get a house salad (hold the croutons and cheese) and use a fork to sprinkle it with low-fat dressing—such as fat-free Tangy Tomato Dressing, fresh lemon juice, or red wine vinegar with olive oil—625, 715, and 775 calories, respectively.
- Chicken on the Barbie: Again, order a baked or sweet potato and a house salad—640 calories.
- Steamed vegetables: Order without butter—75 calories.
- Grilled Shrimp on the Barbie: Order with cocktail or barbecue sauce and no butter—275 calories.
- Sweet potato: Order without toppings and split it with someone because it's large—240 calories.
- Salmon: Order it without butter or seasoning and ask for cocktail sauce or fresh lemon instead of Remoulade Sauce—415 calories.
- Victoria's Center Cut Filet: Order the 7-ounce size with steamed vegetables (no butter) and a baked potato—440 calories.

(All of the above calorie counts have been estimated by a registered dietitian.)

Fit Tip: Almost everything on the menu has butter, seasoning, or some fattening sauce, so make sure to ask that your dish be prepared without. As far as steak is concerned, your best bet would be sirloin (about 700 calories for 12 ounces), one of the leanest cuts you can order. Or go with filet mignon, which is smaller—typically 9 ounces and about 450 calories, with approximately 9 grams of saturated fat. Whatever you do, don't order the Aussie Cheese Fries; they have more than 2,000 calories!

P. F. Chang's China Bistro (www.pfchangs.com)

This is probably the only Chinese restaurant in the country that posts nutrition information for every single dish on its website. Ever wonder how many calories and fat grams you're eating? It's worth taking a peek. There are some great dishes here, but there are also many dieting pitfalls.

- Ginger Chicken & Broccoli: 660 calories, 26 g fat, 45 g carbs.
- Seared Ahi Tuna: 312 calories, 11 g fat, 21 g carbs.
- Shrimp Dumplings (steamed): 290 calories, 9 g fat, 26 g carbs.
- Shrimp with Lobster Sauce (dinner portion): 480 calories, 22 g fat, 24 g carbs.
- Buddha's Feast (steamed): 200 calories, 1.5 g fat, 43 g carbs. The stir-fried version has 230 more calories.
- Cantonese Scallops: 400 calories, 16 g fat, 26 g carbs.
- Cantonese Shrimp: 330 calories, 12 g fat, 21 g carbs.

Fit Tip: Make a meal out of appetizers and sides. Choose Seared Ahi Tuna and Sichuan Asparagus or Shanghai Cucumbers. Avoid all the salads, which have between 610 and 1,230 calories. Steer clear of anything named Kung Pao, such as Kung Pao Chicken (1,240 calories), and avoid Chang's Spare Ribs, which have 1,280 calories and 20 grams of saturated fat (the Northern Style Spare Ribs have 730 calories and 12 grams of saturated fat).

Chili's (www.chilis.com)

The Guiltless Grill menu of low-calorie choices is great. Chili's will also make adjustments to any of the other food items on the menu because they're all made to order. For instance, if you want a house salad as an appetizer, ask for dressing on the side and choose either the fat-free honey-mustard or low-fat ranch dressing.

- Guiltless Chicken Platter with rice, corn on the cob, and steamed vegetables: 580 calories, 9 g fat, 85 g carbs.
- Guiltless Chicken Sandwich with black beans, steamed fresh veggies, and Parmesan cheese: 490 calories, 8 g fat, 63 g carbs. Skip the cheese to save even more calories.
- Guiltless Grill Salmon with steamed fresh veggies and black beans: 480 calories, 14 g fat, 31 g carbs.

Fit Tip: Order your fajitas without the tortillas and save 370 calories. Forget the Awesome Blossom at 2,710 calories! In fact, skip all the appetizers; they're too expensive caloriewise. Avoid the Fajita Steak, Chicken, and Combo Quesadillas, all upward of 1,700 calories each. Steer clear of the margaritas too.

Applebee's (www.applebees.com)

Applebee's has teamed up with Weight Watchers to create some excellent low-calorie choices. Most portions are the same size as those on its regular menu, which means that the chain is using better cooking techniques and healthier ingredients—like whole wheat and low-cal cheeses and sauces, not just giving you half the food.

- Onion Soup au Gratin: 150 calories, 8 g fat.
- Grilled Shrimp Skewer Salad: 210 calories, 2 g fat.
- Teriyaki Steak 'N Shrimp Skewers with rice pilaf and vegetables: 370 calories, 7 g fat.
- Cajun Lime Tilapia with rice pilaf and vegetables: 310 calories, 6 g fat.
- Confetti Chicken with rice pilaf and vegetables: 370 calories, 7 g fat.

Fit Tip: Don't be fooled by the sandwiches and roll-ups: They're high in calories, especially with the fries, cheese, and sauces. Avoid all the "Neighborhood Favorites," which look dangerous. If you order dinner from the Weight Watchers menu and you really want dessert, you can probably fit in the Chocolate Raspberry Layer Cake (230 calories, 3 grams of fat) and not break the calorie bank.

Red Lobster (www.redlobster.com)

Don't think that just because it's seafood it's healthy—there's plenty of unhealthy fried, buttery seafood out there. However, the LightHouse choices at Red Lobster are low fat and low calorie.

- Live Maine Lobster (1¼ pounds) with a baked potato (topped with pico de gallo) and a garden salad with red wine vinaigrette: 432 calories, 8 g fat, 53 g carbs.
- Garlic-Grilled Jumbo Shrimp with seasoned broccoli and wild rice pilaf: 402 calories, 8 g fat, 47 g carbs.
- North Pacific King Crab Legs: 490 calories, 9 g fat, 0 g carbs.
- Grilled Chicken Breast with wild rice pilaf: 518 calories, 13 g fat, 36 g carbs. Replace the rice with broccoli, and it drops to 370 calories, 8 g fat, and 10 g carbs.

Fit Tip: The nice thing about Red Lobster is that you can get the tilapia, rainbow trout, or salmon in full or half orders, so you can save calories on portion size. Make sure to substitute cocktail sauce whenever a dish comes with a side of butter sauce—that saves 115 calories per serving. And pico de gallo (chopped tomatoes, onions, and herbs—like a chunkier salsa) on your potato adds only 6 calories, for a total of 185 calories, which definitely beats butter! Watch out for the salads too; they have high-calorie dressings, cheese, and other unhealthy goodies.

Olive Garden (www.olivegarden.com)

These restaurants are very accommodating and take special requests reasonably well. You can also shave calories by ordering a lunch portion of the Garden Fare meals.

- Minestrone soup: 164 calories, 1 g fat.
- Linguine alla Marinara: 551 calories, 8 g fat.
- Capellini Pomodoro: 644 calories, 14 g fat.
- Chicken Giardino (ask for whole wheat pasta): 560 calories, 15 g fat.

- Pork Filettino with grilled vegetables: 340 calories, 9 g fat (does not include demi-glace or marinade).

Fit Tip: Stick with the Garden Fare choices, designated on the menu with an olive branch, and order Low-fat Italian Dressing (37 calories per serving) or Low-fat Parmesan-Peppercorn Dressing (45 calories per serving) with any salad. You should assume that many of the dishes not designated Garden Fare have more than 1,000 calories, especially those that are creamy, fried, or cheesy. Also, watch out for the bread sticks. At 140 calories apiece, they can make any meal a diet disaster. Put in a "stop order" with your server before they even come near your table.

Ruby Tuesday (www.rubytuesday.com)

One amazing thing this chain has done is to offer full nutritional information on its website. Another is that Ruby Tuesday has asked all of its suppliers to remove trans fat from their products, and it has switched from hydrogenated soybean oil to trans-fat-free canola for cooking. Ruby Tuesday also has a Smart Eating menu with nutritional information printed right on it.

- Petite Sirloin: 206 calories, 5 g fat.
- Garden Vegetable Soup: 183 calories, 7 g fat.
- Asian Spiced Dumplings (appetizer): 130 calories, 6 g fat.

Fit Tip: The salads are high in calories, particularly the Carolina Chicken Salad, at 1,025. Try to stick with an appetizer or soup for your meal or two very low-calorie appetizers and a soup. You should also order from the Smart Eating menu; most of the main dishes are over 1,000 calories. One dish—the Fresh Chicken & Broccoli Pasta—breaks the 2,000-calorie mark!

Family Dining

I know how it feels. You're with your family or friends at one of those "family" restaurants, and you don't want to be a killjoy, but the truth is, these restaurants are not meant for the diet savvy—they are designed for indulgence and value meals. Many of them don't include the nutritional content on their menus, and there's that social aspect of dining with a large group that also encourages more eating. To keep your diet wits about you, try the following suggestions.

Denny's (www.dennys.com)

Denny's is the leading family-style restaurant chain in the United States, with about 1,600 units around the country. They're typically open twenty-four hours a day, seven days a week, and serve breakfast, lunch, and dinner. The menu features a variety of breakfast items along with standards like hamburgers, steaks, salads, and desserts. However, Denny's has developed a Fit Fare menu to help you make healthier choices.

- Grilled Chicken Breast Salad (without dressing): 310 calories, 13 g fat, 13 g carbs.

- Turkey Breast Salad (without dressing): 230 calories, 10 g fat, 13 g carbs.
- Fit Fare Grilled Chicken Breast Dinner: 190 calories, 3 g fat, 12 g carbs. Add sides of plain baked potato (220 calories, 0 g fat, 51 g carbs) and green beans (40 calories, 1 g fat, 8 g carbs).
- Boca Burger with small fruit bowl: 508 calories, 11 g fat, 78 g carbs.
- Vegetable Beef soup: 79 calories, 1 g fat, 11 g carbs.
- Steakhouse Strip Dinner (no sides): 410 calories, 27 g fat, 3 g carbs.

Fit Tip: Watch the sodium content. In most casual dining restaurants, it's usually off the charts. For instance, the Hickory Grilled Chicken has 6,030 milligrams of sodium—more than three times what's recommended for a day. To save calories, if you order the sandwiches, go bare and skip the bread. Also, stay away from the Mini Burgers with Onion Rings: 2,044 calories, 122 grams of fat, and 179 grams of carbs.

Bob Evans (www.bobevans.com/)

With more than 560 family-style restaurants, Bob Evans offers many high-calorie meals but also quite a few healthy items. The best news is that this chain offers nutritional information on its website, so you can plan ahead.

- Grilled Chicken Breast dinner (1 piece): 232 calories, 13 g fat, 0 g carbs.
- Salmon dinner (plain): 287 calories, 13 g fat, 0 g carbs.
- Lite Sausage Breakfast: 469 calories, 21 g fat, 48 g carbs.
- Fresh Fruit & Yogurt Plate: 398 calories, 2 g fat, 92 g carbs.

Fit Tip: For breakfast, avoid the three varieties of Stacked and Stuffed Hotcakes (Roasted Caramel Apple, Chocolate Banana Cream, and Caramel Banana Pecan Cream), with 1,439, 1,466, and 1,553 calories, respectively. Substitute grilled garden vegetables for your fries and have them prepared without margarine or oil. Watch out for the salads (unless that's all you're eating); with the exception of the side salad, at 171 calories, they all have at least 500 calories. The Cranberry Pecan Chicken Salad and the Chili & Cheese Taco Salad top the list at 1,108 and 1,381 calories. For salad dressings, stick with the "side" portion as opposed to the "dinner" portion, which is double the size, and order one of the low-cal choices.

- Hot Bacon Dressing (side portion): 106 calories.
- Lite Ranch Dressing (side portion): 103 calories.
- Or better yet, just have the Vinegar and Oil Dressing side portion: only 27 calories!

Fit Tip: Skip the bakery part of the restaurant, especially the bread bowls, which can be the equivalent of seven slices of bread!

International House of Pancakes (IHOP)
(www.ihop.com)

This company's nearly two thousand restaurants, open twenty-four hours a day, are best known for their high-calorie breakfasts, but they also offer standard family fare (sandwiches, burgers, and salads) for lunch and dinner.

While no nutritional information is available on its website, IHOP claims that the following have fewer than 600 calories:

- Buttermilk Trio: short stack of buttermilk pancakes topped with Promise margarine and sugar-free syrup.
- Garden Scramble: egg substitute, mushrooms, peppers, onions, and tomatoes, two buttermilk pancakes, Promise margarine, sugar-free syrup.

It also lists the Garden Scramble, the Simply Chicken Sandwich, and the Fresh Fruit in the less-than-15-grams-of-fat category.

Fit Tip: Skip the Signature Breakfasts—typically the foods that have the most calories. Don't fall for the Harvest Grain 'N Nut Pancake Combo, which may sound healthy but isn't even whole grain. Also avoid the By the Basketful items, which are basically fried foods plus french fries. And be sure to ask for grilled vegetables without butter or oil.

Friendly's (www.friendlys.com)

There are close to 660 Friendly's family-style restaurants in sixteen states, many in the Northeast and mid-Atlantic regions. Although a Friendly's spokesperson made it clear that it considers itself a chain of ice cream shops—emphasizing that the primary reason to go there is to indulge—Friendly's still manages to have "some lighter selections on the menu." Unfortunately, nutritional information is not available.

The following menu items appear to be the lowest in calories and fat:

- Chunky Chicken Noodle Soup.
- Side Garden Salad with low-fat Italian dressing.
- Grilled Chicken Deluxe Sandwich.
- Gardenburger veggie burger.

Fit Tip: Many of the menu items are fried or have cheese or bacon added and with ice cream everywhere, this place can be a nightmare. Stick to the lighter menu, but if you want to order from the regular menu, make sure that your food is grilled, not fried, and substitute salad for fries.

Cracker Barrel (www.crackerbarrel.com)

If you've ever traveled on a highway, you've surely spotted this neat restaurant chain. There are more than five hundred Cracker Barrel Old Country Store restaurants in forty states. Known for its country design and home-style cooking, Cracker Barrel has a large menu and plenty of healthier options. Breakfast is served all day, and the choices include egg whites (make sure to ask for no oil or butter) and whole wheat bread.

All the following are 400 calories or less:

- Homemade Chicken n' Dumplins Country Dinner Plate with green beans and carrots: 390 calories, 10 g fat, 45 g carbs.
- Grilled Chicken Tenderloin Country Dinner Plate (four tenders) with corn and green beans: 400 calories, 18 g fat, 28 g carbs.
- Country Vegetable Plate with corn, green beans, carrots, and turnip greens: 380 calories, 20 g fat, 37 g carbs.

You can also get a tossed salad (use fat-free Italian or ranch dressing) and a 12-ounce bowl of soup (vegetable, potato, turkey noodle, chicken noodle, chicken noodle & vegetable, cheesy tomato, chicken n' rice) for fewer than 500 calories.

Fit Tip: Cracker Barrel is very helpful and aims to prepare foods the way you like them. Order your grilled dishes prepared with cooking spray instead of oil. Avoid many of the Fancy Fixin's and Daily Dinner Features—pure comfort foods with megacalories. Watch out for all the fried offerings, and make sure to ask for healthier sides such as a baked potato or vegetables made without oil or butter.

Coffeehouses

Every day Americans drink more than 300 million cups of coffee, and, while most are brewed at home, the Specialty Coffee Association of America reports that an ever-growing number are being purchased from coffeehouses like Starbucks. On its own, coffee is not fattening—in fact, it has no calories. The problems start with what we add to it: milk, sugar, whipped cream, chocolate, and more. And as if that weren't enough, we're getting our coffee from places that also offer cakes, croissants, and other treats, making our local coffeehouses more dangerous for dieters than fast-food restaurants.

Think about this: Just one piece of coffee crumb cake and a fancy Frappuccino with whipped cream (1,180 calories total) can add up to more calories than a Big Mac, medium fries, and a soda (1,060 calories). Oh, and if you've heard rumors that caffeine helps you burn calories, let's just say that if it really made much of a difference, Americans would be in pretty good shape, because we're the largest consumers of caffeine in the world.

However, there are choices. As Starbucks claims, there are more than twenty-one thousand beverage combinations to choose from, not to mention the baked goods, sandwiches, and salads. Here are a few hints to help you make better choices the next time you have your cup of java.

Espresso vs. Cappuccino vs. Latte vs. Café Au Lait

At 5 calories per ounce, a shot of espresso is your best deal. A Starbucks cappuccino—an espresso with a small amount of steamed milk and a deep layer of foam—has 150 calories for 16 ounces. A latte is an espresso with more steamed milk than a cappuccino, also topped with foam: it has 260 calories for 16 ounces. Café au lait is a one-to-one mix of coffee and steamed milk and has 140 calories for 16 ounces. Starbucks's Espresso Macchiato, a sweet espresso shot with a small amount of foamed milk, also seems like a good deal at only 10 calories for 1 ounce, if that's all you have.

Fit Tip: Skip the whip. Adding whipped cream to your drink packs on at least an extra 100 calories and as much as a quarter of a day's worth of saturated fat. Your server will probably add it unless you request to have it left off. So go ahead and ask!

Starbucks Hot Chocolate vs. White Hot Chocolate

Yes, you may save a little on caffeine by going with a hot chocolate, but the White Hot Chocolate with whipped cream has 580 calories per 16 ounces with 28 grams of fat (19 of them saturated). Sixteen ounces of hot chocolate with whipped cream, on the other hand, has 450 calories and 24 grams of fat (13 saturated). That's a lot of chocolate. How about having 12 ounces of nonfat chocolate milk or hot chocolate (no whipped cream) for 190 or 210 calories?

Fit Tip: You're better off having a regular coffee with skim milk and Splenda (another sugar replacement or even a tablespoon of sugar is also fine), and if you're at Starbucks, you can get one of those little dark chocolate squares at the front counter to satisfy your chocolate craving. They're small: only 60 calories. Or try the sugar-free flavored syrups for no extra calories.

Dunkin' Donuts Coffee Coolatta with Skim Milk vs. Starbucks Espresso Frappuccino Light Blended Coffee

It's actually a pretty close call. The Espresso Frappuccino Light (140 calories for 16 ounces) wins by 30 calories. The Coolatta with Skim Milk has 170 calories in 16 ounces. Just in case you didn't know, a Frappuccino is coffee and milk blended with ice.

Fit Tip: Always choose skim milk or, at the very least, low-fat milk for coffee and tea drinks. The Coolatta with cream has 180 more calories than the Coolatta with skim milk.

Starbucks Tazo Chai Iced Tea Latte vs. Dunkin' Donuts Caramel Swirl Latte with Soy Milk

The Chai tea is the better option here at 200 calories for 12 ounces; you get 2 more ounces for fewer calories than the 10-ounce latte (210 calories). Tea without sugar and milk has virtually no calories, but when you start to make it fancy, the calories add up. Take a look at Starbucks's 16-ounce Tazo Chai Frappuccino Blended Crème (510 calories), or a Dunkin' Donuts Vanilla Chai: 230 calories for 10 ounces.

Fit Tip: Choose herbal tea—it's flavored and has no calories.

Starbucks Reduced-fat Cinnamon Swirl Coffee Cake vs. Butter Croissant

Surprisingly, the Butter Croissant, at approximately 310 calories (varies by region), is a better choice than the 330-calorie coffee cake. Plus, the coffee cake has 22 more grams of carbohydrates. Neither is a healthy choice (doughnuts, cakes, croissants, muffins, and scones aren't necessarily part of a good diet), but if you're going to have one anyway, at least choose the better option.

Fit Tip: Just because something has fruit in it or is low in fat doesn't mean it's healthy. For instance, Starbucks's Iced Lemon Loaf, with as many as 500 calories a slice, is certainly not a healthy choice. Keep your total coffee shop calories under 350—for both your drink and dessert. Also, watch out for those cookies, because many of them have as many as 500 calories—that's just one cookie! For baked goods, your best bet at most coffeehouses would be a biscotti, at around 110 to 150 calories.

Dunkin' Donuts Strawberry Cheese Danish vs. Chocolate Frosted Donut

The doughnut actually wins. The Danish (320 calories) isn't so bad compared to other potential dieting nightmares, but the doughnut has "only" 200 calories. Doughnuts certainly aren't diet food, but, believe it or not, if you avoid the cake and cream-filled varieties, they might be better than some of the muffins, scones, and Danishes. Even a jelly doughnut has just 210 calories; compare that to the Chocolate Chip Muffin, with a whopping 630 calories, or the Coffee Cake Muffin, at 580.

Fit Tip: All doughnuts are not created equal—and I'm not talking about the difference between Krispy Kreme and Dunkin' Donuts. Cake doughnuts have twice as much fat as yeast doughnuts, and it really does matter whether you have frosting, sprinkles, or a glaze. Just take a look at the difference between the Dunkin' Donuts Chocolate Frosted (Yeast) Donut (200 calories) and the Chocolate Frosted Cake Donut (360 calories).

Dunkin' Donuts Egg Cheese English Muffin Sandwich vs. Bagel with Cream Cheese

The English muffin sandwich (280 calories) wins. The bagel starts out with 280 to 350 calories, and if you add cream cheese (190 calories for 2 ounces), you'll have eaten as many as 500 calories before you even get to your coffee.

Fit Tip: You can save some calories by using low-fat cream cheese (110 calories for 2 ounces), but an even better breakfast option would be low-fat yogurt and fresh fruit, which many coffee places now serve.

Calorie Bargain Spotlight

Calorie Bargain: Holey Donuts (Marble Frosted)

The Why: If you've ever sat in the parking lot waiting for that "Hot Krispy Kreme—Now" sign to light up, this Calorie Bargain is for you. Somewhere over the rainbow, you could eat doughnuts all day long and not get a bellyache. Or a belly. Holey Donuts is here to tell you that "somewhere" is right here, right now.

The Health Bonus: Its proprietary recipe and cooking method give you all the doughnutty taste and texture you love, sans the deep fryer. And that's why the nutritional information on these puppies seems almost too good to be true. Plus, no trans fat.

What We Liked Best: Once cooked, they are flash frozen and shipped via FedEx right to your door. They come with clear and simple instructions on how to defrost and enjoy.

What We Liked Least: Doughnuts must be shipped, so no instant gratification. Also, they're still not super low calorie, so they should be eaten sparingly.

The Price: $23.95 per dozen.

Offerings: Glazed, Coconut Cream Pie, Boston Cream, Apple Caramel, Raspberry Crumb, Jelly, Blueberry Crumb, Strawberry Shortcake, Apple Coffee Cake, Marble Frosted, Classic Vanilla, Caramel Crumb Ring, Dolce Latte Frosted, Caramel Vanilla, Strawberry Swirl.

Website: www.holeydonuts.net.

Where to Buy: company website at www.holeydonuts.net.

Ingredients: wheat flour, niacin, iron, thiamine mononitrate, riboflavin, folic acid, dextrose, soybean oil. Contains less than 2 percent of salt, dairy blend (whey solids, nonfat dry milk, sodium caseinate), leavening (sodium acid pryophosphate, baking soda), soy flour, dried egg yolks, monoglycerides, diglycerides, citric acid added as preservative, sodium stearoyl lactylate (dough conditioner), vegetable color (annatto and turmeric) contains wheat, egg, milk, and soy. Glaze ingredients: sugar, water, cornstarch, corn syrup, modified food starch, wheat starch, agar, guar gum, potassium sorbate (as preservative), citric acid, silicon dioxide, artificial flavor, dextrose, 101904 (L).

Nutritional Analysis per Serving: 1 Donut
210 calories
3.5 g fat
39 g carbs
4 g protein

Deli Food

There are so many choices when you walk into a deli, but it's not just about the sandwiches—deli food is really an entire category unto itself. See if you can pick the healthier choices below.

Stuffed Grape Leaves vs. Roasted Red Peppers vs. Pitted Greek Olives

Stuffed grape leaves are the worst of the lot: Five leaves have 210 calories. Three ounces of roasted red peppers in oil have about half the calories, at 120. If you have four or five olives, however, you're looking at only 25 to 45 calories—they're about 6 to 9 calories apiece. But the real winner would be simple roasted red peppers that aren't packed in oil: 30 calories for 4½ ounces.

Pesto Pasta Salad vs. Tuna Salad

You might think that all the mayonnaise in tuna salad would make it the worse choice, but the numbers show the opposite: For a ½-cup serving, tuna salad has 230 calories, whereas pesto pasta salad, with ground pine nuts, oil, and pasta, is quite a bit higher at 340 calories for the same amount. Coleslaw might be your best option, but with mayonnaise, sugar, and sometimes additional olive oil or other ingredients, the end result can still have 150 calories per ½ cup.

If you're ordering pasta salad, ask the people at your deli if they have 100 percent whole wheat pasta (not semolina or 100 percent pure durum semolina). The extra fiber will fill you up faster. Another way to fill up without increasing calories is to add lots of vegetables—isn't that the idea of a salad anyway? So look for salads that include lots of vegetables, and if you can request extra veggies, go ahead. At home, make your own fresh bean salad with assorted veggies dressed with vinegar and lemon juice for only 70 calories per ½ cup. Make sure to use low-fat mayo when making tuna, and go light on the oil when making pesto salad.

Potato Knish vs. Sour Pickles

A knish consists of a filling enclosed in dough that is either baked or fried. Fillings range from mashed potato or ground meat to kasha (buckwheat groats) or cheese, among others. A 6-ounce potato knish has about 300 calories—no contest when compared with the calories in a pickle. In fact, if we snacked on pickles more often, we would probably lose weight. Pickles have almost no calories at all; their only downside is that they're typically very high in sodium.

Hummus vs. Baba Ghanoush

Hummus, a popular Middle Eastern spread made from chickpeas, tahini (ground sesame seeds), roasted garlic, and olive oil, has 50 to 70 calories per 2 tablespoons (1 ounce). Baba ghanoush, another popular Middle Eastern dish, is made with eggplant sautéed in olive oil and then pureed with tahini; 1 ounce also has about 50 to 70 calories. Keep in mind that these spreads require something to spread them on—and the calories in crackers quickly add up. Assume that each cracker has at least 10 to 20 calories.

Broccoli and Cheddar Quiche vs. Gourmet Ham and Cheese Wrap vs. Tomato, Mozzarella, and Pesto Sandwich

Your best bet is actually the ham and cheese wrap. A 6-ounce ham and cheese wrap with mayo has 360 calories, whereas a 4.7-ounce piece of broccoli and cheddar quiche (one-sixth of the pie) has about 380 calories—and most likely won't be nearly as filling. The highest of the bunch is the tomato, mozzarella, and pesto sandwich, at about 450 calories for 6 ounces. The problem is, many delis serve 10- or 12-ounce sandwiches, which can contain more than 800 calories, so don't be shy about asking them to wrap up half to take home.

Pastrami vs. Roast Beef vs. Corned Beef

Pastrami is corned beef that's been smoked for added flavor, then salted, dried, and seasoned, and sometimes sugared—which means 4 ounces can have as much as 390 calories and 1,900 milligrams of sodium, whereas 4 ounces of roast beef has 220 to 260 calories. However, lean roast beef drops to 120 to 140 calories per 4 ounces. Same with corned beef: Buy it lean, and it comes in at around 120 to 140 calories for 4 ounces. Another good option is chicken or turkey breast slices, at approximately 120 calories for 4 ounces.

The problem is that these meats are typically packed into sandwiches served on huge rolls, often with coleslaw and Russian dressing, both of which are high in calories (because of the mayo) and can increase the total to as high as 800 calories per sandwich. Ask for ketchup, spicy mustard, salsa, horseradish, pickle chips, and plenty of fresh veggies for garnish. Steer away from extras like cheese, mayo, and oil. If you can't completely forgo them, at least choose the low-fat or fat-free versions.

Salami vs. Bologna vs. Prosciutto vs. Dry Sweet Italian Sausage

At 460 calories for 4 ounces, the dry sweet Italian sausage is your worst choice. Bologna (4 ounces: 280 calories) and regular soft beef salami (4 ounces: 300 calories) are close, but Genoa salami has 360 calories in 4 ounces and is also loaded with sodium. Prosciutto has 280 calories in 4 ounces and is surprisingly low in saturated fat (8 grams) and high in protein—great for low-fat, low-carb diets. Always look for lean cold cuts, such as Hebrew National Lean Beef Salami (only 180 calories for 4 ounces).

Wild Rice with Cranberries vs. Brown Rice vs. Rice Pilaf

This wild rice dish (technically not rice but the seed of an aquatic grass) is actually the lowest in calories, at 190 per cup. Other ingredients typically added include scallions, carrots, celery, raisins, shallots, and olive oil, any of which could bring the fiber content higher than that of famously healthy brown rice. But brown rice isn't a bad deal either: At 220 calories per cup, it's packed with 3.5 grams of fiber and 5 grams of protein. And 1 cup of white rice also has 220 calories, although when you start to add the butter, oil, beef or chicken stock, and some diced veggies to the pilaf, the total can go up to about 280 per cup.

Roasted Potatoes vs. Black Bean Salad vs. Fruit Salad

Black bean salad, typically made with black beans, kidney beans, corn, peppers, onions, cucumbers, cilantro, wine vinegar, and oil, is a pretty good choice both calorie-wise and health-wise. A 4-ounce serving has 130 calories and is packed with fiber, protein, and folate. However, the best choice is the fruit. The same 4-ounce serving, including cantaloupe, honeydew, grapes, and pineapple, has only 50 calories. Roasted potatoes, usually doused in oil, have about 160 calories in 4 ounces.

Convenience Stores

Hitting the road always means stopping to fuel up—our cars and ourselves. According to the National Association of Convenience Stores, there are more than 130,000 such stores in the United States, with more than $330 billion in sales. In fact, convenience stores are becoming quick-service restaurants in our time-starved culture: a phenomenon that can be costly if you're counting calories. Take a look and see if you can make the right choices to stay fit.

7-Eleven Slurpee vs. 1 Pint of Häagen-Dazs Chocolate Ice Cream

Of course the pint of ice cream has more calories, but the difference is smaller than you might think. 7-Eleven sells more than thirteen million Slurpees each month. A Coca-Cola Classic Slurpee has 330 calories and about 88 grams of carbs for about 22 ounces. The 40-ounce Slurpee almost doubles that at 600 calories and 160 grams of carbs. By comparison, a pint of Häagen-Dazs chocolate ice cream has 1,080 calories. But a Häagen-Dazs vanilla & almonds bar has only 320 calories, 12 grams of fat, and 22 grams of carbs.

Fit Tip: Try a 12-ounce Crystal Light Tangerine Lime, Berry Pomegranate, or Peach Mango Ice Slurpee—each has 30 calories per 8 ounces.

Potato Chips vs. Terra Chips vs. Doritos vs. Peanut Butter Sandwich Crackers

They're all pretty much the same caloriewise because the chips usually come in 1½ or 2-ounce bags.

- Terra chips (per ounce): 140 calories, 7 g fat, 18 g carbs.
- Wise Potato Chips (per ounce): 150 calories, 10 g fat, 14 g carbs.
- Doritos Cool Ranch Flavored Tortilla Chips (per ounce): 140 calories, 7 g fat, 18 g carbs.
- Frito-Lay Peanut Butter Sandwich Crackers (one package): 210 calories, 10 g fat, 23 g carbs.

Fit Tip: We tend to eat the entire bag of whatever we buy, so choose the smallest one. Don't pretend that you're going to share or save some for later. Also, what about a piece of fruit? Many convenience stores have fresh-fruit cups or loose apples, oranges, and bananas. A few I checked out even had hard-boiled eggs. All are better snacks.

David Sunflower Seeds vs. Planters Nuts, Seeds, and Raisins Trail Mix

The sunflower seeds are the obvious winner, but if you peek at the calories, you'll see that both are pretty high. A 5¼-ounce bag of sunflower seeds in their shells contains 475 calories, 37.5 grams of fat, 12.5 grams of carbs, and 22.5 grams of protein; a 6-ounce bag of trail mix has 800 calories, 60 grams of fat, 55 grams of carbs, and 30 grams of protein. On the positive side, they're both packed with protein and good heart-healthy fat as well as other nutrients.

Fit Tip: Go for the smaller bags of sunflower seeds if the store has them. Nuts and even trail mix can be good sources of nutrients—as long as you don't eat the entire bag. They can be addictive!

Sausage, Egg, and Cheese on English Muffin vs. Banana Walnut Muffin

The banana muffin may sound safe, but it's really quite calorically expensive at 605 calories (not to mention 30 grams of fat and 72 grams of carbs). The breakfast combo on the English muffin is actually a much better deal at 450 calories, 24 grams of fat, and 37 grams of carbs.

Fit Tip: Most convenience stores have small packages of cereal and skim milk, so if you choose a low-cal cereal (about 90 to 150 calories per box), you'll be OK. If you're getting an egg sandwich or a burrito, choose sausage, ham, or cheese, but don't double your trouble by picking both meat and cheese. And you can always remove one of the links or some of the cheese before you heat it up.

7-Eleven ¼ Pound Big Bite vs. Don Miguel Beef Steak Burrito

The ¼ pound Big Bite Hot Dog has 365 calories, 34 grams of fat, 2 grams of carbs, and 1,138 milligrams of sodium, plus

120 calories for the bun. So you're looking at 485 calories before you even add any condiments. It's close, but the Beef Steak Burrito (7 ounces) is the better bargain at 390 calories, 8 grams of fat, 61 grams of carbs, and 930 milligrams of sodium.

Dash Board Hot Dogs

- Dairy Queen Chili & Cheese Dog: 330 calories, 21 g fat, 22 g carbs.
- Dairy Queen Hot Dog: 240 calories, 14 g fat, 19 g carbs.
- 7 Eleven ⅓ Pound Biggest Big Bite (no bun): 480 calories, 45 g fat, 3 g carbs.
- A&W Coney Cheese Dog (with chili): 350 calories, 21 g fat, 27 g carbs.

Fit Tip: Stick to the 5- to 7-ounce burritos (300 to 500 calories) and avoid the 10-ounce (600 to 700 calories). Or you can go for the ⅛ Pound Big Bite Hot Dog, which has 280 calories, including the bun. Not bad if you have only one. But watch the condiments, because they can add up. Sauerkraut, mustard, ketchup, and relish are OK, but steer clear of butter and mayo, and avoid the cheese and chili: They can add more than 250 calories to your frank.

Ready Pac Chicken Caesar Salad vs. Mediterranean Style Turkey Sandwich vs. Hot Pockets Ham 'n Cheese

Your first instinct is probably to go with the salad, because it just seems healthier. But be careful: The salad package reads

230 calories, but that's for one serving, and the package holds two, so the total is 460 calories, 42 grams of fat, 8 grams of carbs, and 1,220 milligrams of sodium. And the turkey sandwich, normally a healthy choice, could become high in calories because of the dressing. Remember that these are prepackaged sandwiches, so you can't "hold the mayo" or the high-calorie special sauces. In this particular case, however, the turkey is still the winner at 400 calories, 14 grams of fat, 43 grams of carbs, and 1,540 milligrams of sodium. The Hot Pockets Ham 'n Cheese is the worst choice (if you eat both sandwiches), at 620 calories, 26 grams of fat, 72 grams of carbs, and 1,534 milligrams of sodium for two sandwiches.

Fit Tip: Sandwiches are typically good deals, but the sauces can take them over the top, so scrape off any excess—just 1 tablespoon of mayo (the typical base for many sauces) has 100 calories. Another great food bargain is soup. Many times all you have to do is heat it up or simply add hot water. For example, Campbell's Soup at Hand is very low in calories, and the container fits into your car's cup holder.

Nutri-Grain Bar vs. PowerBar vs. Clif Bar vs. Snickers Bar

The Nutri-Grain bar is lowest in calories, but it's also about a third the size of the others. If the Nutri-Grain bar satisfies you, and you don't mind the sugar and processing, it would be your best bet.

- Nutri-Grain bar: 140 calories, 3 g fat, 26 g carbs (contains high-fructose corn syrup).
- Chocolate PowerBar: 230 calories, 2 g fat, 45 g carbs (contains high-fructose corn syrup).

- Chocolate Brownie Clif Bar: 240 calories, 4.5 g fat, 45 g carbs (organic and contains no trans fat).
- Snickers bar: 280 calories, 14 g fat, 35 g carbs (contains sugar, saturated fat, and trans fat).

Fit Tip: Probably the hardest part of leaving a convenience store without buying anything unhealthy is staring at all the candy bars at the counter while you're in line. Stay focused and avoid those impulse buys.

Arizona Black Iced Tea with Ginseng vs. Gatorade vs. OJ

The iced tea has 150 calories and 37.5 grams of carbs for a 20-ounce bottle, while 16 ounces of Tropicana Pure Premium No Pulp Orange Juice has 220 calories and 52 grams of carbs as well as 900 milligrams of potassium and all that vitamin C. In terms of calories, however, Gatorade wins. Gatorade Lemon-Lime sports drink has 50 calories, 14 grams of carbs per 8 ounces, or 200 calories and 56 grams of carbs in a 32-ounce bottle.

Fit Tip: Choose no-calorie flavored coffee, like 7-11's Dutch Apple Crumb coffee, and use skim milk.

Diet Detective's What You Need to Know

High-fructose Corn Syrup (HFCS): HFCS is regular corn syrup that has been treated with glucose isomerase, an enzyme that converts glucose into fructose. The conversion process is attractive for two reasons. The first is that fructose is much sweeter than glucose, so, once converted, the same amount drastically increases the overall sweetness of the food. The second reason is that fructose is more soluble at low temperatures, so more can be concentrated per unit of weight. "The final product is a combination of glucose and fructose, usually either 42 percent fructose or 55 percent fructose, with the rest mostly glucose," says Joanne R. Lupton, PhD, a professor of nutrition at Texas A&M University. The 55 percent HFCS is often used to sweeten soft drinks, and the 42 percent HFCS is used to sweeten baked goods.

"Both of these concentrations of HFCS are 'high' as compared to corn syrup (which has no fructose). " However, when people discuss HFCS, they usually compare it to sucrose (ordinary table sugar). Sucrose is 50 percent glucose and 50 percent fructose, so HFCS is *not* high with respect to sucrose," adds Lupton.

Some experts believe that the higher proportion of fructose to glucose creates unique harm. "It is easier for fructose to be made into fat than for glucose to be made into fat. Additionally, there is relatively strong literature showing negative consequences of fructose compared to glucose with respect to raising fatty substances in the blood," says Lupton.

It's also been suggested that the rise in obesity in the United States is related to the rise in HFCS consumption. "However," says Dr. David L. Katz, "most evidence suggests that the metabolic effects of sucrose and HFCS are pretty similar. What makes HFCS such a hazard is that corn growth is highly subsidized in the U.S., so HFCS is very inexpensive— and thus a tempting additive to many foods."

Therefore, it's been argued that adding HFCS leads to an increased consumption of foods that are less nutrient dense, leading to greater calorie consumption and eventually weight gain.

Bar Food

Sitting at the bar with your friends, having a cocktail or two, and watching your favorite sporting event can make for a fun afternoon or evening. The problem is that just a few drinks can add up to 500 or 600 calories, and if you order food as well, you could reach the 1,500- to 2,000-calorie range in no time. Plus, drinking reduces our inhibitions and awareness, so we tend to order and eat more, and bar food is notoriously high in calories. The following should help you to make better bar choices, or, at the very least, make you more aware of what you're eating.

Onion Rings vs. French Fries vs. Cheese Fries

Obviously, they're all high in calories, but the onion rings and french fries are pretty close at approximately 500 calories (6 ounces) each; adding cheese to the fries makes matters even worse by upping the calories to more than 700. And don't forget that when you're sitting at a bar, you're likely to be served a whole basketful of fries or rings with as many as 1,500 calories.

Pretzels vs. Bar Nuts vs. Asian Rice Crackers vs. Goldfish

Pretzels are the lowest-calorie choice. One ounce (about a handful) of Rold Gold Pretzels has 110 calories. The Asian rice cracker mix is slightly higher at 130 calories per ounce, and then there's the Pepperidge Farm Goldfish crackers: Fifty-five of them are 150 calories. An ounce of peanuts (again, about a handful, or thirty to thirty-five) has about 160 calories, but peanuts offer more nutrients than pretzels, including protein and healthy fat. If the bar serves cashews instead of peanuts, you're looking at eighteen nuts for about the same number of calories. Whatever your choice, try not to keep the bowl in front of you; take a handful, put it on a napkin, and move the bowl far away.

Olives vs. Hard-boiled Eggs

As far as calories go, olives are the better deal. Four jumbo olives have about 30 calories, whereas one hard-boiled egg has 75 calories. But both are really good choices. Eggs serve up plenty of nutrition: One egg has 6 grams of protein, and olives are a good source of monounsaturated ("good") fats and vitamin E.

Personal Pan Pizza vs. Garlic Bread with Cheese vs. Wings

A single slice of pizza is actually not bad, but at the bar you're typically served a 6-inch personal pizza (a regular pizza is about 14 inches across and has eight slices), which has about

600 to 700 calories—not counting added toppings. Nonetheless, pizza might be your best bet. One 2½-ounce piece of garlic bread (probably dripping in oil) has 140 to 170 calories without any cheese. Add another 75 to 100 calories for each ounce of cheese, and you're looking at about 240 calories for one piece—not a very good deal. As far as wings go, they're deep fried and they're small. Four chicken wings with hot sauce (4 ounces) have at least 220 calories, but the real calorie buster is the blue cheese dressing: 305 calories in 4 tablespoons.

Potato Skins with Cheese vs. Fried, Breaded Mushrooms

A 10-ounce potato is packed with nutrients (fiber, potassium, and vitamin C), and has only 270 calories, but watch out for the extras—sour cream, butter, bacon, and cheese—which add up to at least 500 or 600 calories. Potato skins are even worse. A typical 12-ounce serving with cheese and bacon comes in at more than 1,000 calories and 80 grams of fat (at least 40 grams saturated). And here's the kicker: That's before you add sour cream. Fried mushrooms are not a great option either: Five fried mushrooms have about 200 calories and 13 grams of fat. Your best bet is to order a plain baked potato and add salsa.

Fish Sticks with Tartar Sauce vs. Fried Clams vs. Oysters vs. Poppers

Each 1-ounce fish stick has about 70 calories, and 1 tablespoon of tartar sauce has about 75 calories (it's made with mayo). So an average serving of five fish sticks with tartar sauce can easily run you about 700 to 800 calories. Fried clams, which are also breaded, are a little better at 380 calories for twenty small clams. Two jalapeño poppers (about 2 ounces) made with cream cheese have 140 calories—if you can stop at just two. Raw oysters have about 40 calories each, so even if you eat five or six, they'll be your best option, with only 200 to 240 calories.

Cheese Quesadillas vs. Chicken Strips vs. Mini Burgers

A 5-ounce mozzarella cheese quesadilla has 450 to 500 calories. Five chicken strips (10 ounces) have approximately 700 calories. In contrast, a single mini burger (sold by the half dozen) contains around 230 to 250 calories, including the bun, and add an extra 30 to 50 calories if you have it with cheese. So if you have three minis with cheese, you're looking at at least 800 calories—not to mention the fact that they usually come with fries or onion rings, tacking on an extra 500 calories or so. Share your mini burgers with a couple of other people—and limit yourself to no more than two.

Chips and Salsa vs. Nachos

Go with the chips and salsa. One ounce of tortilla chips with ½ cup of salsa has 175 calories, whereas an order of nachos with cheese costs 1,100 calories. So if you must have the nachos, spread the wealth among lots of friends. And what if you add guacamole? Just 1 tablespoon—probably the amount you use on each chip—adds 20 calories. Sour cream has about 30 calories per tablespoon.

Mozzarella Sticks vs. Fried Calamari vs. Fried Zucchini

Fried calamari usually comes in a hefty 3-cup serving—that's about 900 calories before you even start using the mayonnaise-based dipping sauce. And although each 1-ounce mozzarella stick has about 90 calories, you'll probably wind up eating at least four or five; that's 360 to 450 calories. The better choice is a 5-ounce serving of fried zucchini, which has 320 calories.

Diet Detective's What You Need to Know

Tips to Keep Those Calories Down While Snacking at the Bar:

- Have a snack before you get to the bar. Don't go hungry!
- Set food limits before you get there; having a plan helps you stay on track.
- Order your food before you start drinking.
- Drink wine or light beer.
- After your first round, order a diet soda or ask for water.
- Choose the foods that are most satisfying in the smallest quantities.
- Don't waste calories on foods you don't really like.
- Try asking for half orders.
- Share your order with your friends.
- If the bar serves popcorn, that's always your best bet.
- Move bowls of nuts or other high-calorie snacks on the bar out of reach.

At the Stadium

Whether you go to watch baseball, football, hockey, or basketball, there is nothing like spending the day at the stadium or arena. No matter if your team wins or loses, you can forget about everything else for the moment and immerse yourself in the experience. Part of the fun, of course, is the food you eat while enjoying the game, and I'm certainly not going to ruin it by telling you not to eat—or to bring along a bag of baby carrots.

However, I do believe that some foods, like the doughnut burger (basically a Krispy Kreme doughnut sliced in half and used as a bun to hold a burger, a pile of cheddar cheese, and two slices of bacon) that's served at one minor league baseball team's concession stand, ought to be illegal and should certainly be avoided at all costs if you're trying to eat healthfully.

That one is probably a no-brainer, but some of the other better—or worse—snacks may be less obvious, so here's the lowdown on what you need to know:

Cracker Jack vs. Cotton Candy

Cotton candy is just sugar that's been heated, colored, and spun into threads with added air. Cotton candy on a stick (about 1 ounce) has 105 calories, but when bagged (2 ounces), it has double that number: 210. Cracker Jack is basically candy-coated popcorn with some peanuts scattered throughout. A stadium-size box has 3½ ounces and 420 calories, so the cotton candy is clearly a better deal. If you must buy Cracker Jack, you may be happy to know that it at least has 7 grams of protein and 3.5 grams of fiber.

Hamburger vs. Chicken Sandwich

A 6-ounce hamburger with a bun has about 490 calories without even counting cheese or other toppings. A 6-ounce grilled chicken sandwich has only 280 calories—a much better deal.

Another alternative, and an even healthier choice, is the 4-ounce turkey burger offered at many of the stadiums serviced by Aramark Sports & Entertainment. At only 147 calories, it's a great bargain. At some stadiums, Aramark also offers salads with a choice of light dressings, including light creamy Italian, country French, ranch, and fat-free honey Dijon.

Chicken Tenders vs. Wrap Sandwich

A typical wrap sandwich (6 ounces) has 345 calories and is usually the smarter choice, depending on the ingredients. Six ounces of chicken tenders, on the other hand, have 446 calories, not even including the barbecue dipping sauce, which can have as many as 30 calories per tablespoon.

Hot Dog vs. Pizza vs. Sausage and Peppers

Most sold-out stadiums sell as many as sixteen thousand hot dogs a day. A regular hot dog with mustard is your best bet, totaling about 290 calories: 180 for the 2-ounce dog, 110 for the bun, and virtually no calories for regular yellow mustard. Sauerkraut adds another 5 to 10 calories (2 tablespoons), ketchup adds 30 (2 tablespoons), and relish, another 40 (2 tablespoons). However, many stadiums also serve foot-long hot dogs, which can double the calories in the frankfurter and bun, bringing the grand total to 580 without any toppings. Pizza at the stadium is a bit larger than a typical slice; about one-sixth of a 16-inch pie (rather than one-eighth), which comes to 435 calories per slice. And the sausage-and-pepper sandwich is about the same: 430 calories for 5 ounces, including the bun.

Super Nachos with Cheese vs. Fries vs. Corn

A 12-ounce serving of super nachos with cheese (forty chips, 4 ounces of cheese) has more than 1,500 calories. Wow! You're better off with a 6-ounce serving of french fries at about 500 calories. Corn on the cob, however, is your best option: 80 calories for the corn and about 100 calories for the butter topping. You could even have two (360 calories) and still save 140 calories.

Peanuts in the Shell vs. Popcorn vs. Soft Pretzel vs. Fruit Cup

Nothing says a day at the game better than a bag of peanuts. Stadiums sell as many as six thousand bags on game days, depending on attendance. The only problem is that an 8-ounce bag has 840 calories, and a 12-ounce bag has 1,260. The upside is that peanuts are high in magnesium, vitamin E, niacin, folate, and monounsaturated (heart-healthy) fats. The popcorn comes in a huge tub, often heaping with more than 120 ounces, which have roughly 1,500 calories. A plain soft pretzel (5½ ounces) at about 400 calories is a much better deal—but stay away from those huge pretzels (7 to 8 ounces), which have about 700 calories. However, your best bet, and definitely the healthiest choice, is a 6-ounce fruit cup—only 80 calories.

Snow Cone vs. Draft Beer vs. Soda

Even though snow cones use 1 to 2 ounces of flavored syrup (at almost 60 calories an ounce), they aren't too bad compared with other game-time snacks. A 12-ounce snow cone has about 120 calories. Beer is not that bad either, but the draft beer served at the stadium comes in 20-ounce cups, which means about 240 calories. Get a light draft if you can, and you'll save 60 calories for a 20-ounce serving. Soda is definitely not a bargain, at about 230 calories for 20 ounces.

Diet Detective's What You Need to Know

Ball Game Nutrition Tips

- Eat before you leave home so that you're not starving when you see the vendors selling enticing treats.
- It's OK to purchase some food, but make sure you also bring along healthy snacks like oranges, apples, energy bars, 100-calorie snack packs, and so on.
- Share the snacks—which shares the calories.
- Be realistic about what you buy; don't overbuy just to have extra.
- Watch out for unconscious eating. When you're focused on the game, you can consume massive amounts of calories without paying any attention. Try not to eat directly from the bag—ask the concessionaire for an extra container or plate and split things up.

What about Healthier Options?

Previously, health-conscious sports fans either had to bring their own snacks or satisfy themselves with basic ballpark fare. Today many stadium food-service providers such as Aramark offer healthier options. For instance, at Atlanta's Turner Field, you can buy freshly made salads; at Anaheim's Angel Stadium, there's corn on the cob; at Baltimore's Oriole Park at Camden Yards, you can find frozen yogurt and fruit smoothies; and at Boston's Fenway Park, enjoy a fresh fruit salad. There are even veggie hot dogs and burgers at Oakland's McAfee Coliseum and baked potatoes at Pittsburgh's PNC Park at North Shore (source: www.ballparkfoods.com).

At the Movies

One of my favorite places to kick back, relax, and enjoy is at the movies. But in order to get that extrasensory excitement, my mouth wants to be entertained as well as my eyes, and eating at the movies is one pleasure I refuse to deny myself. There's nothing like a nice box of Raisinets and a big tub of popcorn, right? After all, don't those Raisinets have "30 percent less fat"? And didn't they change the popcorn oil to make it healthier?

It's been more than twelve years since the Center for Science in the Public Interest (CSPI) came out with the surprising news that going to the movies can pack on the pounds. We learned that movie popcorn, one of the prime suspects, was, in fact, very high in calories and fat—much higher than we thought. Since then, many theater chains decided to change to healthier oils. But even if a "good" oil is used, the popcorn is still loaded with calories and fat.

These days, a large popcorn with butter, soda, and a bag of candy could add up to 2,500 calories and more than three days' worth of saturated fat. Even if you go to the movies only once a month, you could gain as much as 8½ pounds per year.

But if we know it's so bad, why do we continue to eat so much when we go to the movies? How about because as we walk through the theater door, the smell of the popcorn and candy permeates the air?

"Something happens when the lights go off," says Dan Griesmer, director of concession operations for Loews Cineplex. "It's unexplainable. I've seen people who have obviously just come from the gym sit down and eat a big popcorn and oversized candy." What if theaters were to offer healthier snack choices? Many claim they've tried. In fact, Loews Cineplex has attempted to sell fruits, cold sandwiches, salads, and even energy bars to keep their captive audiences away from the evils of high-calorie treats, and each time its efforts have failed. Apparently, fruits are not appetizing when placed next to big containers of popcorn.

You may be telling yourself, well, if my theater would just let me bring my own food from home, I wouldn't eat so poorly. "Not so," remarks Griesmer. "Even though most theater policies do not allow audiences to bring in their own foods, the snacks coming in are definitely not diet friendly. At the end of a movie we're always finding outside candy wrappers, KFC boxes filled with chicken bones, and other fast-food remains. Health foods are not the contraband food of choice."

Here are some tips for the brave audience member who is willing to break the concession-stand "addiction" cycle:

Sneak Attack

OK, it's not exactly cool with theater owners to sneak in foods (they make a huge chunk of their profits, about 40 percent, from concession sales), but until they start offering the good stuff, it may be your only option. Many theaters have a "don't ask, don't tell" policy when it comes to bringing in healthy snacks. "Our goal is not to police the theater for healthy foods," says Dick Westerling, director of communications for

Regal Cinemas. "We're there to serve the guest, and our primary concern is providing foods that people like."

If you're new to snack sneaking, start by bringing foods that don't smell and won't get crushed when they're hidden in the bottom of your bag. Focus on foods that are filling and low in calories so that you can mindlessly munch on them throughout the movie, just like popcorn. Since we're probably not really paying attention to the taste anyway, I wonder how many of us would know the difference if our movie popcorn were replaced by Kashi cereal or even a bag of cut-up vegetables? Try it just once and see if you notice. But even if you brought in a candy bar, it would be a lot smaller, and lower in calories (not to mention less expensive) than the giant bars and packages sold at theater concession stands.

The following are a few snacks that might be worth sneaking into your theater:

- Homemade air-popped popcorn in a Ziploc bag: At only 30 calories per cup, it's a good deal.
- Cereal: Kashi (a variety of healthy versions) or Cheerios are both low-calorie choices that are pretty durable.
- Beef jerky: Especially if you're an Atkins fan.
- Fruit: Apples are not easily crushed when hidden in your bag. Cut them into slices at home because crunching on a big apple can be annoying to other theatergoers. Grapes are another convenient fruit to bring. Avoid bananas, which are more fragile and can get very mushy, not to mention the peel you'd need to deal with.
- Rice cakes: Be careful because calorie and fat content varies widely.
- Energy bars: Although they are not the greatest in terms of calories and fat, they are still a bit better than those king-size chocolate bars (which are made for two) at the candy counter.

DON'T BRING:
- Trail Mix: It's very high in calories and fat.
- Potato chips or stix: They're also high fat, and there's the crush factor, too.
- Nuts: Nibbling on these will send your calories through the roof.
- Crackers: You'll just be left with crumbs once you're inside, and lots of calories when you leave.
- Sandwiches: Too messy, but if you do, watch the mayo!

Eat Before

What a novel idea! Stuff yourself with healthy, low-calorie foods before you go to the movies so you just can't eat another bite. You can also drink water during the movie, but all those bathroom breaks could impact your enjoyment of the entire film.

Calorie Bargain Spotlight

Calorie Bargain: Glenny's Soy Crisps, Bar-B-Que

The Why: I received a number of emails from readers recommending these crisps; plus my family and friends swear by them. In fact, most people who eat them regularly are a bit fanatical. I was reluctant to try them at first. I thought, "Soy—how good could they taste?" I finally broke down and had some, and I was impressed.

The Health Bonus: They really are an excellent snack, especially if you're in a "chips mood."

What We Liked Best: You can eat an entire bag without any guilt— the company actually calls it a "portion control" bag.

What We Liked Least: The soy can upset your digestive tract if you eat too many.

The Price: $35.76 for twenty-four 1.3-ounce bags.

Offerings: Bar-B-Que, Creamy Ranch, White Cheddar, Sea Salt, other flavors.

Website: www.glennys.com.

Where to Buy: Company website, local grocery stores, health food stores.

Ingredients: Low-fat non-GMO soy flour, rice, evaporated cane juice, sea salt, mid-oleic sunflower oil, onion powder, garlic powder, calcium carbonate, tomato powder, extractives of paprika, natural smoke flavor, spices, citric acid, folic acid, vitamin D, vitamin K.

Nutritional Analysis per Serving: 1.3 Ounces:
70 calories
1.5 g fat
9 g carbs
4.5 g protein
1.5 g fiber
260 mg sodium

Don't Assume You'll Share

We rationalize our snack food purchases by saying we'll share them. How much harm can a pack of M&M's do if it's divided among three or four people? But when the lights go out, automatic eating is in full color, and we tend to be less altruistic about sharing our popcorn and candy. We end up eating whatever we buy, and just because there are two or three people in a group doesn't mean the food is dispersed equally. Buy smaller quantities at the beginning of the show. If you happen to run out, and you're really desperate, you can miss part of the movie and get more—at least you're getting some exercise. Let your movie partner hold onto the package; you'll end up eating less if it's not right there in your lap.

Calorie Bargain Spotlight

Calorie Bargain: Jolly Time Yellow Pop Corn and Smart Balance Low Fat Microwave Popcorn

The Why: I'm still amazed at how few calories there are in popcorn. I'd always assumed it was a no-no, but that was probably because of all the oil and butter in movie popcorn. But popcorn is a perfect snack whether you're watching your favorite TV show or just looking for something to munch on.

The Health Bonus: It gives the appearance of loads of food yet is still low in calories. And if you use yellow corn, it has plenty of fiber, which also has health benefits.

What We Liked Best: Jolly Time Yellow Pop Corn is simply a bag of unpopped kernels you can make in a hot air-popper. Or if, like me, you don't love air-popped corn and don't mind the hassle (or occasionally burnt popcorn), pop yours on the stovetop. Put the kernels in a deep pot, coat them with Pam or cooking spray, cover, and pop. "Make sure to occasionally release the steam by slightly opening the cover, and be careful not to burn yourself," advises Tom Elsen, vice president of marketing for Jolly Time. He also recommends shaking the pot throughout the process; the shaking spreads the heat and allows the unpopped corn to pop.

Smart Balance tastes great, is low in sodium, has absolutely no trans fat (which is important because almost all microwave popcorn does), and offers a microwave-friendly, fast, and easy solution for late night munchies that will leave you satiated. Five cups is more than enough for any individual, no matter how much you love popcorn. But if you do eat the entire bag, assume that you're eating about 260 calories (because of the unpopped kernels).

What We Liked Least: If you take up snacking on popcorn, you're gonna need lots of dental floss!

The Price: Jolly Time, $24.95 for twelve 2-pound bags; Smart Balance.

Offerings: Jolly Time—White Popcorn, Yellow Pop Corn; Smart Balance.

Website: www.jollytime.com; www.smartbalance.com.

Where to Buy: local grocery store, company website.

Ingredients

Jolly Time Yellow Pop Corn
Whole-kernel corn.

Smart Balance Low Fat Low Sodium Microwave Popcorn
Corn, natural oil blend (corn and palm fruit oils), salt, natural and artificial flavor (derived from lactose-free milk), colored with annatt, TBHQ for freshness.

Nutritional Analysis per Serving

Jolly Time Yellow Pop Corn—5 Cups, Popped	Smart Balance Low Fat Microwave Popcorn—5 Cups, Popped
100 calories	120 calories
1 g fat	2 g fat
24 g carbs	24 g carbs
4 g protein	4 g protein
6 g fiber	5 g fiber
0 mg sodium	80 mg sodium

Choose the Best of the Worst

It's misleading to just look at the calories per serving on the food label; how many of us actually count out one serving and put the rest away? In all likelihood, you'll eat the whole package, no matter how many people it's supposed to serve. And most theaters keep the candy in those glass cases, so you can't even compare the nutritional content of different types. (And imagine the looks you'll get from the people in line behind you if you start inspecting each one of those candy labels.)

Keep in mind, smaller is not always better. Although cotton candy comes in the largest size package, it has the fewest calories (300 in a 2½-ounce bag), no fat, and 74 grams of carbs. Compare this to the movie-version of Reese's Pieces (8 ounces), which has a whopping 1,150 calories, 57 grams of fat, 132 grams of carbs. Those Twizzlers look tempting with their claim "As Always a Low Fat Candy," but the 6-ounce package holds 560 calories, 4 grams of fat, and 131 grams of carbs.

And look at that bag of Skittles. It might seem like a healthier option with only 2 grams of fat per serving, but the 6¾-ounce bag has four and a half servings and 765 calories, 9 grams of fat, and 175.5 grams of carbs. Choosing a box of Junior Mints (276 calories, 5 grams of fat, 57 grams of carbs), Milk Duds (387 calories, 15 grams of fat, and 60 grams of carbs), or Sno-Caps (360 calories, 16 grams of fat, and 60 grams of carbs) would be a better bet. And Gummi Bears might be your lowest calorie option, at 319 calories.

Or order a small popcorn without butter—you'll get by just fine. A hot pretzel with mustard can even be a better deal than some of the candy options, and more satisfying too (one large pretzel: 495 calories, 4 grams of fat, and 100 grams of carbs).

If none of these suggestions works, consider one movie-goer's thoughts on the subject: "Why can't we try to shut our mouths for one hundred twenty minutes, instead of stuffing our faces at every possible opportunity? I mean, who wants to listen to a hundred people scarfing chips, popcorn, or baby carrots, for that matter? I'd prefer to sit in the peace and quiet of my home rather than listen to this massive feeding orgy, personally."

Movie Candy

- Cotton Candy (2½ ounces): 300 calories, 0 g fat, 74 g carbs.
- Junior Mints (3 ounces): 276 calories, 5 g fat, 57 g carbs.
- Milk Duds (3 ounces): 387 calories, 15 g fat, 60 g carbs.
- Sno-Caps (3.1 ounces): 360 calories, 16 g fat, 60 g carbs.
- Raisinets (3½ ounces): 409 calories, 16 g fat, 71 g carbs.
- Gummi Bears (4 ounces): 319 calories, 0 g fat, 81 g carbs.
- Goobers (3½ ounces): 508 calories, 34 g fat, 53 g carbs.
- Twizzlers Strawberry Twists (6 ounces): 560 calories, 4 g fat, 131 g carbs.
- M&M's (5.3 ounces): 740 calories, 32 g fat, 106 g carbs.
- Skittles (6¾ ounces): 765 calories, 9 g fat, 175.5 g carbs.
- Reese's Pieces (8 ounces): 1,150 calories, 57 g fat, 132 g carbs.

Appetizers

Watch out! Appetizers can be diet disasters. You might think an appetizer would cut the amount you eat for the rest of the meal, but most research shows that starters actually increase total calories consumed. That's why picking the right starter is important. See if you can pick the healthier options from the following choices:

French Onion Soup vs. Minestrone

If you thought French onion soup would start your meal off healthfully, think again. This starter can have more than 500 calories. However, if you skip the bread and cheese topping, the soup will come in at about 100 to 200 calories per cup, depending on ingredients. A vegetable-packed minestrone soup has about 150 calories (8 ounces), which can increase by as much as 75 calories depending on the amount of pasta and Parmesan cheese. Still, compared with regular French onion, it's healthier and has more nutrients.

Steamed Veggie Dumplings vs. Fried Spring Rolls

If you've learned the key words by now, you've probably internalized the following rule: Steamed is good, and fried is bad.

But when you're talking about calorie-packed Chinese appetizers, steamed options aren't always the ticket to better health. First of all, consider how many you're going to eat. Four steamed vegetable dumplings have about 300 calories—not much less than fried, which have 340. You will, however, save 4 grams of fat by switching from fried (12 grams) to steamed (8 grams).

If the spring rolls are small—about 2 ounces—they are a better calorie bet at 80 to 100 calories as long as you have just one. However, watch out for spring rolls that are the size of egg rolls, which have 250 to 300 calories each.

Crab Cakes vs. New England Clam Chowder

The soup is probably a better choice, because research shows that it can help decrease overall calories consumed during a meal. However, serving size makes a difference. Some restaurants serve chowder in 10-ounce rather than 8-ounce bowls, which immediately adds 100 calories or so to your meal. An 8-ounce bowl of New England–style chowder comes in at around 300 calories. (But watch out for Denny's chowder, which has more than 600 calories in 8 ounces.) An average 3-ounce crab cake contains roughly 220 calories, but make sure you know how many are in one order—and how many you plan to eat—because the calories add up fast.

Mozzarella Sticks vs. Onion Rings vs. Fried Calamari

If you love foods that are breaded and fried, you'd better learn the art of nibbling—and adopt the habit of leaving some on your plate. Otherwise, expect to polish off at least 300 (and often closer to 500) calories before the main course arrives. And that's assuming you split these dishes with at least one other person. Those batter-dipped, deep-fried onions, such as Outback Steakhouses Bloomin' Onion, are a calorie catastrophe. According to the Center for Science in the Public Interest, this dish has about 1,700 calories and 116 grams of fat. But there are other items to be wary of as well. Fried calamari usually comes in a hefty 3-cup serving—that's about 900 calories before you even start using the mayonnaise-based dipping sauce. At about 90 calories per stick, mozzarella sticks are OK, but only if you limit yourself to a couple, which isn't easy when there are eight on the plate right in front of you. Split them with a few friends, and they'll do the least damage to your diet, plus you'll be getting some calcium.

Baked Potato vs. Potato Skins

Although a 10-ounce potato has only 270 calories, is filling, and is packed with fiber, potassium, and vitamin C, you still need to watch out for its sidekicks—sour cream, butter, bacon, and cheese—which can send the calories soaring to 500 or 600. Potato skins are even worse. A typical 12-ounce serving with cheese and bacon comes in at more than 1,000 calories and 80 grams of fat (40 grams saturated).

And here's the kicker: That's *before* you add sour cream. For comparison's sake, a 6-ounce order of french fries has about 500 calories and 25 grams of fat (plus the potential dangers from acrylamide, a byproduct of the frying process and a possible cancer-causing agent). So your best bet—in fact, a healthy option—is a baked potato topped with salsa or ketchup.

Antipasto (Including Pepperoni, Salami, and Prosciutto) vs. Bruschetta

Antipasto usually starts with a selection of deli meats, such as pepperoni, salami, and prosciutto. Then throw in an assortment of olives, some cheeses, deviled eggs, roasted vegetables in olive oil, and a variety of crackers. The meats, cheese, olives, eggs, and even the vegetables are full of fat and calories.

- Italian grilled peppers (3 ounces): 124 calories, 12 g fat, 3 g carbs.
- Salami (2 ounces): 230 calories, 19 g fat, 1 g carbs.
- Prosciutto (2 ounces): 140 calories, 10 g fat, 2 g carbs.
- Mozzarella (1-inch cube): 85 calories, 6 g fat, 5 g carbs.
- Olives (15 large): 90 calories, 7.5 g fat, 6 g carbs.
- Deviled eggs (2 halves): 145 calories, 13 g fat, 0.5 g carbs.

Bruschetta would seem like a much better option—after all, it's pretty much a piece of bread with some olive oil and tomatoes on top, right? Well, even though it's made with heart-healthy olive oil and tomatoes, which contain the antioxidant lycopene, bruschetta still has loads of calories—sometimes more than 200 in a single slice. In the end, portion size is what counts. Both bruschetta and antipasto are foods we tend to lose track of while we're nibbling. But if you put them side by side in terms of calories, you will probably consume more of the antipasto.

Oysters on the Half Shell vs. Shrimp Cocktail

Both are good options. Although shrimp is high in cholesterol, it's very low in unhealthy saturated fat, so it can still fit into a heart-healthy diet. Not only are shrimp and oysters low calorie, but so is the cocktail sauce or that vinegary sauce that often comes with oysters. However, raw oysters (and raw clams) are at high risk for contamination by microorganisms, so pregnant women and those with suppressed immune systems might want to skip them.

- Large shrimp (6): 146 calories, 2 g fat, 2 g carbs.
- Cocktail sauce: 35 calories, 0 g fat, 9 g carbs.
- Pacific oysters (6): 240 calories, 6 g fat, 15 g carbs.
- Eastern oysters (6): 60 calories, 2 g fat, 3 g carbs.

Caviar vs. Foie Gras

The name says it all: *Foie gras* is French for "fat liver." One ounce comes in at more than 100 calories, and despite the fact that it's an incredibly rich dish, most restaurants will give you at least a couple of ounces. Caviar is usually a better bet at only 40 calories per tablespoon. It's typically served with crackers or bread, which will add more calories, but it also has a very strong flavor, so you won't need much to get your fix.

Salads

Salads are the better meal starter because they have a shot at reducing your total calorie consumption. Recent research by Barbara Rolls, PhD, a nutrition professor at Penn State University, found that eating a low-calorie, large-volume first course, like a large low-cal salad or soup, can enhance feelings of satisfaction and reduce total calorie intake during the rest of the meal. To avoid salad sabotage, ask for low-fat or fat-free dressing and get it on the side. Oil and vinegar is usually one of your better choices (if nothing fat free is available); 3 tablespoons have 134 calories, a savings of about 100 or more calories compared with other dressings. And avoid high-calorie salad add-ons like cheese and croutons.

Here's what can be found in 3 tablespoons (a standard restaurant serving) of some popular dressings:

- Blue cheese: 231 calories, 24 g fat, 3 g carbs.
- Caesar: 210 calories, 21 g fat, 3 g carbs.
- Ranch: 270 calories, 27 g fat, 4.5 g carbs.
- Thousand Island: 195 calories, 18 g fat, 7.5 g carbs.
- Creamy Italian: 165 calories, 18 g fat, 3 g carbs.
- Olive oil and vinegar: 134 calories, 13.5 g fat, 3 g carbs.

Aperitifs

An aperitif is a very specific drink, like Campari, Limoncello, or cassis, but it's alcohol. And alcohol is packed with calories. When you add mixers like soda, juice, cream, or sugar—well, you could be headed for a calorie nightmare. Turning rum into a rum and Coke nearly doubles the calories; the same goes for a gin and tonic (unless you use diet tonic, which has no calories). Soda or juice adds about 100 to 150 calories per drink. So the average mixed drink contains at least 300 calories for an 8-ounce glass.

And to make matters worse, a study in the *American Journal of Clinical Nutrition* reports that when people have cocktails as opposed to water or fruit juice beforehand, meals last an average of fourteen minutes longer, and calorie intake is higher.

To save calories, keep your drinks simple and on the rocks. Avoid anything creamy, frozen, or fruity. Beer and wine are your best choices, but they still have calories. Choose light beers: Regular beer contains 150 calories a bottle, whereas light beer has 100. Low-carb beers are somewhat lower in calories than the light versions, and nonalcoholic beer is still lower at about 70 calories. Five ounces of dry wine or champagne will cost you only 100 calories—not too bad.

Sandwiches

Years ago, when you talked about a sandwich, it meant something fast, filling, and basic. Your options were pretty simple: roast beef, BLT, ham and cheese, peanut butter and jelly, and a few other choices. But nowadays, sandwiches have become an art form, as well as a nutritional minefield. Here are some clues to help you make the right sandwich decisions:

It's All in the Bread

If you talk to most sandwich makers (I used to make sandwiches for a living), you know that the bread is the key to success. And even with the popularity of the Atkins diet these days, bread lovers are still eating their sandwiches, albeit clandestinely. Remember, all breads are not created equal. For instance, a 6-inch Hearty Italian (white) Bread from Subway has 200 calories, whereas two slices of Nature's Own 100% Whole Wheat bread have only 100 calories.

Choose whole-grain breads for maximum nutrients, including fiber, which helps you stay full. But don't be fooled by a brown, healthy-looking appearance! Make sure to check the ingredients list. Whole-grain flour should be the first ingredient (for example, whole wheat, whole rye, whole oats). Watch out for labels boasting multi-grain, seven-grain, unbleached, stone ground, or just plain wheat—these are not necessarily made with whole grains. Pick "light" breads to save calories. Compared to the typical 80 to 100 calories per slice, they generally contain only 40 calories per slice.

Wraps and tortillas make good sandwich choices, but not when they're fried. A large (10-inch) tortilla has 218 calories and 5 grams of fat when it's baked, but it has 286 calories and 15 grams of fat if it's fried.

Pita bread is typically a low-fat, low-sugar sandwich holder, but be wary—it may not necessarily provide calorie savings over regular bread. Check the package label if possible.

At cafés and bakeries, avoid the croissants; they're rich, doughy, and loaded with butter. A large croissant contains 272 calories, 14 grams of fat, and 31 grams of carbs.

Bagels are low in fat but may contain as many as 400 calories, depending on size—and that doesn't even include the spread. To save up to half the calories, hollow out the bagel or have an open-face sandwich. You can do this for large rolls as well.

Go Lean

Choose leaner cold cuts like turkey, chicken, roast beef, and ham. On average, these contain no more than 110 calories and 5 grams of fat for a 2-ounce serving.

- Subway 6-inch Ham: 290 calories, 5 g fat, 47 g carbs.
- Blimpie 6-inch Roast Beef (regular): 450 calories, 13 g fat, 49 g carbs.
- Schlotzsky's Dijon Chicken (small): 390 calories, 7 g fat, 54 g carbs.

Avoid the Fat

Avoid higher fat meats like bacon, bologna, salami, pimiento loaf, and sausage. Steer clear of anything called "Monte Cristo." While this description varies from restaurant to restaurant, it typically has cheese and is dipped in egg and fried in butter.

- Subway 6-inch Pastrami: 540 calories, 26 g fat, 49 g carbs.
- Cousins Subs Italian Special with bologna, ham, salami, and provolone: 817 calories, 51 g fat, 50 g carbs.
- Blimpie Ultimate B.L.T. Wrap: 830 calories, 50 g fat, 60 g carbs.

And what about the traditional peanut butter and jelly sandwich? It's the peanut butter you've got to watch carefully. Just 1 tablespoon contains 95 calories, 8 grams of fat, and 3 grams of carbs.

- Panera Kids Peanut Butter & Jelly on white whole grain bread: 420 calories, 16 g fat, 55 g carbs.

Cut the Cheese

Cheese is a great source of calcium and protein, but it's also a source of excess calories and fat—primarily saturated fat. One ounce of regular cheese usually contains about 100 calories and 8 grams of fat, of which 5 grams are saturated. Delis typically add three to five slices of cheese per sandwich, which sends the calorie and fat content skyrocketing.

- Schlotzsky's Ham & Cheese—The Original-Style (large): 1,423 calories, 50 g fat, 158 g carbs.
- Einstein Bros Bagels Cheese Steak Panini on Ciabatta: 690 calories, 29 g fat, 69 g carbs.
- Au Bon Pain Prosciutto Mozzarella Sandwich: 880 calories, 49 g fat, 71 g carbs.

Don't Join the Club

Rumored to have gotten its name from the large sandwiches served at country clubs, the club sandwich generally includes three slices of toasted bread layered with bacon, lettuce, tomato, mayonnaise, and some type of meat. With the exception of Subway's club sandwich, these trimmings don't typically add up to a trim waistline.

- Subway 6-inch Club: 320 calories, 6 g fat, 47 g carbs.
- Schlotzsky's Deli Turkey Bacon Club (regular): 760 calories, 29 g fat, 77 g carbs.
- Au Bon Pain Turkey Club on Focaccia: 830 calories, 42 g fat, 58 g carbs.

Leave Reuben Home

This sandwich on rye is grilled the same way that a grilled cheese sandwich is grilled, which generally means slathering the outside of the bread with butter, the high-fat meats, Swiss cheese, and Russian dressing put the calories over the top.

- Schlotzsky's Deli Pastrami Reuben (regular): 890 calories, 40 g fat, 74 g carbs.
- Blimpie Panini Grilled Corned Beef Reuben: 630 calories, 33 g fat, 55 g carbs.

Vegetable and Salad Sandwiches

Vegetables add flavor, crunch, nutrients, and fiber to sandwiches. Besides the traditional lettuce and tomato, try these favorites: red onion, bell peppers, roasted red peppers, spicy jalapeño peppers, carrots, celery, spinach, arugula, cucumber, zucchini, yellow squash, and eggplant. But watch out for the extras often added to veggie sandwiches—specifically cheese, salad dressings, and mayo. Again, Subway has a low-calorie version, but take a look at the high calories in some of the others:

- Subway 6-inch Veggie Delite: 230 calories, 3 g fat, 44 g carbs.
- Panera Bread Mediterranean Veggie: 590 calories, 13 g fat, 100 g carbs.
- Au Bon Pain Mozzarella, Tomato, and Pesto: 638 calories, 30 g fat, 66 g carbs.

Also, skip salads mixed with mayo, such as tuna, chicken, or egg—unless they're made with light or fat-free mayonnaise. The fat and calories in the mayo can turn a relatively healthy food into a dieter's nightmare.

- 7-Eleven Big Eats Tuna Salad: 550 calories, 22 g fat, 56 g carbs.
- Au Bon Pain Southwest Tuna Wrap: 541 calories, 25 g fat, 68 g carbs.
- Panera Bread Chicken Salad on Sesame Semolina: 750 calories, 27 g fat, 85 g carbs.

Condiment Culprits

As you've been told time and again, mayonnaise, oil, and full-fat dressings add unnecessary calories and fat to your sandwiches. To get that creamy texture for less fat, try a slice of avocado (about one-eighth of an avocado) for only 45 calories, 5 grams of fat, and 2 grams of carbs. Other relatively innocuous add-ons include mustard, ketchup, barbecue sauce, horseradish (not horseradish sauce), salsa, and balsamic vinegar. Fat-free mayonnaise comes in tangy flavors like wasabi or chipotle that make you forget you're missing the fat. Also try light or fat-free salad dressings, cocktail sauce, teriyaki sauce, or low-fat honey mustard.

Mexican Food

Tortilla chips and guacamole or some nachos with all the fix-ins to start. Chicken quesadillas with refried beans or maybe an overstuffed burrito for the main course. All accompanied by a few margaritas. Ah, there's nothing like a good, hearty meal at a Mexican restaurant!

Unfortunately, a tasty Mexican meal like that can add up to thousands of calories—and the sodium is off the charts. But where there's a will there's a way, and with some planning, you can enjoy food from south of the border without jeopardizing your diet.

Tortilla Chips with Salsa vs. Guacamole

When the waiter brings over that basket of crispy tortilla chips, it's hard to eat just one—or even just one serving. What you need to remember is that *crispy* is just a nicer way of saying *fried*—and that means loads of fat and calories. Keep munching to a minimum. Or better yet, ask your server to take away the chips. But if you can't resist the call of the chips, at least watch what you're dipping them in. If it's a choice between salsa and guacamole, salsa is, hands down, the better choice. Not only is it much lower in calories, but also tomatoes, the main ingredient, are packed with lycopene, a powerful antioxidant. Guacamole contains heart-friendly mono-unsaturated fat as well as other healthy nutrients, but it's still high in calories.

- Tortilla chips (12 to 15 chips): 140 calories, 6 g fat, 19 g carbs.
- Guacamole (3 ounces): 110 calories, 9 g fat, 7 g carbs.
- Salsa (3 ounces): 26 calories, 0 g fat, 5 g carbs.

Enchiladas vs. Nachos

Talk about a fat trap! Enchiladas are tortillas softened in oil, stuffed with meat, and smothered with cheese. Nachos are made with fried chips, fatty cheese, and high-calorie sour cream. It's really a toss-up between the two, but you can make the nachos a bit lighter by ordering them without the sour cream, asking for less cheese, and eating them with salsa instead of guacamole.

- La Salsa Fresh Mexican Grill Cheese Enchilada (with black beans): 666 calories, 38 g fat, 62 g carbs.
- Taco Bell Nachos BellGrande: 730 calories, 41 g fat, 69 g carbs.
- Chili's Classic Nachos: 1,570 calories, 115 g fat, 66 g carbs.
- Sour cream (2 tablespoons): 62 calories, 6 g fat, 1 g carbs.

Chimichangas vs. Quesadillas

Not much of a choice here—this is almost a Mexican standoff (if you'll pardon the expression) between two fried and greasy dishes. A chimichanga is a deep-fried flour tortilla filled with beans, cheese, onions, and chicken or beef—a greasier, crispier cousin of the burrito. Quesadillas, meanwhile, consist of two tortillas stuffed with cheese and other fillings. Although serving sizes vary, typically chimichangas pack about 1,420 calories versus 1,240 calories for a quesadilla. You can lighten up the quesadilla even more by ordering it with less cheese and sour cream—or without cheese if other vegetable or meat fillings are available. Or, to save still more calories, you could go for an oven-baked burrito without cheese, sour cream, or refried beans.

Burritos vs. Fajitas

Fajitas seemed like one of the best choices on any Mexican menu, but much to my dismay, I found that even those are not diet food by any stretch of the imagination. The meat and vegetables are cooked with loads of oil, and the toppings can almost double the calorie count. One plus is that the tortillas are simply warmed, not fried or cooked in oil. So if you can get the beef, chicken, or vegetables chargrilled (it doesn't hurt to ask!), use a minimal amount of guacamole, and leave out the sour cream, cheese, and refried beans, you'll actually have a reasonably healthy dish. Also, choose chicken over beef to save calories and fat. Or, even better, try to pack in extra flavor with pico de gallo (chopped tomatoes, onions, and herbs—like a chunkier salsa) and "beef it up" with vegetables instead of the meat.

Burritos can be relatively healthy, depending on the ingredients. They are typically stuffed with layers of beef, sour cream, shredded cheese, and guacamole, turning a potentially healthy meal into a ticking fat bomb. You can slash calories and get a protein boost by dumping the fatty extras and choosing a black bean burrito without sour cream, cheese, or rice.

Whether it's a burrito or a fajita, the bottom line is to choose your toppings wisely.

- La Salsa Fresh Mexican Grill Bean and Cheese Burrito (with chicken and black beans):
    - Black beans, jack and cheddar cheeses in a flour tortilla, with chicken.
    - 768 calories, 24 g fat, 89 g carbs.
- Rubio's Grill Fajitas Chicken Burrito:
    - Grilled chicken, jack and cheddar cheese, guacamole, and salsa in a flour tortilla.
    - 630 calories, 24 g fat, 58 g carbs.
- Chili's Classic Marinated Chicken or Steak Fajitas (not including tortillas):
    - Chicken or beef, onions, and bell peppers.
    - Chicken: 330 calories, 11 g fat, 23 g carbs.
    - Beef: 790 calories, 49 g fat, 20 g carbs.

Oh, and by the way, choose whole wheat tortillas (if available) over those made with white flour. The whole wheat is higher in fiber.

Taco Salad vs. Taquitos

They're both fried, but the biggest problem with taco salad is the shell. Taquitos are fried corn tortillas filled with meat and/or cheese, as well as guacamole. You'll probably eat way more than one, because they're not very filling. Order the salad instead of those fried taquitos, but dump the shell and ask for some of the fattier toppings on the side.

- La Salsa Fresh Mexican Grill Taco Salad (with chicken and pinto beans): 972 calories, 44 g fat, 108 g carbs.
- Rubio's Chicken Quesadillas Taquitos (3): 290 calories, 11 g fat, 34 g carbs.

Rice and Beans vs. Tacos

Even though they're about equal in calories, beans are a rich source of protein, folate, and fiber. Also, rice and beans are very filling, so you typically eat only one portion. But if the beans are refried and smothered in cheese, forget it. When it comes to tacos, it really depends on how many you eat. They average about 200 calories each, so if you eat two or three, the calories can add up. Also, keep in mind that those taco shells are fried, and you're adding costly calorie extras when you spoon on the guacamole, sour cream, and shredded cheese. You'd be best off with soft tortillas filled with lean meat, low-fat or nonfat sour cream, tomatoes, and lettuce or spinach.

- Baja Fresh Mexican Grill Rice and Beans Plate (side): 420 calories, 5 g fat, 72 g carbs.
- Taco Bell Original (Crunchy) Tacos (2): 340 calories, 19 g fat, 26 g carbs.

Frozen Margaritas vs. Regular Margaritas vs. Beer

A 12-ounce bottle of Dos Equis beer, at about 150 calories, is definitely the best choice. But most people who go to a Mexican restaurant to have a good time are looking for those fancy frozen margaritas, which can pack more than 800 calories in a single pint glass. And if you think having yours on the rocks is any better, think again—they're about the same.

Italian Food

OK, it's confession time. My biggest food weakness is Italian. Not the "froufrou" nouveau Italian, but the classics: spaghetti, pasta primavera, garlic bread, and my favorite, chicken parmigiana. And as long as I'm coming clean here, I'll also admit that I put off researching this topic for years so that I could continue to live in denial. But the time has come to take a magnifying glass to some of the crowning achievements of the food world.

Like other Mediterranean countries, Italy's cuisine is rich in grains, nuts, fruits, vegetables, and olive oil, all of which may play a role in preventing heart disease and cancer. So what's so fattening about the Italian food you're eating? How about *almost everything*. In one meal, you can eat enough food to put on an entire pound of fat, which would take five hours and nine minutes of jumping rope to burn off. Maybe that's why Olive Garden does not give out the nutritional content of its food.

So, unless you know what to look for, an Italian menu can be hazardous to your health.

The Specialty of the House: Pasta

Yes, pasta can be a healthy choice (at times); it's the preparation and what's added that cause complications. Not only are the sauces, sides, and even the vegetables cooked in oil, but sometimes butter and cheese are also added for extra flavor (not to mention extra fat). Your best defense is to ask the waiter to pack half your meal in a doggie bag before it's even brought out, or share your dish with a friend.

- Spaghetti and meatballs (1 serving): 1,086 calories, 35 g fat, 146 g carbs.
- Potato gnocchi (1 serving): 804 calories, 39 g fat, 99 g carbs.
- Stuffed shells (6 jumbo shells): 780 calories, 32 g fat, 82 g carbs.
- Pasta primavera (1 serving): 542 calories, 23 g fat, 62 g carbs.

Sautéed or Fried Foods

The menu doesn't always say whether or not an item is sautéed, so ask. Frying is pretty standard for mozzarella and zucchini sticks, and calamari; and, of course, chicken, veal, and eggplant parmigiana are sautéed in a pan with loads of oil. You might think eggplant is a healthy choice because it's a vegetable, but not when it's sautéed in oil—which is essentially like deep frying. Then, to add insult to injury, it is smothered with cheese. To save calories, skip the cheese and/or get your food grilled. Trust me, you'll still feel satisfied.

- Eggplant parmigiana (1 serving): 1,396 calories, 78 g fat, 141 g carbs.
- Chicken parmigiana (1 serving): 1,340 calories, 78 g fat, 88 g carbs.
- Fried calamari (1 serving): 1,040 calories, 70 g fat, 62 g carbs.

Not to depress you more, but this nutritional information doesn't include the heaping side order of pasta that generally comes with these dishes and can add another 606 calories, 15 grams of fat, and 101 grams of carbs. That brings your grand total to more than 1,600 calories, not including a few pieces of bread dipped in olive oil.

Don't Get Sauced

The sauce on the pasta is the heart of the dish. It's what gives the pasta its "pastabilities." The problem is that chefs are mostly interested in making their sauces taste good, and there is no better guarantee of this than using plenty of cheese, butter, and oil. At least ask for the sauce on the side and add it yourself—sparingly.

Red and white sauces are both loaded with oil, and that includes marinara sauce. You might think pesto sauce made with basil, olive oil, grated cheese, and pine nuts would be a healthy option, but more than half its calories are from fat. Keep in mind that carbonara sauce is made with eggs, ham or bacon, and cream—an obvious artery clogger. Oh, and if you love Alfredo sauce, sorry, it's made entirely of cream, butter, and cheese.

- Linguine with white clam sauce: 910 calories, 29 g fat, 104 g carbs.
- Linguine with red clam sauce: 890 calories, 23 g fat, 130 g carbs.
- Spaghetti with marinara sauce: 850 calories, 17 g fat, 165 g carbs.
- Mussels marinara: 806 calories, 17 g fat, 71 g carbs.
- Capellini with tomatoes and basil: 860 calories, 30 g fat, 119 g carbs.

- Spaghetti carbonara: 1,067 calories, 34 g fat, 143 g carbs.
- Pasta with pesto sauce: 1,075 calories, 69 g fat, 81 g carbs.
- Fettuccine Alfredo: 1,078 calories, 41 g fat, 137 g carbs.
- Shrimp scampi: 932 calories, 67 g fat, 4 g carbs.
- Spaghetti Bolognese: 975 calories, 24 g fat, 135 g carbs.

Lasagna

Who doesn't love a nice homemade lasagna? The classic lasagna contains way too much cheese and ground meat for a single serving. But even the meatless version is no calorie bargain. Again, halve your entree so that you're eating only half the calories.

- Lasagna with meat and spinach: 1,116 calories, 44 g fat, 114 g carbs.
- Meatless lasagna with spinach: 978 calories, 30 g fat, 127 g carbs.

Appetizers, Sides, and Condiments

Garlic bread? *Fuggedaboudit!* Bread drenched in olive oil? Skip it; it's more fattening than healthy. And that plate of antipasto? All those cheeses and cured meats, such as pepperoni and salami, are full of saturated fat and cholesterol.

- Garlic bread (4 slices): 545 calories, 21 g fat, 75 g carbs.
- Antipasto: 630 calories, 47 g fat, 18 g carbs.
- Roasted peppers in olive oil (½ pepper): 504 calories, 54 g fat, 4 g carbs.

- Bread dipped in olive oil (2 slices): 528 calories, 42 g fat, 30 g carbs.
- Minestrone soup (2 cups): 468 calories, 26 g fat, 44 g carbs.
- Parmesan cheese (1 tablespoon): 23 calories, 2 g fat, 0 g carbs.
- Italian bread (2 slices): 162 calories, 2 g fat, 30 g carbs.
- Olives (10): 91 calories, 10 g fat, 1 g carbs.

Desserts

If you're lucky, your restaurant will serve fresh fruit. Otherwise, cool Italian ices are probably your best bet.

- Tiramisu (1 piece): 400 calories, 29 g fat, 30 g carbs.
- Italian ice (1 cup): 123 calories, 0 g fat, 31 g carbs.

Although it's a challenge, there are some excellent recipes out there for chefs or anyone who wants to cook healthy Italian food that still tastes amazing. I was even able to create a recipe for chicken parmigiana that's low in fat and tastes great. Basically, take a paper-thin cutlet, spray the pan with cooking spray, use Healthy Choice sauce, sprinkle on a tablespoon of Parmesan cheese, and you're all set. But do I ever eat the oil-and-cheese-laden restaurant version? I think I've already confessed enough.

Chinese Food

I grew up eating Chinese food; my favorite dish was General Tso's chicken. That changed about ten years ago when a study from the Center for Science in the Public Interest revealed just how unhealthy Chinese food really is. The study was especially important because an earlier survey had shown that the average consumer thought Chinese food was "more healthful" than typical American fare.

The Chinese diet, long known for its emphasis on grains, legumes and other vegetables, and fruits, has fueled the perception that Chinese food is healthy. Unfortunately for our waistlines, however, we have significantly altered this healthy diet, adding lots more fat and meat with less rice, the end result being what we currently see on the menu at our local Chinese restaurant.

So how can you still enjoy Chinese food without packing on the pounds? Here are a few pointers to help you navigate the menu.

Avoid the Fried: I know this sounds obvious, but the point is that you can enjoy Chinese food without going for fried foods. If you do anything, avoid anything "deep fried" completely. Deep-fried dishes like sweet-and-sour chicken, sesame chicken, and my old favorite, General Tso's, can pack more than 1,000 calories and about 70 grams of fat! While you're at it, be wary of stir-fried dishes, too. Trust me, they're not using a tablespoon of oil as you do at home. Aside from the oil, however, these dishes are usually fairly nutritious.

Speak Up: Most Chinese food is made to order, so ask for your food steamed. If you can't bring yourself to take it that far, ask the server to have the dish prepared with little or no oil. If you're clear and insistent, you can get them to leave out a majority of the oil. You can also request that chicken or fish be used in place of red meat in your favorite dishes, and ask for extra steamed green veggies as a side. Avoid meals that are described as breaded or contain eggs or nuts, or at least ask to have these high-calorie items left out.

Keep It Brown and Steamed: If it's available, choose brown rice instead of white rice for extra fiber and vitamins, and ask for it steamed, not fried. Aside from the obvious, fried rice also contains a lot of egg, which adds more calories, fat, and cholesterol. Choosing steamed rice trims 13 to 20 grams of fat (about 3 to 4 teaspoons of oil). But just because it's brown doesn't mean you can go to town—it still has calories. The steamed stuff packs about 217 calories per cup, so watch those portion sizes!

Watch the Sauce: Don't just dump the main dish onto the rice. Use chop sticks or a fork to get the veggies and meat while leaving the pool of fatty sauce behind. Try not to "drink" the sauce that comes with your dish; this is the primary source of fat, in most instances. Or even better, how about ordering the dish steamed with garlic and herbs, and have the sauce on the side? That way you can dole it out sparingly. A cup and a half of brown sauce typically has about 255 calories, 7.5 grams of fat, and 41 grams of carbohydrate, whereas the same serving of black bean sauce contains as much as 358 calories, 30 grams of fat, and 14 grams of carbohydrate.

Extra Veggies: Order a few sides of vegetables steamed in garlic and herbs. You can mix them with your main dish—a welcome addition to any stir-fried food. And because the veggies increase the portion size, the entree will serve more people while also cutting back on overall calories.

Cut the Crispies: Watch out for those crispy things they put on the table. Whether it's colorful shrimp toast or crunchy Chinese noodles, they've all been fried. Three pieces of shrimp toast contain 222 calories and a whopping 14 grams of fat plus 16 grams of carbohydrate. A single cup of chow mein noodles has 237 calories with nearly 14 grams of fat and 26 grams of carbohydrate—and you can probably eat significantly more than 1 cup while you're waiting for your main dish to arrive. Also, watch where you dip those noodles. Saucy Susan Duck Sauce has 80 calories, 0 grams of fat, and 19 grams of carbohydrate in just 2 tablespoons.

Don't Go Nuts: While many nuts have health benefits, they are very high in fat and calories. Ten peanuts have about 51 calories, 4 grams of fat, and 2 grams of carbohydrate. Ten cashews (which are bigger than peanuts) have about 91 calories, 8 grams of fat, and 4.5 grams of carbohydrate. Since most Chinese dishes are already fattening, it's a good idea to stay away from any that include nuts. At the very least, ask the kitchen to go light on the nuts; even just a few can go a long way toward enhancing taste and flavor.

Add Soup: Unless you need to keep your sodium down, soup can be a great way to fill up as long as you choose carefully. Plus, the servings tend to be small, so you are less likely to overdo it. Start your meal with a bowl of hot-and-sour soup. One cup contains only 160 calories, 8 grams of fat, and 5 grams of carbohydrate. Wonton soup is slightly higher at 182 calories, 7 grams of fat, and 14 grams of carbohydrate per cup. And despite its name, egg drop soup (without noodles) is the best deal of all, with only 70 calories, 3 grams of fat, and 3 grams of carbohydrate per cup.

Portion Distortion: Most Chinese restaurants in America are independently owned, and therefore portions vary from place to place. Keep in mind that many dishes are meant to be shared with at least one other person. A typical order of Chinese food can be more than 4 cups!

Sodium: Chinese food tends to be very high in sodium. Stay away from anything made with soy sauce; even reduced-sodium soy sauce contains over 500 milligrams of sodium per tablespoon.

Watch the Fruit: This means anything orange or lemon flavored. These fruity names might imply a nutritious choice, but, in fact, these types of dishes usually involve deep-fried meats covered in a citrus-flavored sauce, which may also contain oil.

The Good (Based on 2-cup Servings Unless Otherwise Noted)

- Fortune cookie (1): 30 calories, 0 g fat, 7 g carbs.
- Steamed vegetable or seafood dumpling (1): 65 calories, 1.5 g fat, 8 g carbs.
- Steamed brown rice (1 cup): 217 calories, 1.8 g fat, 45 g carbs (contains 3.5 g fiber, compared to white rice's 0.6 g fiber). Keep in mind, a typical takeout container has 2 cups.
- Steamed chicken and broccoli (no sauce): 280 calories, 12 g fat, 13 g carbs.

- Steamed tofu and veggies: 293 calories, 12 g fat, 28 g carbs.

The Bad (Based on 2-cup Servings Unless Otherwise Noted)

- White rice, steamed (1 cup): 205 calories, 0.4 g fat, 44.5 g carbs (a typical serving is 2 cups).
- Szechuan shrimp: 730 calories, 37 g fat, 55 g carbs.
- Stir-fry veggies and tofu: 473 calories, 32 g fat, 28 g carbs.
- Meatless chop suey: 497 calories, 14 g fat, 80 g carbs.
- Chicken chow mein: 690 calories, 16 g fat, 84 g carbs at P. F. Chang's.
- Egg roll (1): 190 calories, 11 g fat (spring rolls typically have half the calories and fat).

The Ugly (Based on 2-cup Servings Unless Otherwise Noted)

- Spare ribs (5): 1,280 calories, 79 g fat, 47 g carbs.
- Sweet-and-sour pork: 1,100 calories, 46 g fat, 106 g carbs.
- General Tso's chicken: 1,173 calories, 68 g fat, 65 g carbs.
- Sesame chicken: 1,318 calories, 74 g fat, 68 g carbs.
- Fried rice: 1,483 calories, 56 g fat, 186 g carbs.
- Orange peel beef: 1,580 calories, 85 g fat, 115 g carbs.
- Anything kung pao; for example, kung pao chicken: 1,240 calories, 80 g fat, 58 g carbs.
- Vegetable lo mein: 1,340 calories, 94 g fat, 96 g carbs.

Steak Houses

Having a good steak is not just about eating, it's about indulgence. It's going to a steak house and stuffing yourself until you can't eat any more. Steak houses have proliferated in the last ten years. I'm sure you can name many of them: Morton's, Ruth's Chris, Outback, LongHorn, Lone Star, Ponderosa, Smith & Wollensky, and, of course, the famed Peter Luger Steak House in New York.

It's funny: When I called a number of their corporate communications offices, they seemed very defensive, as if they had something to hide. And I guess they do, because steak houses are not exactly known for serving up "health" food. But there are a few tricks that can help you navigate the menu next time you visit one.

Bread and Butter

Boy, is the bread good at these steak houses! A bit of irony for low-carb dieters: They come to eat a low-carb, high-protein steak and are faced with the best bread on earth. My advice is, if you can't limit yourself to just one slice, have the basket removed from the table. Or, better yet, refuse it before it arrives. You can try asking for a plate of veggies to snack on instead.

But, if you must have a slice of bread, at least don't slather it with butter.

- French bread (4 slices): 384 calories, 4 g fat, 72 g carbs.
- Garlic bread (4 slices): 545 calories, 21 g fat, 75 g carbs.
- Butter (2 pats): 72 calories, 8 g fat, 0 g carbs.

Appetizers

Watch out! These can be a nutrition disaster. Among the more obvious calorie catastrophes are those batter-dipped, deep-fried onions, such as Outback's Bloomin' Onion. It has about 1,700 calories and 116 grams of fat! But there are other items to be wary of as well. Sautéed mushrooms or crab cakes can pack more than 200 calories per serving—and that's without any sauce. And if you thought you were getting your meal off to a healthy start with French onion soup or lobster bisque, think again. Either one can have more than 500 calories per serving. As always, avoid anything fried, creamy, or served with a sauce. Look for the words *broiled* or *steamed*. And if you're not sure how it's prepared, ask.

Some of the healthy choices to try are oysters on the half shell (only about 10 calories per oyster), shrimp cocktail (about 22 calories per shrimp, including the sauce), or a broth- (not cream-) based soup. To avoid salad sabotage, ask for the dressing on the side and sprinkle it on with a fork. Or ask for fat-free or low-fat dressing—at least give it a try. With the new focus on health these days, many restaurants do carry it. And avoid high-calorie salad add-ons like cheese and croutons. Most of all, try to resist the blue cheese salad dressing some steak restaurants are known for. With a ½ cup (or more) of blue cheese, you'd be better off serving yourself up another steak.

The Steak

While beef is high in saturated (unhealthy) fat, it's tasty as well as a good source of protein, iron, and other nutrients. But there are some nutritional minefields to avoid. For instance, did you know that Outback prepares its steak (as well as Chicken or Shrimp on the Barbie) with butter? Or that Ruth's Chris adds butter to the plate to create a sizzle when served? In fact, many of the steakhouses I called put either butter or oil on their steaks. But don't worry; almost all are willing to make them without if you ask.

Prime Rib: Most restaurants serve this in portions of about 1 pound, which adds up to between 1,350 and 1,400 calories with more than a day's worth (up to 45 grams) of saturated fat.

Rib Eye: The rib eye is not much better. In fact, it's actually just one rib of a prime rib roast. A 16-ounce rib eye contains about 1,100 calories and more than 20 grams of saturated fat—slightly less than the prime rib because the rib eye includes the bone, so there's actually a bit less meat in a 1 pound portion.

T-Bone and Porterhouse: Many restaurants serve their T-bone or porterhouse steaks at over a pound—about 20 ounces—which brings the calorie count to more than 1,200, with 25 grams of saturated fat. It seems like most of these steaks are made for sharing, and some portions—like the mammoth 40-ounce porterhouse served at Ruth's Chris—are specifically dedicated to serving more than one.

New York Strip: An 18-ounce New York strip steak (top loin) contains about 1,050 calories and more than 30 grams of saturated fat.

Sirloin and Filet Mignon: Your best bet would be a sirloin steak (about 700 calories for 12 ounces), which is one of the leanest cuts (lowest in fat) you can order. Or go with the filet mignon, which is smaller—typically nine ounces and about 450 calories, with approximately 9 grams of saturated fat.

Other Tips

Think Ahead: Call beforehand to find out how various dishes are prepared, so that you don't annoy your hungry dinner partners with your pre-ordering questions. Never go to any restaurant without preplanning what you're going to eat.

Avoid the Sauce: Especially béarnaise or hollandaise sauce— only 2 tablespoons have about 140 calories, so go for the au jus.

Make It Smaller: Jayne Hurley, RD, senior nutritionist at the Center for Science in the Public Interest, advises, "Ask yourself, 'Does the prime rib really taste three times better than the sirloin or the filet?' because it often has three times the fat and calories."

Remember that the government recommends a 3-ounce portion of beef, not 20 ounces. Most of the better restaurants don't have a sharing charge, but if you don't have anyone to share with, try ordering the smallest steak—even a children's portion. Or, as soon as you get your steak, try cutting it in half

NUTRITIONAL COMPARISON OF CUTS OF MEAT

CUT	OUNCES	CALORIES	SATURATED FAT
Prime Rib	About 16 ounces	1,350–1,400	Up to 45 grams
Rib Eye	16 ounces	1,100	More than 20 grams
T-Bone and Porterhouse	About 20 ounces	1,200	25 grams
New York Strip	18 ounces	1,050	More than 30 grams
Sirloin	12 ounces	700	More than 15 grams
Filet Mignon	9 ounces	450	9 grams

and taking a portion home. Better yet, ask the waitperson to do that in the kitchen, so you won't have to struggle with the knife or your willpower. Also, find out if the restaurant offers any variety in its portion sizes, "especially for the prime rib and filet," says Hurley.

Trim the Fat: Make sure to trim off any visible fat, which can save you as much 25 percent in calories. "This is key for the fatty cuts like prime rib, porterhouse, and T-bone, but you won't save much fat from the sirloin or filet," adds Hurley.

Order Shrimp or Chicken: Barbecued chicken and shrimp are usually the healthiest items on the menu, especially if you can get the sauce on the side and they're not cooked in butter.

The Sides

"These can make or break your meal," cautions Hurley. "For example, if you order your potato with bacon, butter, cheese, or sour cream, you can kiss good-bye to a day's worth of saturated fat."

Know your suspect sides, which can add up to anywhere from 250 to 800 calories: creamed spinach (about 300 calories per cup), mashed potatoes (200 calories per cup), french fries (600 calories for a large order), and vegetables sautéed in butter or oil (more than 200 calories per cup). Order your vegetables steamed, with steak seasoning added for flavor.

Even a plain baked potato can present a problem since, at most steak houses, they weigh in at approximately 1 pound. That's 450 calories without any butter (100 calories per tablespoon) or sour cream (25 calories per tablespoon). So if you're going to have a baked potato, which is normally a good choice, have it cut in thirds and split it with others at the table, or ask your waitperson for a takeout container.

Drinks

For many people, steak and potatoes go hand in hand with a martini or wine. The good news is that red wine and even martinis are lower in calories (120 to 160) than most other alcoholic beverages, but they still add up. Plus, after a few martinis, when it comes to dessert time, your typical "no" can easily turn into a "yes."

Bottom Line

You can dine out at a steak house and still eat relatively healthfully. Truth is, I ate at Outback about twice a week during a four-month book tour and managed to have a healthy meal each and every time.

Seafood

Fish and shellfish can be very healthy whether or not you're watching your weight. They're low in carbs, packed with protein, and don't have the high quantities of saturated fat contained in many meats. But without some careful planning, even seafood can pack on the calories when you're ordering it in a restaurant.

Clam Chowder vs. Lobster Bisque

You might think that all clam chowders are equal, but the Manhattan version is tomato based, whereas the New England kind is made with milk or cream, which means it's much more fattening. But when it comes to calories, lobster bisque, which is made with heavy cream, is the highest of all. Bisque, after all, means thick and creamy, so what would you expect?

- Manhattan clam chowder (2 cups): 256 calories, 8 g fat, 32 g carbs, 14 g protein.
- New England clam chowder (2 cups): 543 calories, 40 g fat, 29 g carbs, 16 g protein.
- Lobster bisque (2 cups): 710 calories, 58 g fat, 32 g carbs, 16 g protein.

Oysters on the Half Shell vs. Shrimp Cocktail

Both are good options and probably among your best choices. Although shrimp is high in cholesterol, it's very low in unhealthy saturated fat. Not only are the shrimp and oysters low in calories, but the cocktail sauce and that vinegary sauce the oysters come with certainly beat the butter that comes with lobster. However, raw oysters (and raw clams too) are at high risk for contamination by microorganisms, so pregnant women and those with suppressed immune systems should proceed with caution.

- Large shrimp (6): 251 calories, 3 g fat, 2 g carbs, 54 g protein.
- Medium oysters (6): 240 calories, 6 g fat, 15 g carbs, 27 g protein.

Broiled Halibut vs. Shrimp Scampi

Yes, shrimp can be a low-calorie alternative, but not when made with scampi sauce. *Scampi* usually describes large shrimp that are split, often brushed with oil or butter, broiled or sautéed with wine or sherry and lemon juice, and then served with pasta. Keep the shrimp, but without the butter and pasta. The broiled halibut is really the winner here, but then, almost any broiled fish, including cod, sole, flounder, and salmon, will be a winner. Just be careful of side dishes (fries, a baked potato with sour cream and butter, a side salad with fatty dressing) that can pack on calories even when you've ordered a healthy, low-cal main course.

- Shrimp scampi with pasta (8 large shrimp): 830 calories, 26 g fat, 75 g carbs, 74 g protein.
- Broiled halibut (8 ounces): 317 calories, 7 g fat, 0 g carbs, 60 g protein.

Crabs vs. Salmon

If you order crabs, you're typically getting about five or six large crab legs, which add up to about 650 calories' worth of crabmeat. Not only that, but many restaurants have all-you-can-eat crab dinners that eliminate any kind of portion control. And don't forget that the Dijon mustard sauce (often made with mayonnaise) and other buttery dips can add on loads more calories.

Although salmon is relatively high in fat, it's heart-healthy "good" fat, and even a large portion of grilled salmon is lower in calories than the crab. Remember to tell your server that you want your fish grilled dry, not in oil. Just because the menu says "grilled" doesn't mean the restaurant doesn't use butter, oil, or both—how do you think the salmon makes it off the grill without sticking? Perhaps the chef can use a cooking spray if you request it.

- Crab legs (5): 650 calories, 10 g fat, 0 g carbs, 129 g protein.
- Grilled salmon (8 ounces): 466 calories, 27 g fat, 0 g carbs, 50 g protein.

Lobster Roll vs. Fried Clams vs. Popcorn Shrimp

Here it's about choosing the least of three evils, but the lobster roll is best. As far as fried clams go, I know people who eat twenty or more at a sitting with a very high-calorie chipotle mayonnaise sauce and end up breaking the 1,000-calorie barrier. And popcorn shrimp is also a deep-fried diet disaster.

- Fried clams (10 large): 438 calories, 23 g fat, 27 g carbs, 28.5 g protein.
- Lobster roll: 547 calories, 35 g fat, 31 g carbs, 27 g protein.
- Popcorn shrimp (includes chips and slaw): 741 calories, 25 g fat, 96 g carbs, 33 g protein.

Tuna vs. Catfish

Knowing that catfish has a reputation for being high in fat, I was surprised to see that it's very close to tuna in calories—assuming the catfish is broiled or blackened rather than fried. The tuna actually contains about 20 more grams of protein than the catfish, but even though the catfish has more fat, it's the healthy, unsaturated kind. And keep in mind that tuna can be high in mercury, which means that women who are pregnant or attempting to have children should avoid tuna steaks and go for the catfish, which tends to be very low in mercury.

- Fried catfish (8 ounces): 520 calories, 30 g fat, 18 g carbs, 41 g protein.
- Blackened catfish (8 ounces): 345 calories, 18 g fat, 0 g carbs, 42 g protein.
- Broiled tuna (8 ounces): 350 calories, 9 g fat, 1 g carbs, 62 g protein.

Tartar Sauce vs. Cocktail Sauce

Tartar sauce is made with mayonnaise—do I have to say any more? Cocktail sauce is the clear winner. Keep your condiments in check; be wary of sauces made with butter or mayo and try using lemon or malt vinegar instead.

- Tartar sauce (1 tablespoon): 74 calories, 7.5 g fat, 2 g carbs, 0.2 g protein.
- Cocktail sauce (1 tablespoon): 15 calories, 0.1 g fat, 4 g carbs, 0.2 g protein.
- Butter (1 tablespoon): 102 calories, 11.5 g fat, 0 g carbs, 0.1 g protein.

Mercury vs. Omega-3 Fatty Acids

Fatty fish like mackerel, lake trout, herring, sardines, albacore tuna, and salmon are high in two kinds of omega-3 fatty acids, eicosapentaenoic acid (EPA) and docosahexaenoic acid (DHA), both of which have been shown to reduce the risk of heart attacks and strokes. On the other hand, many fish, "specifically large, ocean-dwelling fish like shark, swordfish, tuna, king mackerel, and tilefish, are likely to have high quantities of toxic methylmercury," says Caroline Smith DeWaal, food safety director at the Center for Science in the Public Interest. Young children and women who are pregnant, planning to become pregnant, or nursing should not eat these fish. However, she adds, "Fish is still a great choice. There are many types that don't pose problems with mercury, like salmon and catfish, and the benefits of omega-3s are pretty strong."

Japanese Food

I'm amazed to find that many people believe sushi is basically calorie free. Sure, research has found that a diet high in omega-3 fatty acids (abundant in fish) can help prevent heart disease, diabetes, and even ease arthritis pain. But while traditional sushi made with raw fish is nutritionally impressive, it's a mistake to think that it's a total dietary bargain.

Just for the record, *sushi* does not mean raw fish. The word specifically refers to dishes made with vinegared rice, which traditionally includes fish (often raw) and/or vegetables, wrapped in seaweed. So the basic ingredients in sushi make it sound healthy and calorically light, but that just isn't the case when you take American eating habits into account.

The good news is that most Japanese restaurants don't serve very large portions. The bad news is that we are a nation of supersizers, so we compensate for small portions by over-ordering. I don't know about you, but a single spider roll just doesn't cut it for me. Add to that a Philadelphia roll and part of my friend's eel and avocado roll (just to taste), not to mention the vegetable tempura appetizer, a few dumplings, the miso soup, two or three shots of sake, and, of course, fried ice cream, and I'm on my way to becoming a sumo wrestler.

To make matters even worse, the trend in sushi is away from the traditional rolls and slices, which are usually healthier options. Chefs at sushi restaurants are creating more "interesting" choices these days to satisfy consumer curiosity and demand for innovative culinary treats. This generally means adding more "good tasting but bad for you" ingredients and sometimes omitting the healthful ones.

"These less traditional rolls contain some amazing flavors and new ideas," says Takanori Wada, executive sushi chef at Sushi Samba, an upscale chain of sushi restaurants, "although that doesn't necessarily mean fish or other standard ingredients are involved. Some of our most popular rolls contain ingredients such as smoked duck, braised short rib, and even fried onion and mozzarella cheese."

A smoked duck sushi roll could contain up to 350 calories and 12 grams of fat. Having just one wouldn't be so bad, but that wouldn't satisfy most sophisticated "foodies." (Leave it to us to take a relatively healthy cuisine and turn it into a delicious high-calorie, high-fat food!)

So, how can you keep sushi healthy?

Watch What You Eat, Literally: Japanese menus offer a wide variety of options. Steer clear of fried or battered foods, including dumplings, anything tempura, and spider rolls. The key is to look for anything broiled, grilled, or steamed. Typically, miso soup and sashimi (raw fish without the rice) are low in calories too.

Avoid "Nouveau" Sushi: Be especially careful when it comes to rolls with duck, cheese, or other high-fat ingredients. Also, stay away from eel; its rich taste comes from the fact that it's high in calories and fat.

Keep Sodium Down: I have a friend who gets a "sodium hangover" every time she eats at a sushi restaurant. Use less or request low-sodium soy sauce. Also, note that miso is quite high in sodium.

Limit the Extras: Mayonnaise, cream cheese, and even that traditional Japanese dressing on that little green salad can add significant calories to what you're eating.

Avoid the Feeding Frenzy: Yes, there are many good choices when it comes to sushi, but try to stick to just one or two of the lower-calorie rolls. Order steamed veggies, hijiki (cooked seaweed), or oshitashi (boiled spinach with soy sauce) to help fill you up.

Keep Your Food Safe: Aside from the mercury found in many fish, sushi—or any raw fish or shellfish, for that matter—can contain parasites, parasite eggs, and other microorganisms that cause diseases, including hepatitis. Check the U.S. Food and Drug Administration Center for Food Safety and Nutrition's website for regular updates: www.cfsan.fda.gov.

For the Record:
- Avocado roll: 246 calories, 11 g fat, 33 g carbs.
- Spicy tuna roll: 290 calories, 11 g fat, 26 g carbs.
- Shrimp tempura roll: 544 calories, 13 g fat, 75 g carbs.
- Philadelphia roll (salmon, cream cheese, avocado): 319 calories, 5 g fat, 30 g carbs.
- Spider roll (fried soft shell crab): 317 calories, 12 g fat, 38 g carbs.
- California roll: 266 calories, 8.5 g fat, 36 g carbs.
- Cucumber roll: 136 calories, 0 g fat, 30 g carbs.
- Eel and avocado roll: 372 calories, 17.5 g fat, 31 g carbs.
- Tuna nigiri (2 pieces over rice): 240 calories, 1 g fat, 27 g carbs.
- Salmon sashimi (2 pieces, no rice): 164 calories, 6 g fat, 0 g carbs.
- Beef teriyaki with sauce (2 cups): 870 calories, 37 g fat, 22 g carbs.

- Vegetable tempura appetizer: 255 calories, 15 g fat, 22.5 g carbs.
- Steamed pork dumpling appetizer (6): 174 calories, 6.5 g fat, 21 g carbs.
- Miso soup (1 cup): 85 calories, 3 g fat, 11 g carbs.
- Green salad (with 3 tablespoons of sesame dressing): 260 calories, 24 g fat, 3.5 g carbs.
- Edamame, shelled (4 ounces): 160 calories, 7 g fat, 12 g carbs.
- Fried ice cream (1 cup): 358 calories, 18 g fat, 46 g carbs.

For Your Reference:
- Rice (½ cup): 121 calories, 0 g fat, 26 g carbs.
- Avocado (2 slices): 77 calories, 7.5 g fat, 3 g carbs.
- Tuna (2 ounces): 60 calories, 0 g fat, 0 g carbs.
- Salmon (2 ounces): 82 calories, 3 g fat, 0 g carbs.
- Seaweed (1 slice): 10 calories, 0 g fat, 1 g carbs.
- Mayonnaise (1 tablespoon spicy sauce): 99 calories, 11 g fat, 0 g carbs.
- Jumbo shrimp, battered and fried (1): 74 calories, 4 g fat, 4 g carbs.
- Cream cheese (1 tablespoon): 51 calories, 5 g fat, 0 g carbs.
- Soft-shell crab, fried (2 ounces): 186 calories, 12 g fat, 10 g carbs.
- Crab, imitation (2 ounces): 58 calories, 1 g fat, 6 g carbs.
- Smoked eel (2 ounces): 164 calories, 10 g fat, 0 g carbs.

Desserts

Call them desserts, treats, goodies, even "sin foods," but whatever name you give them, we love them. Why? Probably because these foods include our two favorites: fat and sugar. Just so you know, I'm not going to lecture you about giving up dessert or an occasional treat, but some desserts are better than others. And if you pay attention and choose the right ones, you might prevent some of the weight gain that can come with eating desserts.

Brownie vs. Chocolate Layer Cake vs. Chocolate Mousse

Your best bet is probably the chocolate mousse or the layer cake; both have about 550 calories for a 6-ounce portion. (Incidentally, if you thought flourless cake was lower in calories, a 6-ounce portion has about 800 calories—not exactly diet food.) A typical 6-ounce brownie has about 600 calories. However, many restaurants serve brownies that are 7 ounces or more (for example, a 7-ounce caramel-pecan brownie from Boston Market has 900 calories). Plus, restaurants don't stop with the basic square of chocolate fudge. A brownie dessert is often the biggest treat on the menu, with everything but the kitchen sink thrown in: ice cream, whipped cream, chocolate syrup, pecans, chocolate chunks, and a cherry on top. All this can add up to more than 1,200 calories.

Fit Tip: To satisfy your desire for chocolate, try sugar-free pudding made with skim milk. Drop in a few chocolate chips while it's still hot or top it with light whipped cream. You can also make your own fat-free brownies using No Pudge! Fudge Brownie Mix, which substitutes yogurt for eggs and milk (www.nopudge.com). When eating out, ask your waitperson if there are any healthy desserts; some places have offerings in the 200- to 250-calorie range. For instance, Applebee's has a chocolate raspberry layer cake that's only 230 calories. Or, if you must have the brownie, at least forgo some of the toppings.

Cheesecake vs. Carrot Cake vs. Pound Cake

Plain cheesecake is your best bet at about 430 calories for about 4 ounces, and because it's dense and rich, you'll be satisfied with less. Don't be fooled by the "carrot" in carrot cake—it isn't just a slice of sweetened baby carrots. A 4-ounce portion has about 500 calories, but that can vary, depending on the amount of frosting used.

And what about pound cake? The name says it all. The original recipe calls for a pound each of butter, sugar, eggs, and flour. That's why it's about 550 calories for 4 ounces. Plus, because pound cake is kind of plain, it's often served with ice cream and/or a sauce on top, which adds another 250 to 400 calories. Believe it or not, other types of pound cake, such as banana bread, may actually be lower in calories (470 calories for 4 ounces) because the banana replaces some of the butter and sugar.

Fit Tip: If you choose carrot cake, remove some or all of the cream-cheese frosting (more than 100 calories per ounce). Also, check the menu for a low-carb cheesecake; Ruby Tuesday makes one. If you're staying in, look for low-fat cheesecakes in your supermarket—they have about 200 calories for a 3-ounce portion. If you decide to bake your own cheesecake, make sure to use low-fat or nonfat cream cheese as well as low-fat or non-fat cottage or ricotta cheese. You can also substitute Splenda (or another sugar replacement) for the sugar. Or if you have a craving for pound cake, try zucchini bread instead, which has about 360 calories for a 4- to 5-ounce portion, depending on preparation. Because the main ingredient is zucchini, there is typically less "bread," plus zucchini is a high-moisture vegetable, which allows you to use less oil in the preparation without sacrificing moistness (just add extra zucchini).

Tiramisu vs. Tapioca

They may both seem like blandly colored, strangely textured treats, but in terms of calories they couldn't be more different. Tiramisu is the clear loser at 400 calories for 5 ounces. The primary ingredients are usually some mixture of creamy fats, processed sugars, and alcohol. A typical recipe calls for eggs, mascarpone cheese, ladyfingers, cream, espresso coffee, liquor (such as brandy, Marsala, or rum), sugar, and cocoa or shaved chocolate.

Tapioca, on the other hand, is essentially a root starch taken from the yucca plant (also called cassava) and has only 120 calories for 4 ounces. It can also be used to thicken soups and sweeten baked goods.

Fit Tip: If you do order the tiramisu, get forks for everyone and share.

Key Lime Pie vs. Strawberry Shortcake

Strawberry shortcake (300 to 350 calories for 4 ounces), even though it's made with heavy cream and sugar, is a bit better because, unlike its key lime counterpart (440 calories for 4½ ounces), it doesn't have a buttery crust or a processed, sugar-packed filling.

Fit Tip: Try ordering fresh strawberries (45 calories for ½ cup) without the cake and sprinkle them with Splenda (or another sugar replacement or even a tablespoon of sugar) for added sweetness. Go with plain angel food cake, which is fat free and has only about 300 to 375 calories in 4 ounces, and add your own fresh or frozen berries and low-fat whipped cream. If you're home, you can make angel food cake (it's already made with egg whites) with Splenda for even fewer calories. Or just enjoy a half cup of strawberries, which adds up to only 45 calories. Top the berries with a dollop of light whipped cream at 10 calories per tablespoon, and you're getting a filling dessert for 55 calories.

Apple Pie vs. Blueberry Pie

Either one has about 60 to 70 calories per ounce. So with a typical restaurant serving at 6 to 7 ounces, you're looking at about 420 to 490 calories. However, not all apple pies are created equal. For instance, there's apple crumb pie and apple crisp, which add another 100 calories or so per serving. In fact, stay clear of anything with the word *crumb* in the name—it translates to additional calories (for example, Starbucks Lemon Crumb Bar, 460 calories for one 112-gram bar). And many times the pie is served with whipped cream, which adds another 80 to 100 calories per serving. Oh, and a scoop of vanilla ice cream to make it à la mode can tack on another 270 calories.

Fit Tip: Resist the temptation to go à la mode. Try eating the filling and leave the crust to save almost 100 calories. And, whatever you do, ask your server to hold the whipped cream. Don't think that you'll just scrape it off. Or, if you're craving something sweet at home, try baking your own apple pie and reduce the calories by using baking Splenda and a reduced-fat margarine or butter. Better yet, enjoy a baked apple: Take out the core, dab the apple with a bit of reduced-fat margarine and a tiny bit of brown sugar or Splenda, add some apple juice, and cook for about ninety minutes at 350 degrees. Then top it with low-fat whipped cream and some chopped walnuts before serving. You can even bake apples in the microwave. Or try fresh apple slices and blueberries in Jell-O or frozen blueberries topped with low-fat or nonfat whipped cream. Also, look for reduced-calorie frozen apple pies at the grocery—they're great because they're pre-portioned.

Baskin-Robbins Classic Banana Split Sundae vs. Starbucks Caramel Chocolate Frappuccino Blended Crème with Whipped Cream

OK, a Baskin-Robbins Classic Banana Split sundae has 1,030 calories and is by far the worse of the two. But the Frappuccino, one of the highest-calorie beverages Starbucks offers, weighs in at 730 calories for 24 ounces. Train yourself to recognize desserts when you see them—even if they're disguised as drinks and sold in a coffee shop.

Fit Tip: If you need a cool caffeine jolt, opt for a regular iced coffee. Add skim milk and sugar (or Splenda) if you like it light and sweet. You can even throw it all in a blender and make your own frappuccino. Just remember to skip the whip.

Starbucks Frappuccino Light Blended Coffee vs. McDonald's Triple Thick Shake

A Triple Thick Shake sounds like it will give you triple thick thighs, but be wary of the new Starbucks Frappuccino Light too. If you order it with the whipped cream, it's pretty close to the shake. Instead, go for the plain Coffee Frappuccino.

- Starbucks Java Chip Frappuccino Light Blended Coffee with whipped cream (16 ounces): 400 calories, 19 g fat, 50 g carbs, 9 g protein.
- Starbucks Frappuccino Light Blended Coffee (16 ounces): 150 calories, 1 g fat, 30 g carbs, 7 g protein.
- McDonald's Triple Thick chocolate shake (16 ounces): 580 calories, 14 g fat, 102 g carbs, 13 g protein.

Soft-serve Yogurt vs. Soft-serve Ice Cream

If you are ordering the fro-yo to watch your waistline, don't bother. Although frozen yogurt has less fat (1.5 fewer grams per serving and 1 fewer gram of saturated fat), both contain approximately 140 calories per serving. If you're going to get soft-serve, order nonfat frozen yogurt, which is approximately 110 calories. Oh, and if you decide to have your soft-serve dipped in chocolate, it can double your calories.

- Dairy Queen Vanilla Ice Cream (½ cup): 140 calories, 4.5 g fat, 3 g saturated fat, 22 g carbs, 3 g protein.
- TCBY Hand-scooped Frozen Yogurt (96 percent fat free) (½ cup): 140 calories, 3 g fat, 2 g saturated fat, 23 g carbs, 4 g protein.

Calorie Bargain Spotlight

Calorie Bargain: Sugar-free Jell-O with Added Blueberries and Banana (All Flavors)

The Why: My wife actually purchased this a few weeks ago, and my first response was "Jell-O? You have to be kidding me!" I even tried to take it out of the shopping cart. Then I tasted it and was amazed.

The Health Bonus: Putting in the fruit may add a bit of calories, but it makes it a great package, especially since blueberries are a good source of antioxidants—those age/cancer-fighting substances.

What We Liked Best: It takes only a minute or so to prepare and stick in the fridge. Then just wait for it to set.

What We Liked Least: Unless you add the fruit, it has no nutritional value.

The Price: 89 cents.

Offerings: Black Cherry, Cherry, Cranberry, Lemon, Lime, Mixed Fruit, Orange, Peach, Raspberry, Strawberry, Strawberry-Banana, Strawberry-Kiwi.

Website: www.kraftfoods.com/jello.

Where to Buy: local grocery store.

Ingredients: gelatin, adipic acid, disodium, maltodextrin (from corn), fumaric acid, aspartame, contains less than 2% of artificial flavor, acesulfame potassium, salt, Red 40.

Nutritional Analysis per Serving: 8 Cups: The nutrition information below is the total amount for two entire packages, all eight servings; so if you want to, you can really stuff yourself and still not pack on the pounds.

Sugar-free Jell-O
80 calories
0 g fat
0 g carbs

½ banana
63 calories
0 g fat
16 g carbs

⅔ cup of blueberries
54 calories
0 g fat
14 g carbs

Total for the entire batch: 197 calories, 0 grams of fat, 30 grams of carbohydrate. (Yes, that's it for all that Jell-O.)

Part Three

AT THE SUPERMARKET

There are actually thousands of Calorie Bargains to be found in the supermarket, including snack foods, condiments, dressings, and desserts, as well as prepared and frozen meals. Before you sleuth them out, however, you need to separate the hype from the truly healthy and understand what the terms on those food labels really mean. The Diet Detective has done the legwork for you so that you won't have to spend so much time trying to separate the good from the bad and the ugly.

The Basics: What's Healthy and What's Not

Looking for Calorie Bargains and losing weight are as much about being healthy as they are about looking good, so I thought it would be useful for you to know just what all the health claims for organic, fresh, and natural foods really mean, and whether seeking them out is actually cost effective for the Calorie Bargain shopper. Walk into any supermarket, especially the newer types such as Whole Foods, and you'll see an array of "better for you" promises on the packages. These terms may make the foods seem healthier, but are they really? "Just because they sound better doesn't necessarily mean they are better. These terms are more about food safety and consumer perceptions than about nutritional quality," says Jane Kolodinsky, PhD, a professor of nutrition economics at the University of Vermont.

So why do we feel more comfortable eating "fresh," "natural," or "organic" foods? "We are less afraid of any risk when it's natural and more afraid when it's man-made," says David Ropeik, a lecturer on risk perception and risk communication at the Harvard School of Public Health. He cites two reasons for this. One, there is an "implicit lack of trust by the consumer in businesses that are out for their own profit, and we trust nature a lot more." Two, when we encounter things we don't understand, we don't trust them, or at least we proceed with caution.

According to Ropeik, there is not necessarily any reason to fear processed foods. He argues that there is a much higher risk associated with food poisoning or an allergic reaction to the food itself than with the chemicals or pesticides used in foods. Still, these terms do make us feel good about the foods we buy, so it's helpful to know what they actually mean.

Fresh

Fresh makes me think that the food was recently made, produced, or harvested, but that's not what it means to the FDA or the USDA. "It's more about the fact that the food was never frozen," says Kolodinsky. "A consumer could easily misinterpret the meaning," she adds.

So although it's not mandated by the Nutrition Labeling and Education Act of 1990, as other nutrient content claims are, the FDA has issued a regulation for the term fresh in order to avoid its possible misuse on food labels. The regulation defines fresh to mean that a food is raw, has never been frozen or heated, and contains no preservatives (except for low-level irradiation to kill bacteria, approved pesticides before or after harvest, FDA-approved food additive wax on raw fruits and vegetables, pasteurization of milk, or a mild chlorine or acid wash on produce). Refrigeration is also OK.

The terms *fresh frozen, frozen fresh*, and *freshly frozen* can be used for foods that are quickly frozen while still fresh. Blanching (brief scalding before freezing to prevent nutrient breakdown) is allowed.

In terms of meat and poultry, which are regulated by the USDA, the term fresh can be used only on foods that have never reached temperatures below 26 degrees Fahrenheit. Despite the fact that this is below freezing, the USDA has stated that the product still remains "fresh" and pliable at this temperature.

"And don't confuse the dating system with the term fresh," says Gail Frank, RD, a professor of nutrition at California State University, Long Beach, and spokesperson for the American Dietetic Association. Fresh food may have a "sell-by date" (the last day recommended to sell) printed on it, but it's not required by the USDA. Some labels may also have a "use-by date," which means the food should be consumed by that time.

Natural

Natural seems to be the term for the new millennium. It implies made by nature, unchanged, nothing artificial, and healthy. " 'Natural' is probably the least trustworthy of all the label terms," says Kolodinsky. While it sounds attractive, it truly doesn't say much about the nutritional quality of the food or its safety.

Although the FDA has not established a regulatory defini-

Diet Detective's **What You Need to Know**

Functional Foods: "This is a nutrient or a food that may provide additional health benefits beyond basic nutrition—for example, yogurt with added bacteria," says Fran Grossman, MS, RD, a nutritionist at Mount Sinai Medical Center in New York City.

"Nearly all whole foods are 'functional' in some way. A functional food is not necessarily a healthy one, so make sure to read the fine print," advises Amy Joy Lanou, PhD, an assistant professor at the University of North Carolina at Asheville. "For example, the egg industry describes eggs as a functional food, yet whole eggs are very high in cholesterol and should be limited in a healthy diet."

tion for natural, its policy regarding the use of the term is that nothing artificial or synthetic has been included in or added to a food that would not normally be expected to be in it (for instance, any chemical). The same applies to use of the terms *100% Natural* and *All-Natural.*

The USDA allows meat and poultry products to be labeled natural if they do not contain ingredients, colors, or preservatives considered artificial and not natural to the product.

"Keep in mind that the term is a passive description," says Frank. "It tells you what the food is not, but that doesn't mean it's better for you. Yes, it might have no preservatives, but that isn't always a good thing."

And don't confuse the term *natural* with *organic.* They're not interchangeable. Natural foods are typically made without additives or preservatives, but they may still contain chemicals, pesticides, or genetically engineered components. Certified organic food has none of these things.

Ditto for *free-range* and *hormone-free.* The chicken at the supermarket labeled free-range may have been exactly that, but it's still not the same as organic.

Organic Foods

For years I'd been pretty skeptical about the value of eating organic food. I believed that there probably wasn't much difference between organic and nonorganic foods. However, with organic foods becoming mainstream, big corporations getting into the act, and more people wondering if they should be eating organic, I wanted the answers to a few key questions.

What Are Organic Fruits and Vegetables?

Only food producers who comply with federal organic rules can call their food "certified organic." The USDA requires that certified organic crops "be produced without pesticides, herbicides, synthetic fertilizers, sewage sludge, bioengineering, or ionizing radiation." Farmers must use organic seeds and may not apply "prohibited substances" such as pesticides and synthetic fertilizers to the land for at least three years before harvest. Accredited USDA certifying agents approve farmers' "organic system" plans and make sure farms adhere to standards. Organic products can be labeled several ways:

- *100% Organic:* products made entirely with organic ingredients.

- *Organic:* products with 95 percent organic ingredients. The remaining 5 percent or less must be listed on the label and can consist of synthetics approved by the USDA.
- *Made with Organic Ingredients:* The product must contain at least 70 percent organic ingredients and can display the phrase "Made with Organic . . ." followed by a listing of up to three specific ingredients.
- Products that have less than 70 percent organic ingredients cannot use the term organic anywhere on the display label but can put specific organic ingredients on the ingredients list.

That said, the USDA makes no claims that organic food is safer or more nutritious than conventionally produced food. The term organic foods refers to the method used to produce food rather than to the characteristics of the food itself. You can view all the organic standards on the USDA website at: www.ams.usda.gov/nop/NOP/standards/ProdHandReg.html.

Are Organic Foods More Nutritious?

The impact of farming practices and food processing on the antioxidant content of food is one of the hottest areas of investigation in the food and nutrition sciences. It's difficult to make a blanket statement that organic fruits and vegetables are more nutritious. Nevertheless, some preliminary evidence indicates that certain specific organic foods are more nutritious. A few studies suggest, for example, that organic fruits may contain a higher level of antioxidants (e.g. vitamin C). Beyond that, the evidence that these foods are significantly healthier is not clear, although some scientists are optimistic.

"On average, organic produce contains marginally higher

levels of vitamin C, antioxidants, and certain minerals compared to conventional foods grown under the same soil and climatic conditions," says Charles Benbrook, PhD, chief scientist of the Organic Center. "For people wanting to prevent disease by increasing their intake of these health-promoting components of food, organic food delivers on average more nutrition per serving and per calorie consumed than does conventional food." After an extensive review of the scientific literature, he asserts that organics have about one-third more antioxidants. (You can read the entire text of the Organic Center's review on antioxidant levels in organic food at www.organiccenter.org/reportfiles/Antioxidant_SSR.pdf.)

One theory explaining the higher antioxidant content of organic foods is that they need to produce more antioxidants to fight off pests and diseases. Because the plants aren't treated with pesticides, they must work harder to stay healthy, which increases stress and creates a higher level of antioxidants.

But does the higher antioxidant content make a real difference in terms of health? Is it "biologically meaningful"? "Science cannot predict nor necessarily prove that a 30 percent or 80 percent increase in antioxidant or vitamin intake will prevent some disease from afflicting a given person, but across the whole population, strong evidence demonstrates that increased nutrient and antioxidant density of food promotes incremental progress in disease prevention and health promotion," argues Benbrook.

On the other hand, says Anthony Trewavas, PhD, a professor and plant scientist at the Institute of Molecular Plant Sciences in Edinburgh, Scotland, "The common belief that 'If a little of anything does you good, a lot more will do even better' has no basis in our understanding of toxicology. Virtually all vitamins and minerals are dangerous if too much is consumed."

Additionally, many of the studies have not taken into consideration differences in soil, weather, and other variables, says Joseph Rosen, PhD, a professor of food science at Rutgers University in New Jersey.

Most experts agree that increased nutrient content is not necessarily the primary reason to buy organic. According to Urvashi Rangan, PhD, an environmental scientist at the nonprofit advocacy group Consumers Union, "While preliminary evidence does suggest, for example, that an organic orange has four times the antioxidants of a conventionally grown orange, if that's why you're buying them, you may want to wait until there is stronger scientific proof."

Is It True That Organic Foods Taste Better?

Organic food has a reputation among many people for tasting better. The reason? For a long time it was mainly available at roadside stands and, therefore, was fresher than the conventional produce sold in supermarkets, says Rosen. However, he doesn't believe there is any difference.

Benbrook offers an alternative reason: "Organically grown food tends to grow a bit more slowly and does not reach the size of conventional produce. Conventional fruits and vegetables grow faster, tend to get bigger, and yield a bit more per acre, but they do so at the expense of nutrient and antioxidant density. As a result, the taste, flavor, and aroma of conventional produce tend to be diluted."

Instead of relying on scientists, why not do your own taste test?

Are There Any Other Reasons to Eat Organic?

One of the most popular and quantifiable arguments in support of organic food is less about the final product and more about the environmental conditions surrounding organic versus conventional farming. By eliminating petroleum-based fertilizers, organic farms could help reduce soil erosion, climate change, and water contamination. And if you are concerned about genetically modified foods, for the most part you can avoid them by purchasing organic.

When it comes down to it, buying organic is an individual decision on many levels. "Some people focus on environmental issues; others care about health issues, worker issues, animal issues, cost issues—there are all kinds of value decisions a consumer can make," says Rangan.

Am I Avoiding Dangerous Chemicals by Eating Organic?

There is no question that more dangerous chemicals are used on fruits and vegetables that are not grown organically. "There are absolutely fewer pesticides used on organic foods," says Rangan. "Some natural pesticides and even a few synthetic pesticides have been approved, but if you look at the list of approved substances, there are only about thirty-five options, and one of them is baking powder."

In fact, many organic proponents claim that the major benefit is avoidance of commonplace toxic contaminants, particularly carcinogenic and neurotoxic pesticides. "These are certainly a concern to healthy people, but more so to the unhealthy, and even more so to toddlers and infants, who are extremely sensitive to carcinogens," says Samuel S. Epstein, MD, a professor emeritus of environmental and occupational medicine at the University of Illinois School of Public Health and chairman of the Cancer Prevention Coalition.

However, not everyone agrees. " 'The dose makes the poison' is a cardinal rule of toxicologists," argues Rutgers's Dr.

Rosen. "Yes, some agricultural chemicals are dangerous, but humans do not ingest enough to threaten their health."

Nevertheless, a glimpse of the effects of these chemicals on agricultural workers may make you want to reduce your exposure as much as possible. One analysis, published in *Reviews on Environmental Health,* determined that agricultural and industrial workers are at high risk for developing cancer following pesticide exposure. Children of farmworkers can be exposed to pesticides through their parents, and maternal exposure can pose a health risk to the fetus and the newborn.

Do Government Regulations Protect Our Food from Harmful Chemicals?

"We rely on a 'proof of harm scale' in this country," says Rangan. "We tend to believe that something is safe until it's proven otherwise. In Europe, they work the other way—they don't believe anything is safe until they see proof that it is. Right now, we don't have a lot of hard proof demonstrating that conventionally grown foods could be considered dangerous. But we do know that chemicals could be harmful. The EPA [Environmental Protection Agency] is constantly reevaluating and reexamining allowable levels of chemicals in food. And science is not static—we know more in 2005 than we knew in 1975. So just because we don't have all the evidence to explain the danger doesn't mean the danger isn't there." The bottom line is that eating organic food is a way to be "safer than safe."

And according to Dr. Epstein, "The USDA and FDA have a statutory obligation to inform the public of risks from carcinogens and contaminated foods, but both have abysmally failed to do so. Both agencies are more protective of agribusiness industry interests than consumer safety interests."

How Does the Food and Drug Administration View Its Responsibilities to Protect Citizens from Harmful Chemicals?

"The FDA has an extensive program and commitment to protect the public health from chemical contaminants, such as acrylamide, dioxins, methylmercury, furan, perchlorate, mycotoxins, and lead," says an FDA spokesperson. "This program, depending on the contaminant, includes setting action and guidance levels; action plans aimed to minimize exposure to harmful contaminants; public meetings both to inform the public and solicit input; food advisory committee meetings; posting of activities and data on the FDA website; surveillance; consumer advice; and enforcement actions."

Some would say that eating organic isn't necessarily better because natural pesticides can be as bad as synthetic ones. "There is a common assumption that natural chemicals are somehow safe to eat, whereas synthetic chemicals are dangerous. That is completely untrue," says Dr. Trewavas. "In fact, some natural pesticides kill insects by precisely the same chemical mechanism as synthetic pesticides. And there is no difference in the overall toxicological stability of natural and synthetic chemicals in the human body. But while the daily consumption of natural pesticide is equivalent to about a quarter of a teaspoon, the synthetic pesticide trace is the equivalent of one-quarter of a grain of salt—about 10,000-fold lower. That amount of synthetic chemicals is toxicologically irrelevant."

Nevertheless, even die-hard cynics like Dr. Rosen agree that if you can afford to buy organic, "Why not do it?"

How Likely Is It That an Organic Food Will Contain Pesticides?

It depends on the crop and where it is grown. When organic vegetables are grown in the midst of conventional crops, pesticide drift is hard to prevent. Low levels of pesticides can remain in the soil thirty years after the product was applied, and sometimes pesticides in irrigation water lead to detectable levels in an organic field.

"For most organic fresh fruits and vegetables," says Benbrook, "there are fewer pesticides found, less frequently, and at lower levels. The pesticide risk posed by organic food is one-tenth to one one-hundredth that of conventional produce."

What Do Organic Farms Use in Place of Chemical Pesticides?

There are several kinds of natural pesticides and chemicals that certified organic farms are allowed to use, including ladybugs (which kill many plant-eating insects) and various kinds of insect pheromones—hormones extracted from insects and then sprayed over crops. However, one study (which has since come under a good deal of scrutiny and controversy) suggests that people who eat organic foods may be up to eight times more likely than those who eat nonorganic foods to get *E coli*.

Should You Avoid All Nonorganic Foods Even If You're on a Tight Budget?

Not necessarily. According to Rosen, an average family of four would probably spend between 50 percent and 300 percent more to be completely organic. However, there is a middle ground.

Not only do the amounts of pesticides used on different kinds of produce differ, but the physical makeups of the fruits and veggies themselves change the level of pesticides you're likely to ingest. For example, even heavily sprayed bananas are low risk because you remove a majority of the pesticides when you peel them. Therefore, Tufts University researcher Kathleen A. Merrigan, PhD, is less concerned about bananas than strawberries, which could have as many as sixty-five chemical treatments by the time they get to the consumer.

If you're concerned about contamination but don't want to go completely organic, here are the "Dirty Dozen": the twelve foods with the highest chemical levels, according to a USDA analysis of data regarding pesticide residue in food:

- peaches
- strawberries
- apples
- nectarines
- pears
- cherries
- red raspberries
- imported grapes
- spinach
- celery
- potatoes
- sweet bell peppers

To find out the level of pesticides on your produce, go to www.foodnews.org, the website of the Environmental Working Group, which lists government findings on the amounts of pesticides used on fruits and vegetables. According to the EWG, the six fruits least likely to have pesticide residues are pineapples, mangoes, bananas, kiwis, avocados, and papayas. And the vegetables least likely to have pesticide residues are sweet corn, cauliflower, asparagus, onions, peas, and broccoli.

Calorie Bargain Spotlight

Calorie Bargain: Wha Guru Chews (Energy Bars)

The Why: *Smothered.* It's almost a dirty word. It's reminiscent of a time in our lives when we used to be able to chow down on anything whether it was smothered in butter, syrup, gravy, or fudge. So it's not every day that we "healthy eaters" get to bite into something smothered—but today is our lucky day.

Wha Guru Chews are sort of like an all-natural PowerBar: soft, chewy, and full of fresh nut crunch and flavor. Not only that, but every ingredient on the label is readable, even without a PhD in chemistry. It figures something so perfect would come from an Oregon company called Golden Temple, founded by a yogi, no less.

The Health Bonus: Wha Guru Chews are all-natural, handmade, vegan—and portable.

What We Liked Best: The taste is off the charts, and they are only 160 to 190 calories each, a great value.

What We Liked Least: They make your fingers a little sticky, so don't forget the Wet Ones.

The Price: about $1 each.

Website: www.whaguruchew.com.

Where to Buy: Amazon.com, www.tealand.com.

Ingredients: The Cashew Almond flavor contains: barley malt syrup, cashews, sunflower seeds, brown rice syrup, almonds, maple syrup, high-oleic safflower oil, wheat germ, cashew butter, almond butter, natural maple flavor, sea salt, soy lecithin.

Offerings: They are available in five flavors: Sesame Almond, Almond Ginger, Cashew Almond, Peanut Cashew, and Cashew Vanilla—all nice and smothered in a special caramel to hold them together.

Nutritional Analysis per Serving: 1 Bar

Cashew Almond
160 calories
10 g fat
9 g carbs
4 g protein

Sesame Almond
160 calories
11 g fat
10 g carbs
3 g protein

Almond Ginger
150 calories
9 g fat
16 g carbs
2 g protein

Cashew Vanilla
150 calories
9 g fat
16 g carbs
3 g protein

Can't You Simply Rinse off Pesticides, Fertilizers, and Other Allegedly Harmful Chemicals?

Washing can substantially reduce the amount of pesticides left on the skins of fruits and vegetables, although how much residue you remove is dependent on myriad factors, including the amount of exposure to chemicals, the skin of the food, and the kinds of chemicals used. Generally speaking, your best bet is a thirty-second rinse, a fifteen-second soak, and then a final rinse. This process, however, works a lot better for a tomato than it does for something like a raspberry, which has a complicated and fragile skin. Always pay attention to any bases or stems, as dirt and pesticides tend to lodge themselves in these places. Conventional apples are pretty heavily sprayed; you might want to also cut out the belly buttons and wash the rest, offers Joan Dye Gussow, EdD, a professor emeritus of nutrition at Columbia University.

Diet Detective's What You Need to Know

Enriched Foods: Technically a food can be enriched if it naturally contains important vitamins and minerals but in amounts so low as to fail to provide consumers with any noticeable benefit. Higher levels of these trace components are then added to the food until it becomes a viable source of these nutrients. However, according to Dr. Lupton of Texas A&M University, the most generally accepted definition of an enriched food is one in which nutrients that were lost in processing have been replaced. For instance, when certain foods, such as grains, are refined, they lose many of the nutrients they had in their original form. Once the food has been processed, manufacturers reintroduce (usually at higher levels) the vitamins and minerals that have been leached. In flour, for example, thiamin, riboflavin, iron, and niacin lost in the translation from wheat to white are often added again to the final white flour. This process is technically called "restoration" but appears most often on food labels as "enriched."

Omega-3 Basics

Health claims on foods are proliferating, and one that's particularly popular is using omega-3 fatty acids to improve cardiovascular health in addition to other health benefits. Here's the lowdown on this healthy type of fat.

Are Omega-3s Absolutely Necessary in Our Diets?

It depends. "There's needed, and there's needed," says Debra Palmer Keenan, PhD, a nutrition professor at Rutgers University in New Jersey. They're essential fatty acids—meaning our bodies don't manufacture them. "You can probably live without eating any omega-3s, but you may not function as well. Your health outcomes might not be as good."

Additionally, omega-3s are found in breast milk and have been shown to be important in brain and eye development. According to Keenan, "It's been documented that healthier children are born to women who get the proper amounts of the omega-3s DHA and EPA."

Omega-3 and omega-6 fatty acids share the same pool of enzymes and go through the same oxidation pathways while being metabolized. Omega-6s are typically found as linoleic acid (LA), which is in many processed foods as well as meat, egg yolks, and cooking oils, including sunflower, safflower, corn, cottonseed, and soybean oils. According to Jay Whelan, PhD, a professor of nutrition and omega-3 researcher at the University of Tennessee, "A typical American diet tends to contain approximately fifteen times more omega-6 than omega-3 fatty acids." This is one of the reasons some researchers say we need more omega-3s to make up for this imbalance. And although we need both, the imbalance can increase risk for long-term health problems such as cardiovascular disease. Why not just reduce omega-6 consumption and close the ratio? "We don't know to what extent high intake of omega-6 fatty acids compromises any benefits of omega-3 fatty acid consumption," says Whelan.

What Are Omega-3s, and Is There a Difference Between the Omega-3s in Fish and Those in Walnuts?

Omega-3 fatty acids are a type of polyunsaturated fat. There are a few types of omega-3s: EPA (eicosapentaenoic acid), DHA (docosahexaenoic acid), and ALA (alpha linolenic acid).

"They are not the same thing," says Keenan. "We have to stop talking about omega-3s and talk about DHA and EPA and ALA as separate fatty acids. All three are long-chain fatty acids, but EPA and DHA are longer. They can be formed from ALA, but it's not a process that the human body performs efficiently," she adds.

EPA and DHA, which come from fish oils, are the most valuable to health and wellness. Both play an important role in normal function of the heart, brain, eyes, nervous system, kidney, and liver. These essential fats have also been proved to reduce the risk of cardiovascular disease and inflammation.

ALA is found in leafy, green vegetables and some commonly used oils, including canola and soybean. Some less commonly used oils, such as flaxseed oil, contain relatively high concentrations of ALA, but these oils are not commonly found in the food supply. "If you get ALA from walnuts, flaxseed, or canola oil, it can be beneficial because it gets converted to DHA and EPA, but that's only if ALA is already lacking in your diet, which it probably isn't," says Whelan. Eating more ALA just for it to be converted to EPA and DHA is not recommended. "The amounts converted are very small," he explains, "and in the long run, ALA starts to replace the needed DHA in the tissues, which is not a good thing."

According to most research, ALA is not a viable source of EPA and DHA and cannot replace fish and fish oils in the diet. "ALA is still a good guy with its own benefits, even if it's not converted," says Whelan, who believes that ALA, while not as effective as EPA and DHA in reducing risk of cardiovascular disease, might work independently, helping reduce risk in other ways.

Why Are Omega-3s Getting So Much Attention?

One of the key health benefits of omega-3 fatty acids is that they significantly reduce the risk for sudden death caused by cardiac arrhythmias and decrease all-cause mortality in patients with coronary heart disease. In addition to helping regulate the heart, omega-3s prevent the formation of clots and act as anti-inflammatories.

In fact, the U.S. Department of Health and Human Services Agency for Healthcare Research and Quality studied omega-3s and concluded, "Overall, a number of studies offer evidence to support the hypothesis that fish, fish oil, or ALA-supplement consumption reduces all-cause mortality and various cardiovascular disease outcomes, although the evidence is strongest for fish or fish oil." If you look at the studies, many with thousands of participants, the research looks very strong. Keep in mind, this is not like the herbal remedy echinacea, where one day you wake up and read that it has no effect; this is based on strong, well-documented research. It should be noted that although there are certainly studies showing benefits for primary prevention, the research into EPA and DHA indicates that they are most valuable—in helping to slow the progress of heart disease in patients already diagnosed.

Last year the FDA allowed the following claim to be placed on certain foods: "Supportive but not conclusive research shows that consumption of EPA and DHA omega-3 fatty acids may reduce the risk of coronary heart disease. One serving of [name of food] provides [x] grams of EPA and DHA omega-3 fatty acids. [See nutrition information for total fat, saturated fat, and cholesterol content.]" The label must state how much omega-3 fatty acids the product contains; however the FDA doesn't require the food to contain a minimum amount of omega-3s to carry the claim.

Are There Other Health Benefits?

"This could be one of those nutrients that becomes a 'magic bullet,' but we don't say things are conclusive until there have been many studies. And with heart disease, we say it's conclusive. There are many other things that they're looking at that are looking strong but are not quite there yet," says Professor Keenan.

Omega-3s (specifically DHA and EPA) are being examined for other health benefits, including: treating rheumatoid arthritis, ulcerative colitis and Crohn's disease (because of their anti-inflammatory properties); treating depression and other psychological disorders (because they may boost levels of the brain chemicals serotonin and dopamine, decreasing depression and violent behavior); reducing the risk of diabetes, insulin resistance in people with diabetes, psoriasis and other skin conditions; helping osteoporosis (because they may enhance bone density); and fighting cancer (they may inhibit proliferation of cancer cells in the breast, prostate, and colon). In infants, omega-3s may improve cognition and visual acuity.

What Are the Sources of Omega-3s?

Sources of ALA include soybeans and soybean oil, canola oil, walnuts and flaxseeds and their oils, whereas sources of EPA and DHA are fatty fish, such as salmon and tuna, and their oils.

For a complete list of omega-3s (broken down into DHA, EPA, and ALA) and where to find them, check out www.ncbi .nlm.nih.gov/books/bv.fcgi?rid=hstat1a.table.38454.

What about Omega-3 Supplements?

There are new products on the market made with encapsulated fish oil, so they don't smell or taste like fish. However, Dr. Whelan is not so sure that the benefits will match those from eating the actual fish. If you're not getting omega-3s from any other sources, supplements are a good option, but we don't know enough to say that the fish doesn't have other properties working in conjunction with omega-3s to bring about these purported health benefits.

That said, if you don't like fish, supplements are always a possibility. Some research has shown positive outcomes for omega-3 fish supplements over a placebo. "Fish oil supplements are an excellent way to get EPA and DHA," says Tod Cooperman, MD, president of the supplement research group ConsumerLab.com. "So far, they have lacked contaminants such as mercury and PCBs [polychlorinated biphenyls], probably because smaller fish are used to make the oils, and contaminants tend to stay with fish muscle and not the oil. Furthermore, most products also undergo distillation, which removes contaminants." Take them at night just before bed, advises Professor Keenan. "This way, if and when you burp the fish taste, it will be in your sleep."

However, adds Cooperman, "The real quality concerns with both fish and seed oils are that they not be spoiled and that they contain all the oils that they promise. This is not always the case."

For information about the best omega-3 from fish oil supplements, visit www.consumerlab.com/results/omega3.asp for omega-3 seed oils, visit www.consumerlab.com/results/flax seed.asp.

What Are the Other Food Sources of Omega-3s Besides Fish?

Some of the foods fortified with omega-3s (DHA and EPA) include:

- Arnold Smart & Healthy Omega-3 DHA/EPA bread (1 slice): 33 mg omega-3 (DHA and EPA).
- Smart Balance Omega Plus Spread (1 tablespoon): 150 mg.

I tried the Arnold bread and a bread made from National Starch (it manufactures the encapsulated fish oil), and they were very good. I could not detect any fish taste. Also becoming popular are foods fortified with ALA such as Barilla Plus pasta and Health Valley Organic Golden Flax Cereal.

Omega-3s in fish oils, algal oils, and linseed oil can be highly susceptible to oxidation, which deteriorates flavor, increases the risk of rancidity, and reduces shelf life. However, the food industry is working around these issues, and—according to the Institute of Food Technologists—it expects to see omega-3 fortification in the future in the following products: frozen food entrees, soups, refrigerated foods, salad dressings, yogurts, spreads, juices, egg products, and cheeses.

How Much Omega-3 Do I Need to Consume in Order to Reap the Benefits?

Using the estimates from USDA's special analysis, 8 ounces of high omega-3 fatty-acid fish would provide approximately 3,250 milligrams of EPA and DHA a week—an average of slightly less than 500 milligrams per day, which is about a twofold increase over current intake. Adverse effects are not observed until intake exceeds 3 grams per day.

The American Heart Association's recommendations state: "Patients without documented coronary heart disease (CHD) should eat at least two servings of fatty fish per week along with other foods rich in omega-3 fatty acids. Persons with CHD are encouraged to eat at least one daily meal that includes a fatty fish or take a daily fish-oil supplement to achieve a recommended level of 0.9 grams per day of EPA." The association also recommends, "People who have elevated triglycerides may need 2 to 4 grams of EPA and DHA per day provided as a supplement." The AHA recommends the supplements because "even the 1-gram-per-day dose recommended for patients with existing CVD [cardiovascular disease] may be more than can readily be achieved through diet alone." The association also suggests, as do most experts, consulting your physician before taking this or any other supplement.

Also keep in mind that if you're eating fish, you certainly don't want to get it battered and fried, which would pretty much defeat the purpose.

Recommendations for Omega-3s from Experts Around the World

- American Heart Association: 2 servings of fish (preferably fatty) per week (Krauss et al., 2000; Kris-Etherton et al., 2002).

Diet Detective's What You Need to Know

Fortified Foods: A food that is "fortified" is used as a vehicle to get underconsumed nutrients into the food supply. Fortification is the process by which nutrients and minerals are added to a food that never had them to begin with. This can serve two purposes: to increase the amount of nutrients in the food and to help our bodies better absorb the natural nutrients that were there originally. One of the most popular examples is milk fortified with vitamin D. In addition to providing milk drinkers with an extra vitamin, the added ingredient increases the rate at which the body absorbs the calcium naturally found in milk.

Some experts suggest that fortified foods should be treated like supplements—only to help you meet nutrient needs you cannot otherwise meet. Karen Collins, MS, RD, a nutritionist at the American Institute for Cancer Research, says, "Fortified foods should not replace the goal of a balanced plant-based diet—a plate comprised of at least two-thirds fruits, vegetables, grains, and beans—as the crucial step to supply the nutrients and protective phytochemicals we need."

- National Cholesterol Education Program: Choose fish as a food more often (NCEP, 2002, table V.2–6).
- World Health Organization: regular fish consumption (1 to 2 servings per week; each serving should provide the equivalent of 200 to 500 mg of EPA and DHA) (WHO *Technical Report,* 2003).
- European Society of Cardiology: Oil fish and omega-3 fatty acids have particular protective properties for primary CVD prevention (De Backer et al., 2003; Priori et al., 2003; Van de Werf et al., 2003).
- United Kingdom Scientific Advisory Committee on Nutrition: Consume at least 2 portions of fish per week, of which 1 should be oily and provide 450 mg per day of EPA and DHA (Scientific Advisory Committee on Nutrition, 2004).
- American Diabetes Association: Consume 2 to 3 servings of fish per week to provide dietary omega-3 polyunsaturated fats (Franz et al., 2004).

(Source: U.S. Department of Health & Human Services and U.S. Department of Agriculture. *Dietary Guidelines for Americans, 2005,* 6th Edition, Washington, DC.)

Calorie Bargain Spotlight

Calorie Bargain: Annie's Naturals Low-fat Honey Mustard Vinaigrette

The Why: It can be tricky to find a low-cal, low-fat alternative to regular salad dressing, anyone who's had a typical low-cal version of a ranch or Italian dressing can attest to that. That's why Annie's Honey Mustard Vinaigrette is such a treat.

The Health Bonus: Many of her organic dressings are as good as marinades as they are on salads, and this low-cal version is no exception. Compare it to Maple Grove Farms Honey Mustard Dressing, which comes in at 120 calories for the same 2 tablespoons, and you'll see why Annie's is such a deal.

What We Liked Best: All Annie's dressings are safe bets in terms of flavor.

What We Liked Least: All of our tasters really liked this, and we struggled for something that "we liked least." Hopefully you can find it in your local supermarket!

The Price: $2.49 for an 8-ounce bottle.

Offerings: Artichoke Parmesan, Balsamic Vinaigrette, Cowgirl Ranch, Honey Mustard Vinaigrette, Raspberry Vinaigrette, others.

Website: www.consorzio.com.

Where to Buy: Whole Foods Market, Wild Oats Marketplace, The Fresh Market, company website.

Ingredients: water, organic Dijon mustard (organic apple cider vinegar, organic mustard seed, salt, organic turmeric), honey, cider vinegar, expeller-pressed canola oil, sea salt, xanthan gum.

Nutritional Analysis per Serving: 2 Tablespoons
45 calories
2 g fat
6 g carbs
0 g protein
0 g fiber
200 mg sodium

Keeping Healthy Foods Healthy

While it's true that some foods may fight disease and help you live longer, many of us forget that just because a food is healthy doesn't mean it's calorie free. In fact, eating too much of even a healthy food might cancel the very benefit it provides. Here are a few foods along with their health benefits and ways to keep them healthy.

Avocados and Guacamole

The Good: Avocados are nutrient dense and packed with antioxidants, vitamins B_6, C, and E, as well as folate and potassium (60 percent more potassium per ounce than bananas). They're also a great source of monounsaturated fat, which studies have shown reduces serum cholesterol levels when used in place of saturated fats.

The Bad: The calories add up; a 7-ounce avocado has about 360 calories. That's about 50 calories per 1-ounce slice or 110 calories in just 3 ounces of guacamole. Plus, guacamole doesn't keep very good company. Its best friends—cheese, chips, and refried beans—can really pack on the pounds.

- Tortilla chips (7 to 10 chips): 140 calories, 6 g fat, 19 g carbs.

- Sour cream (2 tablespoons): 62 calories, 6 g fat, 1 g carbs.

Fit Tip: Keep avocados and guacamole in your diet, but avoid the fried tortilla chips and other unhealthy foods that tag along. Serve it in small dishes for portion control, and have baked, low-fat chips. Also, you can use avocado slices to replace other high-calorie foods that contain saturated fat, such as whole-fat cheese, which has 100 calories per ounce/slice.

Figs

The Good: There was a fig tree in the Garden of Eden, and the fig is the fruit (actually it's a flower inverted into itself) most mentioned in the Bible. You can eat them fresh or dried. High in antioxidants, figs are a top source of fiber as well as potassium, manganese, and vitamin B_6. They are fat free, sodium free, and, like all plant foods, cholesterol free. A ¼ cup serving provides 244 milligrams of potassium (7 percent of the daily value), 53 milligrams of calcium (6 percent of the DV), and 1.2 milligrams of iron (6 percent of the DV).

The Bad: Ever look at the calories for one Fig Newton? Fifty-five calories. The average fig has 40 to 50 calories. And to make matters worse, fresh figs are rare because they last only about a week after harvesting. As a consequence, about 90 percent of the world's fig harvest is dried. One dried fig has about 58 calories, and they're as easy to pop down as M&M's.

Fit Tip: Chop some figs to scatter over oatmeal or any cold cereal. Skip the sugar and enjoy the fig flavor and crunch. Sweeten up mashed or cubed winter squash or sweet potatoes with chopped California figs. The figs add a richness of their own, so you can skip the butter or margarine.

Dried Plums (Formerly Known as Prunes)

The Good: It's a delicious fruit that serves multiple purposes. Dried plums are a source of dietary fiber, sorbitol, potassium, copper, magnesium, iron, boron, and phenolic compounds, which are active in a web of interrelated physiological and health-promoting functions, and they're also packed with vitamin A.

Dried plums are also high in antioxidants, which help neutralize the damaging effects of oxidation that are believed to play a role in the aging process and the development of cancer, heart and lung disease, and cataracts. It takes about 1¼ pounds of fresh plums to equal the antioxidant capacity of 3½ ounces of dried plums.

The Bad: There are about 22 calories per dried plum. So if you want to get your daily dose, you need to use them as a replacement for other, less healthy foods—like a bag of potato chips, for example. Another issue: If you eat too many prunes, well, they have a laxative effect.

Fit Tip: Combine one or two with a variety of other lower-calorie fruits. Or chop the prunes and use them as topping on cereal and other foods.

Raisins

The Good: Raisins are basically sun-dried grapes. They're low in sodium and fat free. In addition, they provide many necessary vitamins and minerals, including iron, potassium, and fiber, and they're loaded with antioxidants.

In fact, raisins rank among the antioxidant-richest fruits. For 100 grams (about 3½ ounces), raisins have about 2,830 ORAC units (oxygen radical absorbance capacity, a measure of the antioxidant power of foods). Antioxidants help neutralize the damaging effects of oxidation, which is thought to play a role in the aging process and the development of certain cancers as well as heart and lung diseases.

Raisins can also be stored for a long time, and we don't have to eat as many of them as other fruits to gain all their health benefits.

The Bad: Because they're dried, their nutrients are very concentrated, and so are their calories. There's about one calorie in every raisin. At that rate, even a very small box can be costly at 45 calories. To get the same antioxidant benefit as 3½ ounces of raisins, you would have to eat almost four times as many (13½ ounces) red grapes (ORAC, 739 units), but you'd still be consuming roughly the same number of calories— about 320. In fact, ounce for ounce, all dried fruits are much higher in calories than their fresh equivalents because of the water that's lost and the concentration of sugar that occurs during the drying process. Eating grapes will also leave you more satiated because of their high water content. Raisins have about 73 percent less water than grapes. Interestingly, raisins are made from green grapes, not red (their color results from the reaction between the proteins and the sugar that occurs as the grapes are dried), and green grapes have fewer antioxidants.

Fit Tip: Eating raisins is a real treat, so use them as a replacement for other sweet foods in your diet. For instance, if you typically sprinkle sugar on your cereal, try using ten or fifteen raisins instead. Or, if baking, try them in low-fat muffins and cookies instead of chocolate chips.

Yogurt

The Good: Yogurt has gained a reputation for being a healthy food for a variety of reasons. It improves digestion, prevents intestinal infection, and reinforces your immune function. Yogurt is a fermented dairy product made by adding bacterial cultures to milk, which transforms the milk's sugar, lactose, into lactic acid. This process gives yogurt its tart flavor and distinctive puddinglike texture. It's high in vitamins and minerals such as calcium, potassium, riboflavin, magnesium, and phosphate, and it's low in fat. One cup of fat-free yogurt contains 50 percent more calcium than the same-size serving of milk, providing one-third of your recommended daily requirement. It also provides a milk alternative for those who are lactose intolerant, since it is virtually lactose free.

The Bad: The truth of these health claims notwithstanding, we can't ignore the fact that yogurt still contains calories and quite a lot of sugar. So eating too much of it may negate any potential benefits by increasing the health risk of being overweight. For instance, a 10-ounce bottle of Stonyfield Farm Organic low-fat Yogurt Smoothie has 250 calories, as well as added sugar. And then there's frozen yogurt (even low-fat or no-fat), which is typically on a dieter's shopping list but is really more like ice cream and may not have the same health benefits as regular yogurt. Two examples: A cup of Ben & Jerry's Chocolate Fudge Brownie Low Fat Frozen Yogurt contains 380 calories, while Häagen-Dazs's Vanilla Raspberry Swirl Low-fat Frozen Yogurt has 340 calories.

Also, keep an eye on yogurt-covered snacks: Some varieties

are more like candies in disguise. One cup of yogurt-covered raisins contains over 900 calories, and one cup of yogurt-covered pretzels has more than 1,000 calories.

Fit Tip: Stick with the low-fat or no-fat yogurts, and try to find a brand with no added sugar. If you normally eat high-calorie foods like ice cream or cheese, it's great to replace them with low-fat or no-fat yogurt.

Olive Oil

The Good: The Food and Drug Administration recently granted olive oil a qualified health claim. Manufacturers are now allowed to state on the label: "Limited and not conclusive scientific evidence suggests that eating about 2 tablespoons (23 grams) of olive oil daily may reduce the risk of coronary heart disease due to the monounsaturated fat in olive oil."

Diet Detective's What You Need to Know

Q: Is it true that cooking sprays like Pam and Mazola have no fat at all?

A. No. First of all, to qualify as fat free, a food must have fewer than 0.5 grams of fat per serving. The key words here are *per serving*. These claims are based on standardized serving sizes, which can be unrealistic or confusing. And even though Pam has fewer than 0.5 grams of fat per serving, technically qualifying it for the fat-free claim, the Food and Drug Administration thought such an assertion would be misleading for a product that is essentially 100 percent fat (that's right—it's full of fat). The compromise was to allow Pam and similar products to put the words "for fat-free cooking" on the label.

I'm still a fan—as long as you're careful about how long you're spraying!

Diet Detective's What You Need to Know

Q: Which is the best oil?

A: They're all pretty much equal in terms of weight control, meaning that all oil has about 120 calories per tablespoon. Yes, regular vegetable oil has the same number of calories as olive oil. Just because an oil is heart healthy doesn't mean it's calorie free. The best oils? While most of the vegetable oils are pretty low in saturated fat, technically, canola and soybean are the best. They are both high in omega-3 fatty acids, and soybean oil is high in polyunsaturated fat, while canola is high in monosaturated fat—both of which are heart healthy. Does that mean olive oil isn't good? Olive oil tastes great and is a very good oil, and it is important to actually enjoy your food.

The Bad: The allowable claim goes on to say: "To achieve this possible benefit, olive oil is to replace a similar amount of saturated fat and not increase the total number of calories you eat in a day." Why? Because oil has about 120 calories per tablespoon. So if you don't use it as a replacement, you could put on about 25 pounds in a year by following only the first part of the advice. Oh, and keep in mind that "light" olive oil does not have fewer calories—it's just lighter in color.

Fit Tip: When using olive oil as a dressing, drizzle it on with a fork. For cooking, use olive oil misters, available at most cooking stores, such as Williams-Sonoma.

Oatmeal

The Good: You've probably seen food labels or TV commercials touting oatmeal as a food that lowers your cholesterol. That's because oats contain soluble fiber. According to research, soluble fiber (beta-glucans) may help lower blood cholesterol levels and reduce the risk of heart disease when included in a diet that is also low in saturated fat and cholesterol. The 3 grams per day of oat beta-glucan needed to lower cholesterol can be obtained by eating 1½ cups of cooked oatmeal (¾ cup of uncooked oatmeal), or roughly three packets of instant oatmeal. Eating this amount on a regular basis typically lowers total cholesterol by up to 23 percent.

Besides lowering your cholesterol, oats are just plain healthy, providing protein, iron, insoluble fiber, and other nutrients—and they have only 145 calories per cup (cooked). Also, in terms of weight control, studies show that an increase in either soluble or insoluble fiber intake helps you feel full longer, thereby decreasing your subsequent hunger.

Finally, oats are naturally cholesterol free and low in saturated fat and sodium.

The Bad: The problems start when we add the extras: brown sugar, butter, salt, honey, whole milk, and/or fruit (which is not bad in moderation). Too many add-ons bring up the total fat, cholesterol, and calories beyond what would be considered a healthy breakfast.

Fit Tip: Stick to a cup and a half of cooked oatmeal (218 calories) and throw in a half cup of frozen blueberries (35 calories), which are also high in antioxidants. Or toss in ¾ of a cup of frozen mixed berries for 70 calories. Also, add your own cinnamon or nutmeg to plain oatmeal rather than buying the flavored versions, which come with added sugar.

Soy Crisps

The Good: With about two-thirds the calories of potato chips and no saturated fat, soy crisps make a good snack. And they're made from soy, which means they contain a complex mix of phytochemicals, including isoflavones, which can help fight or prevent heart disease, cancer, and osteoporosis, as well as other diseases.

Experts recommend integrating a total of 11 grams of soy protein (two 8-ounce glasses of soy milk or 1 ounce of soy nuts) from food sources—not supplements—into your diet each day. Glenny's Onion & Garlic Soy Crisps have 10 grams of soy protein per 1.3 ounce bag.

The Bad: The calories still add up, so if you weren't a chip eater to begin with, this isn't the best way to start adding soy to your diet. But even if you are making the switch from potato chips to soy crisps, you might not come out ahead. For instance, Glenny's Soy Crisps have 130 calories per 1.3-ounce bag, and since we almost always eat what's in the bag, that would be only 10 to 20 calories less than an equal serving of potato chips.

Plus, soy might not be good for everyone. For instance, adding soy is controversial for postmenopausal women who happen to be at high risk for breast cancer, so be sure to check with your doctor before you start on soy.

Fit Tip: Look for soy chips in packages with 110 calories or less for the entire bag. Choose them only to replace higher-calorie chips already in your diet. Or you can try opening the package and dividing the chips in two sealable bags, which will give you the recommended serving size and only 70 calories.

Calorie Bargain Spotlight

Calorie Bargain: Vermont Sugar Free Syrup and Maple Grove Farms Sugar Free Maple Flavor Syrup

The Why: If you enjoy pancakes, waffles, and French toast, and you're counting calories, these sugar-free syrups are a great idea.

The Health Bonus: The calorie reduction is huge. A regular serving of maple syrup comes in at 200 calories. Given that the foods to which we add syrup tend to be fairly high in calories to begin with, trimming the number you get from the additions can make a big difference.

What We Liked Best: Syrups that are low in calories, fat free, and tasty—what more could we ask for?

What We Liked Least: It's not all natural. Also, if you don't like using artificial sweeteners, both products are sweetened with Splenda (sucralose).

The Price: $11.95 for three 12-ounce bottles, $36.60 for twelve 12-ounce bottles.

Offerings: Vermont Sugar Free Syrup, Maple Grove Farms Sugar Free Syrup.

Website: www.maplegrove.com.

Where to Buy: www.maplegrove.com.

Ingredients

Vermont Sugar Free Syrup
Water, sorbitol, natural and artificial maple flavor, cellulose gum, sucralose (Splenda brand), salt, citric acid, potassium sorbate and sodium benzoate (to preserve freshness), zinc lactate, niacinamide (vitamin B_3), D-calcium pantothenate (vitamin B_5), pyridoxine

hydrochloride (vitamin B_6), thiamine mononitrate (vitamin B_1), cyanocobalamin (vitamin B_{12}), caramel color.

Maple Grove Farms Sugar Free Syrup

Water, sorbitol, cellulose gum, natural and artificial maple flavor (sulfites), salt, sucralose (Splenda brand), sodium benzoate (to preserve freshness), phosphoric acid, acesulfame potassium, sorbic acid, and potassium sorbate (to preserve freshness), caramel color, citric acid.

Nutritional Analysis per Serving

Vermont Sugar Free Syrup—¼ Cup	Maple Grove Farms Sugar Free Syrup—¼ Cup
10 calories	30 calories
0 g fat	0 g fat
4 g carbs	11 g carbs
0 g protein	0 g protein
0 g fiber	0 g fiber
120 mg sodium	110 mg sodium

Calorie Bargain Spotlight

Calorie Bargain: Garden-in-a-Bag

The Why: Because there is a wonderful group of people working at Potting Shed Creations, based in Troy, Idaho. Their products—and the biggest key to their success—are based on one simple premise: "Develop exciting, high-quality products that offer a fresh approach to gardening." The Garden-in-a-Bag collection provides a great selection of herbs, fruits, and veggies that can be grown indoors, right in the leakproof bag. All you need to do is mix in the enclosed packet of seeds and add water. The seeds germinate in seven to fourteen days, and you can start using the leaves in about eight weeks.

The Health Bonus: You can add flavor to your food with your very own herb garden. It's certainly an encouraging way to get you to cook and eat more healthfully. Plus, if you have kids, it's a great way to get them to eat better foods—they get to eat what they grow.

What We Like Best: How simple and cute they are, plus they make wonderful gifts.

What We Liked Least: They're not available everywhere, but at least you can order them online.

The Price: $7.50 per plant, plus shipping.

Offerings: chives, cilantro, oregano, basil, thyme, dill, mint, parsley, sage, tomatoes, and strawberries. They also offer an herb Garden-in-a-Pail and mixed-herb hanging baskets, which we think are fabulous too.

Website: www.pottingshedcreations.com.

Where to Buy: Order online or call 800-505-7496.

Ingredients: seeds, soil wafer, drainage peanuts, and leakproof bag.

Wonder Foods: Fruits

Everyone is trying to get us to eat more fruits—as if they were the Holy Grail of better health—touting their abilities to help us lose weight, fight cancer, and even prevent the common cold. Unlike some other "wonder cures," much of what we're hearing in this case is actually true.

In fact, all fruits have amazing disease-fighting substances called antioxidants, which come mostly from phytochemicals (chemicals in plants), which may prevent the harmful oxidation from both inside and outside the cell that leads to disease and signs of aging. And in terms of cancer prevention, fruits (and vegetables) are extremely powerful, says Mehmet Oz, MD, a professor of surgery and director of the Cardiovascular Institute at Columbia University Medical Center. "Ninety percent of the population has cancer at any given point; it's just that our bodies are constantly fighting it off, which is exactly why cancer-fighting foods are so important," says Oz, adding, "I would estimate that as much as 50 percent of your ability to fight off cancer on a daily basis comes from the foods you eat."

Keep in mind that the natural combinations of phytochemicals in fruits cannot simply be reproduced in pill form. Plus, there are literally thousands of phytochemicals in whole foods, some of which we haven't even discovered yet.

Yet another benefit of fruits is their ability to help you lose weight. Since they're high in both fiber and water, you get a lot of food for relatively few calories. The trick is to substitute them for higher-calorie foods you normally eat, not simply to add fruit to what you're already eating.

So while experts recommend eating a variety of fruits, here are the best of the best, based on the following criteria: taste, nutrients (biggest bang per gram), fewest calories (compared with other fruits and vegetables), antioxidant (disease-fighting) value, portability, ease of use and storage, mouth feel, and cooking and eating flexibility.

Oranges

Why: Oranges are jam-packed with nutrients, low in calories, and easily transported because of their protective peel. And there are multiple varieties from which to choose. Oh, and if you think you can simply drink your oranges, think again. Orange juice is not a terrible choice, but it doesn't have anywhere near the impact of the actual fruit in terms of hunger satisfaction, nutrient content, and disease-fighting ability.

Nutrients: Packed with vitamin C and fiber, oranges also contain thiamin, folate, vitamin A (in the form of beta-carotene), potassium, and calcium. A medium orange has about 60 calories.

Health Perks: Researchers have found more than 170 phytochemicals in oranges, including more than 20 carotenoids, antioxidants that reduce risk of disease. Regular consumption of oranges is associated with a significantly lower risk of lung and stomach cancers. According to Karen Collins, nutrition adviser to the American Institute for Cancer Research, "Oranges are among the few major sources of a group of flavonoid phytochemicals called flavanones, including the one called hesperidin. Because the white membranes separating the segments have an especially high concentration of this phytochemical, a whole orange may contain up to five times as much as a glass of orange juice." The flavonoids help to prevent DNA damage from cancer-causing substances and decrease inflammation throughout the body. In addition, compounds called limonoids—which give citrus fruit its slightly bitter taste—appear to be highly active anticancer agents as well.

Purchasing Tips: According to Aliza Green, author of *Field Guide to Produce* (Quirk Books, 2004), choose oranges that are firm, heavy for their size (they will be juiciest), and evenly shaped. The skin should be smooth rather than deeply pitted. Skin color is not a good guide to quality because some oranges are artificially colored with a harmless vegetable dye (this is permitted in Florida, but not in California or Arizona), while others may show traces of green even though they are ripe. Avoid any with serious bruises or soft spots or those that feel spongy.

Uses: Oranges are very versatile; pack one in your gym bag, pocketbook, briefcase, or suitcase. Use oranges in salads, cooking, or mixed with your morning cereal.

Apples

Why: How great are apples? They come in hundreds of varieties, they taste wonderful, you can bake them, and they are very low in calories. I know it's a cliché, but it's partially true that "an apple a day keeps the doctor away." While apples aren't bursting with vitamins, they make up for that with their disease-fighting ability and portability. Apples are high in fiber, which not only decreases cholesterol but also helps protect against cancer.

Nutrients: A good source of vitamin C and fiber, apples are known mainly for their disease-fighting capabilities. A medium apple has 80 calories.

Health Perks: Apples are loaded with flavonoids such as quercetin, which is important for keeping blood vessels healthy, reducing inflammation throughout the body, preventing DNA damage that can lead to cancer, and slowing cancer-cell growth and reproduction. According to Rui Hai Liu, MD, PhD, a professor of food science at Cornell University, the antioxidant concentration in apples is among the highest of all fruits. "In fact, it's similar to that of store-purchased blueberries (vs. wild blueberries—the highest), which are often touted as the highest in antioxidant activity." According to Liu, the antioxidant content of apples was originally underestimated because bound phenolics (phenolics that survive stomach digestion) weren't included. And make sure to eat the peel; it's very rich in phenols and flavonoids.

Additional research from Cornell recently suggested that apples could fight Alzheimer's disease as well.

Purchasing Tips: Apples can be bought year-round but are in their prime during the fall. Choose apples with smooth, clean skin, and good color for the particular variety. An apple's skin should be shiny, says Aliza Green. Avoid apples with dull skin or bruises and punctures. Store apples in the refrigerator for up to two weeks.

Uses: Throw an apple in your bag as you leave the house and have it as a daily snack. For a delicious, low-cal dessert, dust an apple with cinnamon and Splenda (or a bit of sugar) and bake it. Ever get the craving for something crunchy? Grab an apple instead of that bag of chips.

Blueberries

Why: If blueberries were packaged in a colorful box and sold at the movies, we would think they were candy. Their taste is both sweet and tart, and they are filled to the brim with nutrients and antioxidants.

Nutrients: Blueberries are a good source of vitamin C, manganese, and dietary fiber. A cup of blueberries has 82 calories.

Diet Detective's What You Need to Know

Macronutrients: These are the nutrients that we need to consume in relatively large amounts in order to stay healthy. They also provide us with the energy we need to survive. They include carbs, fat, and protein, the three nutrients that constitute the majority of our diet. Macronutrients supply calories, whereas micronutrients do not. As a result, recommendations for macronutrients take calories into consideration and must be balanced against one another. The general recommendation for adults (which varies according to weight) is 45 percent to 65 percent of total daily calories from carbs, 20 percent to 35 percent from fat, and 10 percent to 35 percent from protein.

Micronutrients: These are the nutrients in foods that are in quantities too small to see. They include vitamins, which are organic compounds our bodies need to function normally, and minerals, which are inorganic compounds our bodies need to function normally. In addition, there are some related compounds that have not been placed in either category, such as coenzyme Q10.

Health Perks: Blueberries protect against heart disease, weak eyesight, cancer, and aging. According to a study at Tufts University, the antioxidant activity of blueberries consistently outscores that of other fruits and vegetables. Anthocyanin, the antioxidant that gives the blueberry its deep blue pigment, appears to make it one of the healthiest food choices in the fight against aging. In addition, blueberries contain potassium and vitamin C, both of which play a role in lowering blood pressure. Keep in mind that while store-bought blueberries are high in antioxidants, wild blueberries are higher.

Purchasing Tips: Choose firm, large, plump, full-colored blueberries that are free of moisture and with few stems in dry, unstained containers. Blueberries should be a deep purple-blue to blue-black color with a silver frost. Refrigerate for five or six days. To prevent mold, don't wash them until just before they're used.

Uses: They're great as a finger food but also added to muffins, smoothies, yogurt, breads, waffles, and so on. Cut back on the amount of cereal in your bowl to make room for a handful of blueberries. It's also great to add frozen blueberries to hot oatmeal.

Calorie Bargain Spotlight

Calorie Bargain: Smucker's Sugar Free Red Raspberry Preserves

The Why: Now you can wake up looking forward to your breakfast toast and jam without the guilt. They keep the calories down by using a carbohydrate called polydextrose, which has only 1 to 2 calories per gram. The choice is definitely a no-brainer, so dump the sugared jam and pick up this sugar-free version.

The Health Bonus: It's very low in calories; makes it easy to stay on your diet.

What We Liked Best: I was completely impressed with this product's fresh, sweet taste.

What We Liked Least: This is not an all-natural fruit product.

The Price: $3.59 for 12¾ ounces.

Offerings: apricot, boysenberry, concord grape, orange, seedless blackberry, strawberry, others.

Website: www.smuckers.com.

Where to Buy: local grocery store, company website.

Ingredients: water**, red raspberries+, polydextrose**, maltodextrin**, fruit pectin, locust bean gum**, natural flavor**, citric acid, potassium sorbate (preservative), sucralose (nonnutritive sweetener)**, calcium chloride**, Red 40**, Blue 1**.

Nutritional Analysis per Serving: 1 Tablespoon
10 calories
0 g fat
5 g carbs
0 g protein
0 g fiber
0 g sodium

** Ingredients not in regular preserves. + adds a trivial amount of sugar, <.5 g per serving.

Wonder Foods: Veggies

I recently saw a public health advertisement that featured a photo of a mother pointing and saying, "Remember when your mom told you to eat your vegetables?" Well, Mom was right—and she didn't have the results of all the research that now supports eating plenty of vegetables. Veggies help you lose weight because they're high in both fiber and water, which means that you get a lot of food for very few calories. But even more importantly, they fight disease.

While experts recommend eating a variety of vegetables, here are the best of the best, based on the following criteria: taste, nutrients (biggest bang per gram), fewest calories (compared with other vegetables), antioxidant (disease-fighting) value, portability, ease of use and storage, mouth feel, and cooking and eating flexibility.

Broccoli

Why: Broccoli is one of the tastiest, healthiest, low-calorie, inexpensive vegetables, and it's readily available year-round and easy to prepare.

Nutrients: It's high in vitamins A, C, and K and is also a great source of iron and folate, both of which are at less-than-optimal levels in most American diets, according to David

Katz, MD, MPH. One cup of steamed broccoli contains 44 calories.

Health Perks: Broccoli's ORAC value (measure of antioxidant content) is a very high 890. It contains some very important phytochemicals—beta-carotene, indoles, and isothiocyanates—which have significant anticancer effects. Indole-3-carbinol has been shown to suppress not only breast-tumor-cell growth but also cancer-cell movement to other areas of the body. Indoles also block carcinogens before they ever create the damage that starts the process of cancer development, and they promote cancer-cell self-destruction.

According to Karen Collins, nutrition adviser to the American Institute for Cancer Research, "Cruciferous vegetables such as broccoli have been linked with a lower risk of colon, prostate, lung, and other cancers. Phytochemicals in cruciferous vegetables may also offer some protection from substances in grilled and broiled meats linked with colon cancer." In addition, scientists have found that another substance in broccoli, sulforaphane, boosts the body's detoxification enzymes, thus helping to clear potentially carcinogenic substances more quickly.

Broccoli also helps battle diabetes because of its high fiber content. Eating a diet high in fiber may improve the control of blood sugar, thereby decreasing the need for insulin and other medications. In addition, broccoli has as much calcium, ounce for ounce, as milk. Calcium is essential for building and maintaining bone mass as well as controlling muscle function.

Broccoli also contains lutein and zeaxanthin, both of which are concentrated in large quantities in the lens of the eye and can lower the risk of developing cataracts.

Purchasing Tips: Choose dark green bunches; good color indicates high nutrient value. Florets that are dark green, purplish, or bluish green contain more beta-carotene and vitamin C than paler or yellowing ones. Choose bunches with stalks that are very firm. Stalks that bend or seem rubbery are of poor quality. Avoid broccoli with open, flowering, discolored, or water-soaked bud clusters and tough, woody stems. "Refrigerate unwashed in an airtight bag for up to four days," advises Aliza Green.

Uses: Super versatile, broccoli can be used fresh in salads, cooked in soups, or sautéed with garlic and a little olive oil for a wonderful accompaniment to many foods! Add a side of broccoli and cut back on your main-dish portion to save calories.

Spinach

Why: Spinach is packed with an amazing quantity of nutrients for very few calories, and it tastes great either hot or cold.

Nutrients: This is where spinach shines. It's a great source of vitamins A, B$_2$, C, and K (which helps keep bones strong), as well as folate, potassium, magnesium, beta-carotene, and fiber. One cup of steamed spinach contains 42 calories.

Health Perks: "Spinach is helpful in controlling blood pressure, keeping blood vessels healthy, reducing cancer risk, and slowing the development of age-related eye damage (macular degeneration)," says Karen Collins. "Spinach also seems to protect against breast cancer risk linked to excess alcohol." No wonder. With an ORAC level higher than broccoli (1,260), spinach has thirteen different flavonoid compounds that function as antioxidants and anticancer agents. Vitamin C, beta-carotene, and lutein reduce the risk of heart disease by preventing buildup of oxidized cholesterol in the artery walls.

Lutein and zeaxanthin also seem to protect the eyes from ultraviolet light damage.

The lutein and folate in this leafy, green wonder food protect against birth defects and heart disease. And according to one recent study, a carotenoid found in spinach called neoxanthin helps destroy prostate cancer cells.

Purchasing Tips: Aliza Green recommends looking for "deeply colored, crisp, perky leaves that are unbroken. Avoid spinach with yellowed leaves." Spinach is tender and will spoil quickly. She also recommends checking for any unpleasant odor if you are unsure if the leaves are still good. Store bunched spinach in a plastic bag in the refrigerator for two to three days.

Uses: Spinach can be a great addition to pastas, soups, casseroles, and salads. Substituting spinach for lettuce can be an "eye-opening" experience. Try substituting spinach, onions, or mushrooms for one of the eggs or half the cheese in your morning omelet or even in lasagna—they'll add volume and flavor with fewer calories than the egg or cheese.

Garlic

Why: Garlic can ward off vampires, and it can give you horrific bad breath, but it's also one of the tastiest, healthiest, and most useful vegetables. (Yes, it's a vegetable.)

Nutrients: Garlic is an excellent source of manganese, a very good source of vitamin B_6 and vitamin C, and a good source of selenium. One garlic clove has about 4 calories.

Health Perks: Garlic protects against cancer through several mechanisms. "Substances in garlic block formation of ni-

Top Ten Tips to Increase Vegetable and Fruit Intake:

1. Add on: Start by eating your favorite fruits and vegetables—at least one serving every day—and gradually add new varieties. Try a new fruit or vegetable every month.

2. Think soups and sauces: Vegetables give these foods texture and flavor, plus sauces and soups will "mask" the taste of vegetables, allowing you to ease into eating them. Next time you open a can of soup or a jar of sauce, add some frozen spinach or mixed veggies for a quick, easy, and complete meal.

3. Sandwiches: Can you imagine your BLT sandwich without the *L* and *T*? In addition to lettuce and tomato, experiment with other veggies. Try adding some peppers, onions, cucumbers, mushrooms, or sprouts to your next sandwich or burger.

4. Breakfast: Breakfast is perfect for fruits and vegetables. How about some banana in your cereal or on your pancakes, berries in your yogurt, mushrooms and onions in your omelet, or tomato slices on your bagel with cream cheese?

5. Pizza: Skip the pepperoni and order peppers on your pizza instead. Fresh green or roasted red—you can't go wrong! If you feel daring, try a broccoli or salad slice!

6. Snacks: Pack an apple or banana (or another favorite fruit) in your backpack, briefcase, pocketbook, or gym bag. Fruit is nature's portable snack. Baby carrots and grape tomatoes are also great to snack on.

7. Salads: Salads are available almost everywhere food is served. If you don't want one as your main course, order one on the side.

8. Frozen meals: If you can't get fresh, frozen is just as good. Many frozen dinners are prepared with at least a cup of vegetables!

9. Best for last: If you're still working on acquiring a taste for fruits or vegetables, eat them first and save your favorite part of the meal for last.

10. Be adventurous: Besides nutrients, vegetables and fruits add color, texture, and flavor to a meal. Still skeptical? Think about old favorites such as sausage and peppers, strawberry shortcake, western omelets, and apple pie. These dishes wouldn't exist without fruits and vegetables as their "star ingredients."

trosamines, which have been linked to stomach cancer," explains Karen Collins. "In addition, garlic's phytochemicals stimulate enzymes that detoxify carcinogens, potentially stopping cancer before it even starts." Laboratory studies link garlic consumption to the reduced risk of a variety of cancers, particularly colon and stomach cancers in humans.

Garlic is also known to have antitumor properties, owing to the wide variety of organic sulfides and polysulfides it contains. It is also reported to enhance immune function by stimulating white blood cells called lymphocytes and macrophages to destroy cancer cells, and it is reported to disrupt the metabolism of tumor cells.

The compound that produces much of this disease-fighting activity is allicin, which is released when a garlic clove is cut or crushed. Allicin inhibits a wide variety of bacteria, molds, yeasts, and viruses. Research also suggests that regular use of garlic can be effective in reducing the risk of heart attack and stroke because it lowers total and LDL (bad) cholesterol as well as triacylglycerol concentrations without affecting HDL (good) cholesterol.

Garlic's benefits seem to start with a consumption of anywhere from a couple of cloves a week to five cloves a day. Larger amounts are neither necessary nor safe, since too much increases the risk of stomach bleeding, warns cancer nutritionist Collins.

Purchasing Tips: Choose bulbs that are large, plump, and firm with tight, unbroken sheaths, says Green. Avoid soft, spongy, or shriveled bulbs or those with a green sprout in the center. Store up to three weeks in the refrigerator.

Uses: Garlic can make nearly any food taste great. Stir-fry chopped garlic in a bit of cooking spray with cut-up chicken, spinach, and broccoli to make an antioxidant-rich, delicious dish. Chopping garlic activates the enzyme that activates its phytochemicals. Cooking it too much, however, destroys that enzyme, so chop garlic and let it rest for about ten minutes while you prepare other ingredients. "Add garlic toward the end of cooking," recommends Collins.

Calorie Bargain Spotlight

Calorie Bargain: Birds Eye Steamfresh Fresh Frozen Vegetables

The Why: What a great food-packaging idea. You simply take the frozen veggies out of the freezer, put the unopened bag in the microwave for four to five minutes, and you're done. Wow, it's that simple; you have steamed vegetables. And they're great. Vegetables are very filling and extremely low in calories. Steaming is a healthy method of preparing vegetables. There is no need for oil, which means no added fat or calories.

The Health Bonus: Get your daily dose of veggies loaded with antioxidants.

What We Liked Best: It makes eating vegetables and preparing healthy meals so much easier. Our two favorites are the Broccoli, Carrots, Sugar Snap Peas & Water Chestnuts and the Asparagus, Gold & White Corn, Baby Carrots.

What We Liked Least: Almost all of the versions are just vegetables flash frozen, nothing else. However, the four Specially Seasoned varieties are not all-natural (and they're not listed below as part of the offerings). For instance, Asian Medley has added sugar.

The Price: Approximately $2.20 per 12-ounce bag.

Offerings: Broccoli Cuts; Super Sweet Corn; Sweet Peas; Cut Green Beans; Mixed Vegetables; Sweet Mini Corn on the Cob; Broccoli,

Cauliflower & Carrots; Broccoli, Carrots, Sugar Snap Peas & Water Chestnuts; Broccoli & Cauliflower; Asparagus, Gold & White Corn, Baby Carrots; Broccoli Florets; Baby Brussels Sprouts; Whole Green Beans.

Website: www.birdseyefoods.com/birdseye/steamfresh.

Where to Buy: local grocery store, frozen-food aisle.

Ingredients: just vegetables.

Nutritional Analysis per Serving: Broccoli, Carrots, Sugar Snap Peas & Water Chestnuts—¾ Cup
35 calories
0 g fat
6 g carbs
1 g protein
2 g fiber
25 mg sodium

Super Spices

Spices are a wonderful way to add flair and improve taste when taking on new eating habits and cooking healthier. Not only that, but they have a long history of medicinal use. "There have been many recent studies validating the historic habit of using spices for health benefits," says Donna Tainter, a food technologist and coauthor of *Spices and Seasonings: A Food Technology Handbook* (Wiley-Interscience, 2001).

Although the amounts we consume in any given meal are tiny, spices can add up to big health gains. Their key health benefits lie in their pigments, which may help stabilize damage to our cells. "However, their potency rapidly declines when ground. Plus, we still don't know what would be considered an effective dose," warns Mary Ellen Camire, PhD, professor of food science at the University of Maine.

Nonetheless, one of the clearest benefits spices provide is flavor, which allows you to use less butter, oil, and other fattening extras.

Which spices are healthiest, tastiest, and simplest to add to foods? Here are a few that are particularly noteworthy.

Cinnamon

Background: Cinnamon comes from the dried brown bark of the cinnamon tree. There are more than one hundred varieties of this fragrant, somewhat sweet spice.

Purported Health Perks:

Anticlotting Action: decreases unwanted clumping of blood platelets.

Antimicrobial Activity: stops the growth of bacteria as well as fungi, including the yeast *Candida*.

Blood Sugar Control: A December 2003 study in the journal *Diabetes Care* suggested that 1 to 6 grams of cinnamon a day significantly reduce blood sugar levels in patients with type 2 diabetes. In addition, the study showed that cinnamon reduced triglycerides, LDL cholesterol, and total cholesterol. A number of studies also suggest that as little as a half teaspoon a day can improve the insulin response of individuals with type 2 diabetes. And a recent study indicates that cinnamon may stabilize blood sugar even when eating foods high in sugar.

Antioxidant Activity: Of all the spices, cinnamon is among those with the most anti-aging, disease-fighting antioxidants, according to a Norwegian study in the *Journal of Nutrition*.

Brain-Boosting Function: may improve cognitive processing.

Nutrients: manganese, dietary fiber, and iron—all typically lacking in our diets. Two teaspoons have about 12 calories.

Uses: Sprinkle on cappuccino, coffee, or toast, or, for an interesting twist, on chicken; or mix it into ground meat for a Middle Eastern flavor.

Capsicum

Background: The capsicum family includes red and green chilies that add "heat" to all kinds of foods. Paprika is a ground form of capsicum.

Purported Health Perks:
Antioxidant Activity: Capsicum has beta-carotene, which is beneficial to the mucous membranes, eyes, and skin, and wards off infection. It also has antioxidant properties that neutralize the free radicals that damage tissue and cells, and it promotes cardiovascular health by cutting blood pressure.
Anti-inflammatory Action: Topical creams with capsaicin (the heat-producing property of capsicum) may reduce joint pain. Capsaicin also helps treat eczema topically by drawing blood to the skin, and it is in many over-the-counter heat patches.

Nutrients: great source of vitamin A and beta-carotene. Two teaspoons of dried red chili peppers have 25 calories; dried cayenne pepper contains 11 calories in 2 teaspoons.

Uses: common in Mexican, South American, and Asian cuisines to flavor meats, poultry, and vegetables.

Turmeric

Background: This yellow spice has been called the poor person's saffron and is the main ingredient in curry powder. It has a warm, slightly bitter, spicy taste.

Purported Health Perks:
Antioxidant Activity: Turmeric contains high levels of the yellow pigment curcumin, a potent antioxidant and anti-

inflammatory that has been said to inhibit tumor growth. It has been shown to slow the growth of prostate cancer and prevent the activation of genes that cause cancer. "Curcumin shuts off the master switch which controls tumorigenesis (tumor growth); it specifically works against skin and breast cancer metastasis," says Bharat B. Aggarwal, PhD, a professor of cancer medicine at the University of Texas M. D. Anderson Cancer Center. In addition, curcumin has been associated with reduced risk of childhood leukemia and improved liver function.

Anti-inflammatory Activity: The antioxidants in turmeric fight the free radicals responsible for joint inflammation and damage. It may help treat rheumatoid arthritis and cystic fibrosis.

Alzheimer's Disease: Recent research at the University of California, Los Angeles (UCLA), indicates that eating food with low doses of curcumin slashed the accumulation of Alzheimer's-like plaque in the brains of mice by 50 percent.

Nutrients: Turmeric contains calcium, magnesium, dietary fiber, vitamin B_6, iron, potassium, and manganese. Two teaspoons have 16 calories.

Uses: Enhances the flavor of chicken, rice, meat, and lentils.

Ginger

Background: Popular Asian spice, one of the first traded in Western Europe.

Purported Health Perks:
Antioxidant Activity: Ginger is high in disease-fighting antioxidants.
Anti-inflammatory Activity: Inflammation is believed to be a contributing factor in cardiovascular disease, cancer,

Alzheimer's, and arthritis. Like aspirin, gingerols—compounds found in ginger—are said to thin the blood and help reduce pain.

Gastrointestinal Relief: Certain properties in ginger seem to ease motion sickness. It has been shown to inhibit vomiting, and its nausea-fighting properties can be helpful for people suffering the side effects of chemotherapy.

Nutrients: Potassium. One ounce of ginger root has 20 calories.

Uses: Minced fresh ginger is great with all kinds of meat, poultry, vegetables, sushi, and, of course, many desserts. It's also used in tea.

Whole Grains

Whole grains are the new "in" foods—everyone's talking about them. They fit in with many low-carb diets, and even the government is on board. But do you know the ins and outs of whole grains? Check your whole-grain IQ.

Q. Why are whole-grain foods (for example, whole wheat) healthier than "white" refined foods?
A. According to Nicola M. McKeown, PhD, a nutrition professor at Tufts University, whole-grain foods are rich in dietary fiber, vitamins, minerals, and phytochemicals. "The synergistic effect of these nutrients is important to overall health. When grains are refined, fiber and other nutrients, such as vitamin E, vitamin B_6, and magnesium, are removed, and these are not replaced." And research has consistently found that whole grains reduce the risk of several chronic diseases, including cardiovascular disease, diabetes, and certain types of cancer, whereas refined grains do not protect against these diseases. How much protection do you get from eating whole grains? According to Len Marquart, PhD, RD, a nutrition professor at the University of Minnesota, "Epidemiological studies suggest that whole grains reduce risk for coronary heart disease and diabetes by 20 percent to 30 percent versus refined grains."

Calorie Bargain Spotlight

Calorie Bargain: YogaToday.com

The Why: We've all heard about the amazing benefits of regular yoga, but it can be such a hassle (not to mention expensive!) to drag yourself to a studio several times a week. With YogaToday.com you can play free yoga videos right on the site—you don't even have to leave your house. They also tell you the level of each class, and there are typically two students following along: one a beginner and the other experienced.

The Health Bonus: Yoga is great exercise, with health claims ranging from better strength, flexibility, posture, coordination, and balance to stress reduction, stronger bones, cardiovascular conditioning, and the prevention of cancer, heart disease, diabetes, asthma, carpal tunnel syndrome, arthritis, and more. Devotees are pretty emphatic about the benefits on three levels: physiological, psychological, and biochemical.

What We Liked Best: YogaToday.com offers a new class each day. And all the classes are filmed with wonderful backdrops, such as Wyoming's Jackson Hole. Nice. Just watching the video can be a peaceful experience. Also, the video and music are both crystal clear, and you can choose to view them in full-screen mode. And all at no cost. Wow!

What We Liked Least: The site doesn't archive programs (other than the last four days). So, if you're looking for a specific class—like beginning yoga moves—you will not be able to find it. The good news is that there will eventually be a searchable archive, but you'll have to pay a small fee to download from it. And there's advertising in the beginning. I guess they have to pay the bills somehow.

The Price: Free.

Website: www.yogatoday.com.

Where to Buy: www.yogatoday.com (you can view several recent sessions).

Offerings: Daily one-hour videos with wonderful, diverse instructors. You can play in Windows Media, QuickTime/iPod, or Audio Only.

Ingredients: The experienced instructors (www.yogatoday.com/instructors) practice various styles, including: Ashtanga, Vinyasa, Hatha, Anusara, Kripalu, and Kundalini.

Q. Do whole grains help you lose weight?

A. Probably, but evidence is still inconclusive. Basically, foods that contain significant whole grains are rich in fiber. Choosing naturally fiber-rich foods is important for weight loss because they are typically low calorie and low density due to their water content (for instance, fruits and vegetables), which means you get more food for fewer calories. Fiber is also thought to enhance satiety (feelings of fullness). A high amount of soluble fiber is typically found in the whole grains oats and barley. According to Joan Conway, PhD, RD, a scientist at the U.S. Department of Agriculture, "If you experience great satisfaction from food, you might eat less. Eating foods high in soluble fiber that are viscous (gummy) could, therefore, give one a feeling of fullness. Data are not yet in on this, but we are doing a study in this particular area."

McKeown points out, "Observational studies have found that people who eat more whole grains tend to weigh less and also gain less weight over time, but it's important to recognize that these individuals have healthier diets overall, are more physically active, and are less likely to smoke."

Q. Does whole wheat taste better today than it used to?

A. "Yes," says Marquart, "because improved processing methods soften the texture, lighten the color, and reduce grain particle size in the whole-grain product." Also, more white whole wheat is entering the market. According to Julie Miller Jones,

Calorie Bargain Spotlight

Calorie Bargain: Lean Cuisine's Southwest-Style Chicken Panini

The Why: Mesquite-seasoned white-meat chicken strips are combined with green peppers, tomatoes, onions, cheese, and Southwest-style sauce on sourdough bread. I've been taste-testing these for about three weeks now, and they are great! And get this: They're filling and only 280 calories. I still haven't figured out how to get the bread crispy each time even though I've been using the special tray that helps to crisp it—but I'm working on it.

The Health Bonus: Each panini has about 30 percent of your daily calcium needs and 15 percent of your iron as well as 3 grams of fiber and 20 grams of protein. And did we mention they're low in calories?

What We Liked Best: Great-tasting, low-calorie hot sandwiches prepared in a matter of minutes.

What We Liked Least: The bread isn't whole grain, and the crisping tray performs haphazardly. The paninis are also high in sodium, as are most frozen dinners.

The Price: $3.09.

Offerings: Chicken, Spinach & Mushroom; Steak, Cheddar & Mushroom; Southwest-Style Chicken; and Chicken Club. Two more— Chicken Tuscan, which has tender white-meat chicken, peppers, olives, tomatoes, and margherita-style sauce on Italian herb bread (340 calories, 8g fat, 0g trans fat), and Philly-Style Steak & Cheese, with steak, red and green peppers, onions, and cheese sauce on sourdough bread (350 calories, 9g fat, 0g trans fat)—will be available some time in July.

Website: www.leancuisine.com.

Where to Buy: Any supermarket.

Nutritional Information: Serving size one package (6 ounces), calories 280, calories from fat 70, total fat 7g, saturated fat 3g, trans fat 0g, polyunsaturated fat 1.5g, monounsaturated fat 1.5g, cholesterol 30mg, sodium 730mg, potassium 140mg, total carbohydrates 32g, dietary fiber 3g, sugars 3g, protein 20g.

Ingredients: Too many to print—you can go to the following Web page to view: www.leancuisine.com/Products/NutritionInformation.aspx? ProductID=10622.

PhD, CNS, LN, professor of nutrition and food science at the College of St. Catherine in Minnesota, "It is somewhat less bitter than the more commonly used red wheat, so some say it tastes better. In addition, breads in general have been improved, and there are many artisan breads available, some of which have a great whole-grain taste that is nutty, sweet, and interesting."

Q. Why was white bread made in the first place?
A. According to Marquart, "White bread was originally consumed by the upper crust of society, and became popular in the mid-1800s when roller milling allowed for greater production of white refined flour for the masses." It's still easier to make than whole-grain bread, and refined flour is less perishable. The bran in whole-grain flour reduces loaf volume and makes it bitter. "Also, refined flour makes products lighter, flakier, and generally has a texture that many prefer," says Dr. Jones.

Q. As long as it says "wheat" on the bread, you're getting whole wheat, right?
A. Wrong. Almost all bread is made from wheat, so don't be fooled. In fact, it could be white bread with caramel coloring. You want to see "whole wheat" on the label.

Q. Do the words whole grain on the package mean it's 100 percent whole grain?

A. Not necessarily—although it's a start. Even if the package is labeled "whole-grain" bread, you aren't necessarily getting 100 percent whole grains. According to McKeown, you need to be aware of the packaging. "For example, if it says 'made with whole wheat,' check the ingredients list because the food may contain some whole grain but not very much. If the ingredient list starts with 'enriched wheat,' or if 'wheat' is the first ingredient, it is not a whole grain."

Whole grains contain the entire grain kernel—meaning they have the bran, the germ, and the endosperm. (White bread has only the endosperm.) "In order for a food to be whole grain," adds McKeown, "one of the following ingredients should be listed first: whole rye, whole oats, whole wheat, whole barley, whole cornmeal, or graham flour."

Other Tips

Check the dietary fiber content on the Nutrition Facts label. Products made with wheat, rye, or oats should have 2 to 3 grams of fiber per serving. But the fiber level in whole rice and whole corn is relatively low and is, therefore, a poor indicator of whole-grain content, says Marquart.

Another clue is to look for products that carry the FDA-regulated health claim that reads: "Diets rich in whole grains and other plant foods and low in fat, saturated fat, and cholesterol may reduce the risk of heart disease and some cancers." If the product carries the whole-grain health claim, the FDA requires that 51 percent of the weight of the ingredients must be whole grain. "This doesn't mean that half the grain is whole grain; usually it means that virtually all the grain is whole grain," explains Cynthia Harriman, manager of partner services at the Whole Grains Council. "Take bread, for instance. Bread is about 40 percent moisture by weight, so if it's 51 percent whole grain, that only leaves 9 percent for other ingredients, such as sugar, oil, yeast, white flour, flax seed, raisins, whatever."

Be aware that even though dark or brown bread is often a whole-grain food, it may just have molasses or caramel food coloring added. Alternatively, whole-grain foods may be light in color, such as those made from oats or white wheat, says McKeown.

Look for a whole-grain seal from the Whole Grains Council. If it says "Excellent Source," it has one serving of whole grains per portion; "Good Source" indicates a half serving. The USDA guidelines suggest three servings of whole grains per day. Examples of one serving:

- About 5 whole wheat crackers.
- 1 slice of whole wheat bread.
- 1 cup of whole-grain cereal.
- 1 cup of ready-to-eat cereal.
- ½ cup of cooked rice, pasta, or hot cereal.
- 3 cups of popcorn.

Q. If Oreos or other foods (for example, Cocoa Puffs) were made with whole wheat, would they be healthier?
A. This is tough one. "Yes, refined flour is nutritionally inferior to whole wheat flour," says Tufts University's McKeown. "Certainly they'd be higher in fiber, which would be good, but they'd probably also be high in sugar. As a source of whole grains, I think brown rice or whole wheat spaghetti would be better alternatives."

Keep in mind that the words *whole grain* are not a green light for endless consumption. Even a whole wheat doughnut is a doughnut—no amount of whole grains makes up for the

315 calories it packs. Use whole grains as replacements for refined foods you're already eating, *not* additions.

Q. Are seven-grain and multigrain breads better for you than 100 percent whole wheat?
A. Not necessarily. Sure, multigrain breads such as wheat, oat, barley, or seven-, twelve-, or fifteen-grain sound nutritionally impressive, but take a closer look at the label. Most multigrain breads contain enriched wheat flour along with other grain flours—basically, a mixture of whole wheat and enriched flour with caramel coloring.

Q. Are whole-grain foods much lower in calories than refined or processed foods?
A. No, not really. In fact, whole-grain foods are about the same or perhaps a tiny bit higher in calories than refined, or "white," foods. However, the point here is not to save calories but to get all the health benefits whole grains offer.

Sources of Protein

Protein is an important macronutrient for weight control, but eating poultry, meats, and dairy requires a bit of thought before you get to the supermarket. Here are a few guidelines to follow.

Poultry

Choose primarily chicken and turkey, and make sure to select lean cuts. The leanest poultry choice is white meat from the breast without the skin. Although skinless dark meat is leaner than some cuts of beef or pork, it has nearly twice as much fat as white meat. Many grocery stores offer ground chicken and ground turkey, which may have as much (or more) fat as ground beef if they include dark meat and skin. So ask for ground breast meat. Avoid duck, which is very fatty.

Fish

Fish is a great source of both protein and heart-healthy omega-3 fatty acids. However, the FDA advises against eating shark, swordfish, king mackerel, or tilefish because they contain high levels of mercury. Five of the most commonly eaten

Diet Detective's What You Need to Know

Why Protein Works for Weight Control: Many studies are now reporting the positive effects of protein on weight loss. In a recent review published in the *Journal of the American College of Nutrition*, Frank Hu, MD, PhD, MPH, a professor of nutrition and epidemiology at the Harvard School of Public Health, confirmed protein's positive effects on losing weight. "Although most of the high-protein studies have only looked at short-term weight loss, the evidence is very convincing that protein increases satiety and decreases overall caloric intake," says Hu.

First of all, foods that are high in protein slow the movement of food through the digestive tract, and slower stomach emptying means that you feel full longer and get hungrier later (increasing satiety) compared with lower-protein diets. "The evidence also suggests high-protein meals lead to a reduced subsequent calorie intake," says Hu.

Protein also helps keep blood sugar stable, avoiding the quick rises that can occur when you eat carbohydrates that are rapidly digested (for example, white bread).

Also, eating foods that are low fat, low carb, and high in protein will help you avoid other less healthy, high-calorie foods that do not keep you full.

Lastly, the body uses more calories to digest protein than it does to burn fat or carbohydrates. "There is convincing evidence that a higher protein intake increases thermogenesis [generation of heat within the body, which increases caloric burn]," says Hu. He believes that you could burn an additional 30 calories per day simply by eating a diet composed of about 30 percent protein.

fish and seafood products that are low in mercury are shrimp, canned light tuna, salmon, pollock, and catfish. Another commonly eaten fish, albacore ("white") tuna, has more mercury than canned light tuna.

You can take a look at fish mercury levels on the FDA website at www.cfsan.fda.gov/~frf/sea-mehg.html.

Diet Detective's What You Need to Know

Making Your Chicken Healthier: Remove the skin, either before or after cooking, to reduce the fat content by almost half. Leaving the skin on during cooking will keep the meat juicier. But keep in mind that if you remove the skin after cooking, the fat that was under the skin will have melted, and some of it will have been absorbed into the meat—which is also why it is juicier.

- Trim all excess fat from the chicken before cooking.
- Rather than using fat such as butter and oil to enhance the chicken's flavor, try other flavoring ingredients such as flavored vinegars, wines, herbs, spices, or citrus fruit.
- Cook chicken without added fats by baking, roasting, broiling, grilling, or poaching it. Stir-fry in olive or canola oil, or better yet, use a fat-free nonstick cooking spray.
- Chicken breast, skinless (3 ounces): 140 calories, 3 g fat, 26 g protein.
- Chicken breast, with skin (3 ounces): 167 calories, 7 g fat, 25 g protein.
- Chicken drumstick, skinless (3 ounces): 146 calories, 5 g fat, 24 g protein.
- Chicken drumstick, with skin (3 ounces): 184 calories, 9.5 g fat, 23 g protein.

Meats (Including Beef, Veal, Pork, and Lamb)

You can still have meat as long as it's lean, with visible fat removed, and you control portion size and frequency. Just make sure you pick right. Here are some tips from the U.S. Department of Agriculture:

- **Beef:** The leanest beef cuts include round steaks and roasts (eye round, top round, bottom round, round

Calorie Bargain Recipe Spotlight

Calorie Bargain: Charles' Chicken

The Why: There are some excellent recipes out there for chefs or anyone who wants to cook healthy Italian food that still tastes amazing.

The Health Bonus: I was able to create a recipe for chicken parmigiana that's low in fat and tastes great.

Ingredients: 4 (3-ounce) boneless chicken breasts pounded paper thin, ⅓ cup seasoned bread crumbs, Pam or other cooking oil spray, salt, pepper, onion flakes, garlic powder, ½ cup Healthy Choice Garlic & Herb Pasta Sauce, 2 tablespoons Kraft Grated Parmesan Cheese.

Preparation: Pound the chicken breasts as thin as you can get them—basically paper thin (if you've ever heard of the product Steak-umm, think that thin). You'll be surprised how large a 3- to 4-ounce pounded chicken breast can get. How thin they are is critical, because it reduces the cooking time and the amount of cooking spray you need, plus it makes the portion size look bigger. You can even ask your supermarket or butcher to pound them for you. They may charge a bit extra, but it's worth it.

Coat the pounded breasts lightly with the bread crumbs. Lightly spray a 12-inch frying pan with the cooking spray and turn the heat to high. You'll probably have to do this in batches, depending on the size of your pan. Give a quick spray to the tops of the chicken breasts and cook, sprayed side up, for three to five minutes. Look for the "up" side to start turning white. Turn off the burner, flip the chicken over, cover the pan, and let the chicken steam cook for another five or six minutes. This makes the meat tender, ensures moistness, and enhances the flavor. Season with salt, pepper, onion flakes, and garlic powder to taste. Drizzle with the sauce and top with the Parmesan cheese. Makes two servings.

Nutritional Analysis per Serving: 6 Ounces
277 calories
3.5 g fat
15.5 g carbs

tip), top loin, top sirloin, and chuck shoulder and arm roasts.

- **Ground Beef:** Look for at least 90 percent lean. You may even be able to find ground beef that is 93 percent or 95 percent lean.
- **Pork:** The leanest pork choices include pork loin, tenderloin, center loin, and ham.
- **Sandwich Meats:** Choose lean roast beef, ham, or low-fat luncheon meats for sandwiches instead of luncheon meats with more fat, such as regular bologna or salami.

Fat: Avoid meat that is heavily marbled—that is, streaked with fat. Look for meat with the least amount of visible fat.

For cooking:

- Trim visible fat beforehand.
- Broil, grill, roast, poach, or boil meat instead of frying.
- Drain any fat that appears during cooking.

NUTRITIONAL COMPARISON OF DIFFERENT TYPES OF MEAT

	SERVING	CALORIES	GRAMS OF FAT
■ **Beef**			
Eye Round	3 ounces	188	12.8 grams
Top Round	3 ounces	153	8 grams
Bottom Round	3 ounces	191	13 grams
Round Tip	3 ounces	171	11 grams
■ **Ground Beef**			
90 percent lean	3 ounces	180	10 grams
95 percent lean	3 ounces	164	6 grams
■ **Pork**			
Pork Loin	3 ounces	122	6 grams
Tenderloin	3 ounces	116	4.6 grams
Center Loin	3 ounces	169	7.7 grams
■ **Ham**	3 ounces	133	4.7 grams
■ **Sandwich Meats**			
Lean Roast Beef	3 slices	93	4.5 grams
Lean Ham	3 slices	69	1.8 grams
Low-fat Turkey Breast	3 slices	66	1 gram
Bologna	3 slices	261	24 grams
Salami	3 slices	105	9 grams

- Skip or limit the breading; it adds fat and calories, especially since it causes meat to soak up more fat during frying.

Dairy

Dairy is a great source of protein and calcium, and it's particularly important to replace potential lost calcium from eating higher amounts of protein. However, it is full of fat, so always choose low-fat or nonfat milk, yogurt, and cheese.

Calorie Bargain Spotlight

Calorie Bargain: Cabot Cheese 75% Reduced Fat Cheddar

The Why: Many people find it difficult to switch to lower-calorie and lower-fat versions of their favorite cheeses. Lucky for them, the people in Cabot, Vermont, renowned for the exquisitely tasty Cabot Cheddar, have made a light version that tastes as good as the original.

The Health Bonus: With one-quarter the fat, one-third the cholesterol, and half the calories of regular cheddar, this one lights the way for those who want a great tasting, lower-calorie alternative.

What We Liked Best: It tastes 100 percent like cheddar and melts like a dream.

What We Liked Least: Unfortunately, even as a Calorie Bargain, this is still cheese—it has enough calories per serving that it can't be eaten freely. Keep an eye on your serving size, and on how many servings you grab for, or you could blow your budget before lunch.

The Price: 8 ounces for $3.50.

Offerings: 75% Reduced Fat Cheddar.

Website: www.cabotcheese.com.

Where to Buy: Wal-Mart, Whole Foods Market, Giant Eagle, Trader Joe's, Publix.

Ingredients: pasteurized low-fat milk, cheese cultures, cornstarch*, salt, monoglyceride*, enzymes, annatto (if colored), vitamin A palmitate.

Nutritional Analysis per Serving: 1 Ounce
60 calories
2.5 g fat
Fewer than 1 g carbs
9 g protein
0 g fiber
200 mg sodium

*Ingredients not found in regular cheddar cheese.

Diet Detective's What You Need to Know

Q: Which one has the most fiber: steak, skinless chicken breast, chicken breast with skin, or eggs?

A: That's a trick question because animal products contain practically no fiber. Only plant-based foods have fiber. Basically, the term *fiber* refers to carbohydrates that cannot be digested. Fiber is present in all plants, including fruits, vegetables, grains, and legumes.

Egg Whites

Egg whites are virtually fat free, but some people don't like the idea of eating eggs without the yolks. So start off by combining one-third egg whites with two-thirds whole eggs, and then gradually reduce the amount of whole eggs. You can do the same with other foods, such as whole milk and skim milk or low-calorie, whole-grain cereal and regular cereal. Eventually you'll get used to the healthier option.

Other Protein Sources

Nuts, seeds, beans, soybeans, and legumes. Make sure to limit portion sizes, especially of nuts and seeds. They're super healthy but very high in fat (even though it's good fat). Prepare beans and legumes without added fats.

How to Get the Right Protein Mix
Sample Menu and Nutritional Information

Breakfast
Yogurt Crunch
Combine:
1½ cups plain nonfat yogurt
¼ cup low-fat granola
1 cup berries
1 tablespoon walnuts

Midday Snack
15 carrot sticks
¼ cup hummus

Lunch
Spicy Chicken Sandwich
5 ounces grilled chicken breast
1 medium whole wheat or whole-grain roll
2 tablespoons salsa
3 thick tomato slices
Lettuce

After-work Snack
1 small apple
1 tablespoon peanut butter

Dinner
Spinach Pasta Bake
1½ cups cooked whole wheat pasta (measured *after* cooking)
½ cup tomato sauce
⅓ cup low-fat or nonfat cottage cheese
1 cup cooked spinach
1 ounce shredded part-skim mozzarella

Spread the pasta in a baking dish, top with the tomato sauce, cottage cheese, and spinach. Sprinkle the cheese on top and bake in a 350-degree oven for thirty minutes.

Nutrition Information for the Day
Calories: 1,513
Fat: 36 g (22 percent)
Saturated fat: 9 g (6 percent)
Carbs: 199 g (46 percent)
Fiber: 34 g
Protein: 115 g (32 percent)

Eggs

According to the Egg Nutrition Center, about 280 million hens produce some 60 billion eggs each year in the United States. Since a good majority of those eggs get consumed, I thought it would be helpful to unravel some of the mystery surrounding the egg.

NUTRITIONAL COMPARISON OF EGGS AND EGG DISHES

FOOD	SERVING SIZE	CALORIES	FAT	PROTEIN
1 Large Boiled Egg	1 Egg	78	5.3 grams	6.3 grams
Egg White from 1 Large Egg	1 Egg White	17	.06 grams	3.6 grams
Denny's Ultimate Omelette	12 ounces	600	49 grams	34 grams
Scrambled Egg	2 eggs	199	15 grams	14 grams
Egg Beater	¼ cup	30	0 grams	6 grams

I've Heard Eggs Can Raise My Cholesterol. Is That True?
Not really. It turns out that normal intake of dietary cholesterol from foods doesn't elevate blood cholesterol to a point of concern—saturated fat does—a fact of which many Americans are simply not aware. "The type of fat we eat, not cholesterol, is what is correlated with increased blood cholesterol levels," explains Anne VanBeber, PhD, RD, LD, associate professor and chair of the department of nutritional sciences at Texas Christian University. "Most people don't know there is a difference between dietary cholesterol and blood cholesterol. These two things are not the same at all. Our bodies produce cholesterol naturally."

If you are in good health and have total blood cholesterol below 200 mg/dl (milligrams per deciliter), it is probably OK to have one whole egg a day. The American Heart Association recommends an intake of 300 milligrams or less of dietary cholesterol a day, and one large egg contains 215.

On the other hand, if you have total cholesterol over 240 mg/dl, a family history of heart disease, diabetes, or high blood pressure, or you smoke, aim for no more than 200 milligrams of cholesterol per day. You can still eat an egg a day, but rather than large eggs, choose one small or medium egg with 157 and 187 milligrams of cholesterol, respectively.

The bottom line is that dietary cholesterol has some effect on blood cholesterol, but it's not an issue unless you eat a lot of eggs, says Bonnie Liebman, director of nutrition at the Center for Science in the Public Interest. At what level should you be concerned? The fact is, if you take a balanced approach and eat eggs occasionally, it's OK. "However, if you're eating two or more eggs a day, there could potentially be an issue with cholesterol and increased risk factors for disease," adds Liebman.

Remember, eggs aren't the only food containing dietary cholesterol. "On average, an ounce of meat contains about twenty milligrams of cholesterol," advises Andrea Dunn, RD, LD, CDE, of the Westlake Family Health Center at the Cleveland Clinic. "Cholesterol comes only from animal sources, so pay attention to how much meat or cheese you're having on egg days. Why not go meatless and cheeseless for a meal?"

How Do Eggs Compare with Other Common Breakfast Foods?
One egg, 1 ounce of sausage, and 1 ounce of ham each has about 5 to 6 grams of protein. Ham comes in the leanest, with 2 grams of fat, compared with the egg at 5 grams and the sausage at 8 grams. Ham and sausage don't even come close to eggs when it comes to cholesterol: Ham has 17 milligrams of

cholesterol, sausage has 23, and eggs, 211. Surprisingly, eggs are not sodium free, but while a large egg contains 70 milligrams, 1 ounce of sausage has 180 milligrams and ham has 370 milligrams, says Dunn.

Are There Other Reasons Eggs Are Considered Unhealthy?

Yes. They can keep bad company. If you're in the habit of eating one or two eggs a day, you may also be cooking them with butter, sausage, bacon, and cheese, all of which raise blood cholesterol—which affects heart health.

Are There Any Health Benefits to Eating Eggs?

Yes. One egg contains 6 grams of protein (a little more than half in the white). Plus, there are vitamins, minerals, and other nutrients also found in eggs. "The beta-carotene content is high," says VanBeber. "Specifically, lutein and zeaxanthin are found in the yolk of an egg. These two carotenoids have been shown to decrease macular degeneration, which causes irreversible blindness."

Additionally, the *Journal of the American College of Nutrition* has cited the high choline (said to have a role in early brain development) content of the egg. Eggs also contain 15 percent of the daily requirement for riboflavin (an important B vitamin necessary for metabolism) and 17 percent for selenium (an important antioxidant mineral).

Are There Other Reasons to Eat Eggs?

Eggs cook quickly and are ready within minutes. They're very easy to eat (which is especially important for the young and elderly) and store. Plus, eggs are portable when hard-boiled and make a great low-calorie snack. And they're inexpensive. "Today at the supermarket, one dozen large eggs can cost as little as one dollar," says Dunn. "One egg contains the protein equivalent of one ounce of meat—that's a great value for the money."

Eggs are also quite versatile, used in beverages, appetizers, main dishes, sauces, and desserts. They're easy to incorporate into a variety of recipes to add protein and a host of other nutrients. "Eggs are a great vehicle for sneaking in the vegetables most of us are lacking in our diets," says Bonnie Taub-Dix, MA, RD, a New York–based nutritionist and spokesperson for the American Dietetic Association. Try adding chopped fresh or frozen vegetables to omelets, or make a delicious baked veggie frittata.

Since most people need more than one egg to satisfy their hunger, consider whipping up omelets using one whole egg and two or more egg whites. Egg whites add volume and protein to your omelet with few calories and no extra fat or cholesterol. You can find other alternatives like egg substitutes, which scramble and cook up just like eggs. But unlike whole eggs, they are virtually fat- and cholesterol-free.

Do the White and Yolk Have Different Nutritional Values?

Definitely. While both have protein, the albumin (that's the egg white) has a little more than half the total protein in an egg (about 3.5 grams) and none of the fat. This part of the egg can indicate the egg's freshness: As the protein composition of the albumin changes over time, the albumin changes texture. For instance, fresher eggs will remain more upright when cracked, while older eggs spread out more. If whipped, the albumin can increase in volume six to eight times—it becomes airy and light, almost like a weightless whipped cream texture. You'll also find about 55 milligrams of potassium and sodium in the white. In contrast, the yolk has almost 3 grams of protein and about 5 grams of fat, but it also has 0.5 milligrams of iron, 66 milligrams of phosphorus, and 245 IU (international units) of vitamin A.

What Are Good Health-conscious Egg Meals?

There are lots of fast, easy, healthy meals you can make with eggs. Scramble one up with low-cal cooking spray, put it on a piece of toasted whole wheat bread, and add a slice of low-fat or no-fat cheese for a satisfying breakfast. Also, egg-white omelets with lots of veggies make some of the healthiest breakfasts. Chop up anything you like: peppers, mushrooms, onions, broccoli, tomatoes, and toss the ingredients in the center of the omelet. Then fold the eggs and cook briefly on both sides. Get creative and try new combinations to keep things interesting. For instance, try mixing cucumbers and avocado into your eggs for a change. Remember, as you add low-cal veggies, you increase the density and amount of food without noticeably adding calories, so you can increase the amount of food you eat without worrying about the calorie count.

Can You Explain Egg Grading?

According to VanBeber, egg grading is voluntary, but it is done for the benefit of the consumer. "The grade refers to the quality of the egg and what it will look like when cracked open. It has nothing to do with spoilage. Grade AA is best, with a thicker white and a yolk in the center. The yolk will have some height to it when cracked. Grade A, usually less expensive, is second best, with a thinner white and slightly off-center yolk. Grade B eggs are often packaged as liquid eggs for industrial and commercial use, so you won't see them in stores, but they're fine for use in recipes, scrambled eggs, and omelets."

Why Is It That I Can't Always Find the Expiration Dates on the Cartons?

All USDA-inspected egg cartons must carry the date the eggs were packed. That's not the same thing as an expiration date, although many brands voluntarily opt to label their cartons with a date beyond which the eggs should not be sold. That date can be no more than thirty days from the packing date for USDA-inspected eggs. The format of the packing is a little unusual: Each day of the year gets a number (the first day of January is number 1, and the last day of December is 365). So you might not recognize these numbers—the Julian system of dating—as dates unless you know what to look for. Plants not governed by the USDA are governed by their state's laws.

How Should You Store Eggs?

"Eggs have porous shells," says VanBeber, "so it's best to keep them in the carton they come in or in a covered container in your refrigerator. Don't use the egg slots in the refrigerator, or they'll become stale quicker." And according to McNamara, "Fresh shell eggs can last four to five weeks after the expiration date without real loss of quality as long as they're in their cartons in the refrigerator."

Can Eggs Make Me Sick?

It's possible, but highly unlikely. Only one egg in twenty thousand contains salmonella bacteria, according to most experts.

"The literature shows that salmonella food-borne illness from eggs has declined. Most salmonella in eggs is traced to the hen who lays the egg. This has prompted the egg industry to improve sanitation of egg farms," says VanBeber. Home-made foods made from raw eggs (mayonnaise, eggnog, Caesar dressing, and hollandaise sauce) carry a greater risk for salmonellosis (the disease caused by salmonella bacteria). "Be sure to 'coddle' eggs first if you are using them in a recipe—that is, submerge them in boiling water for one minute—to kill some of the bacteria," advises VanBeber. Nonetheless, people with decreased immunity, including the very young or very old, as well as cancer and chemotherapy patients, should avoid any raw eggs.

Cook eggs until the yolk and whites are both firm (160 de-

Calorie Bargain Recipe

Egg-white French Toast
2 pieces of 100 percent whole-grain bread (70 to 80 calories—preferably with no sugar added)
3 eggs
2 tablespoons skim milk

Crack egg whites into a bowl, add 2 tablespoons of skim milk. Spray a frying pan with cooking spray (Pam for example, heat up pan. Dunk bread into bowl, then cook to desired style in pan.

Approximately 200 calories in two slices; margarine spray (10 sprays adds about 10 calories).

---

grees) to eliminate the risk of any bacteria surviving. "Or buy already pasteurized eggs if you like your eggs runny," says Dunn. "You'll pay more but have peace of mind. Egg substitutes are a pasteurized product; you can use them freely without worry of salmonella. You can also buy frozen whole eggs that are pasteurized."

What If You Get a Blood Spot in an Egg?
Blood spots, occasionally called "meat spots," sometimes (albeit rarely) are found in the egg's yolk. Fewer than 1 percent of all eggs have blood spots, which, contrary to popular belief, do not indicate a fertilized egg. They are actually caused by a rupture of the blood vessels on the surface of the yolk while the egg is being formed. If you do happen across one, it is actually a sign of freshness.

What's the Difference between Brown Eggs and White Eggs?
Virtually nothing. White-shelled eggs are produced by hens with white earlobes. Brown-shelled eggs are produced by hens

with red earlobes. There is no difference in taste or nutrition between white and brown eggs, says Rebecca Odabashian, RD, LD, a nutritionist at Levindale Hebrew Geriatric Hospital in Baltimore.

Confused about All the Labels and Claims You're Seeing on Egg Cartons? Here's What They Mean.

CLAIM	MEANING	VERIFIABLE?
Organic	Hens are fed organic feed and are not given antibiotics, pesticides, or animal byproducts.	Yes
Certified humane	Animals are raised without antibiotics or hormones, have a safe living environment, and enough food and water.	Yes
Biodynamic	Hens were raised in the most natural way.	Yes
Natural	Contains no artificial coloring, flavoring, or preservative—not meaningful for eggs, since they typically don't ever have anything added within the shell.	No
Free range	Meaning varies—contact manufacturer for more information.	No
No hormones	No hormones were used for production—but law requires that no egg producers use hormones, so all eggs are hormone free.	Yes

SOURCE: www.eco-labels.org.

Frozen Meals

For people who don't like to cook or just don't have the time, keeping a supply of healthy frozen foods on hand means not having to think about calorie count or portion size, which is exactly why prepackaged food plans like Jenny Craig and NutriSystem are so successful. The idea is to use entrees from Healthy Choice, Smart Ones, Lean Cuisine, and other frozen foods that are prepackaged and healthy.

When shopping for frozen foods, watch out for the sodium levels and look for the word *healthy* on the package. By federal law, any foods that say "healthy" (including the brand Healthy Choice) must meet certain government standards: They must contain fewer than 3 grams of fat per 100 grams and no more than 30 percent of calories from fat. In addition, sodium content cannot exceed 600 milligrams. Weight Watchers Smart Ones also conform to Weight Watchers's own guidelines and cannot contain more than 300 calories or 9 grams of fat per serving.

Research Says It Works

In a study appearing in the journal *Obesity*, Sandra M. Hannum, MS, RD, a research dietitian at the University of Illinois at Urbana-Champaign, found that using prepackaged meals was an uncomplicated method to help study participants lose weight. "The problem is that those who choose to eat out in restaurants on a regular basis are vulnerable to potential weight gain from the excessively large portions. Being served a large portion usually results in overeating because people tend to consume the amount of food that is presented to them," says Hannum.

Because many people eat out for convenience reasons, packaged entrees provide a reasonable alternative to restaurant eating. Preparation requires only a few minutes in a microwave oven, and the portions are controlled. This means you can scarf down the entire meal without any guilt. Not only that, but frozen meals can teach people how to recognize appropriate serving sizes. "When you're familiar with the size of a three-hundred-calorie entree, certainly the next time you go out to dinner, or even when you're eating at home, you'll have a better idea of how much you should be eating," says Susan Bowerman, MS, RD, coordinator for the UCLA Center for Human Nutrition in Los Angeles.

How It Works

The great thing about using frozen dinners as a diet tool is that there are no special diet foods, medications, or extreme measures required for success. Grabbing foods from the supermarket freezer aisle is something anyone can do right now to lose weight.

Just take an extra half hour or so to check out the frozen food section the next time you go to the supermarket. Your research will pay off in the end, and that half hour will translate to saved time, calories, and money. It's more than worth the effort.

My recommendation is to make an initial onetime investment of about $55 to taste-test twenty meals. Pick a variety of healthy entrees and dinners (e.g. Healthy Choice, Lean Cuisine, Smart Ones) that appeal to your tastes and provide a satisfying portion. If a frozen meal tastes great but you need three of them to fill you up and feel satisfied, it's not the one for you.

There is enough variety to please almost anyone. Healthy Choice now offers seventy-six selections, including dinners and entrees; Smart Ones has about fifty-five entrees; and Lean Cuisine offers eighty-eight dinners and entrees.

For about 200 to 350 calories, you get a great entree that really does satisfy your cravings.

Here are a few of my favorites:

- Weight Watchers Smart Ones Fajita Chicken Supreme (9¼ ounces): 260 calories, 7 g fat, 33 g carbs, 3 g fiber, 18 g protein, 650 mg sodium.
- Healthy Choice Beef Merlot (10 ounces): 220 calories, 6 g fat, 22 g carbs, 5 g fiber, 17 g protein, 580 mg sodium.
- Lean Cuisine Chicken Chow Mein (9 ounces): 210 calories, 3 g fat, 35 g carbs, 2 g fiber, 13 g protein, 630 mg sodium.
- Lean Cuisine Dinnertime Selects Grilled Chicken & Penne Pasta (14 ounces): 330 calories, 4.5 g fat, 52 g carbs, 6 g fiber, 20 g protein, 580 mg sodium.
- Healthy Choice Grilled Chicken Marinara (10 ounces): 250 calories, 4 g fat, 32 g carbs, 5 g fiber, 20 g protein, 550 mg sodium.
- Lean Cuisine Cafe Classics Bowl Chicken Fried Rice (12 ounces): 280 calories, 6 g fat, 39 g carbs, 3 g fiber, 17 g protein, 690 mg sodium.
- Weight Watchers Smart Ones Fire-grilled Chicken and

Vegetables (10 ounces): 290 calories, 3 g fat, 47 g carbs, 2 g fiber, 18 g protein, 730 mg sodium.
- Michelina's Lean Gourmet Garden Bistro Asian Style (9 ounces): 180 calories, 6 g fat, 29 g carbs, 5 g fiber, 5 g protein, 590 mg sodium.
- Healthy Choice Country Herb Chicken (11.35 ounces): 240 calories, 5 g fat, 34 g carbs, 5 g fiber, 15 g protein, 600 mg sodium.
- Kashi Pesto Pasta Primavera (10 ounces): 290 calories, 11 g fat, 37 g carbs, 7 g fiber, 11 g protein, 750 mg sodium.
- Kashi Sweet & Sour Chicken (10 ounces): 320 calories, 3.5 g fat, 55 g carbs, 6 g fiber, 18 g protein, 380 mg sodium.
- Amy's Light in Sodium Vegetable Lasagna (9½ ounces): 290 calories, 8 g fat, 41 g carbs, 4 g fiber, 15 g protein, 340 mg sodium.

Lose 20 Pounds

Think about it this way. If you were to get a cheeseburger, fries, and a soda at a fast-food restaurant, that would add up to about 1,500 calories and take at least fifteen minutes with travel, ordering, and waiting time.

These healthy frozen entrees or dinners, on the other hand, are ready to eat in about four to eight minutes, without your having to leave your house. Plus, with the calories you'll save (on average, 300 calories or more per meal), if you simply substitute frozen dinners for five of your twenty-one weekly meals, you could cut out at least 1,500 calories per week. Translation: You could lose 20 pounds in one year! However, keep in mind, this is *only* if you're eating the healthy frozen meals—not the Hungry-Man versions.

Calorie Bargain Spotlight

Calorie Bargain: Twice the Veggies—Lean Cuisine Sesame Stir Fry with Chicken

The Why: As if a convenient frozen meal with veggies wasn't good enough, Lean Cuisine now offers twice the veggies. Which means more food for less calories, plus you'll feel full longer. This is part of its Spa Cuisine Classics line.

The Health Bonus: extra veggies. (Need we say more?)

What We Liked Best: The flavor is great; it's sort of like sweet-and-sour chicken.

What We Liked Least: The sodium count is high, but that's typical of most frozen meals.

The Price: $3.79.

Website: www.leancuisine.com.

Where to Buy: local grocery store.

Ingredients: Cooked chicken white meat (chicken white meat, water, modified tapioca starch, chicken flavor, dehydrated chicken broth, chicken powder, natural flavor), carrageenan, whey protein concentrate (made from milk), salt, blanched whole wheat vermicelli (water, whole durum wheat flour), broccoli, water, yellow carrots, red peppers, edamame soybeans, brown sugar, soy sauce (water, wheat, soybeans, salt), apple cider vinegar, modified cornstarch, chile garlic sauce (chile pepper, chiles, salt, garlic, water, sugar, rice vinegar, modified cornstarch, acetic acid), corn syrup, soybean oil, brown sugar syrup, sesame seeds, garlic concentrate (garlic, salt, natural flavors, sesame oil, canola oil, citric acid), caramel color, spice.

Nutritional Analysis per Serving
300 calories
6 g fat
41 g carbs
20 g protein
5 g fiber
680 mg sodium

Words of Advice

Keep in mind that many of these frozen dinners skimp on the vegetables, so it's important to add a piece of fruit and a salad or frozen vegetables. Pick frozen dinners that have about 20 grams of protein per package to help keep you satisfied.

Another tip: "It's a good idea to serve them on a plate. The volume of food fills it up, making your portion appear larger, and as a result you will be more satisfied."

What about Liquid Meals?

How do these prepackaged meals compare to meal replacement drinks and shakes? With liquid formulas, the downside is the monotony of having the same (or very similar) products one or more times per day. "In addition," says Hannum, "meal replacement products lack some of the benefits of a balanced diet of real foods, such as the nontraditional nutrients and phytochemicals that continually emerge as having health benefits." Also, when you drink liquids, you simply don't get the satisfaction that comes from eating a real meal.

Soups

Unless you're one of the lucky ones who live in a warm climate, a nice cup of hot soup probably sounds like a great idea in the winter. But soup can do a lot more than warm you up; it can also fill you up and help you lose weight. A recent study published in the journal *Physiology & Behavior* found that soups reduced hunger and increased fullness as much as solid foods. And total calorie intake was lower when participants ate soup rather than drinking similar quantities of ordinary beverages.

"Soups have a water base, which keeps the calories down. They tend to make you feel more satisfied, so you eat less," says Barbara Rolls, PhD, of Penn State University. Dr. Rolls led the original groundbreaking research that found that eating soup prior to your meal could reduce mealtime consumption by as many as 100 calories. However, "The soup itself must be fairly low in calories to be the most effective—otherwise you end up eating two meals," she cautions.

Here are a few tips to help you choose the right soup.

French Onion vs. Broccoli-Cheddar Soup

If you skip the bread and cheese topping (which can add 350 calories), your best bet is French onion soup, made with sherry, onions, butter, and beef bouillon, at about 100 to 200 calories per cup, depending on ingredients. For instance, Au Bon Pain's has 80 calories per cup (keep in mind, the serving size is 12 ounces), whereas Panera Bread's has 220 calories per cup (80 without cheese and croutons). And Applebee's French Onion Soup au Gratin has only 150 calories per cup, including crouton and reduced-fat cheese.

On the other hand, broccoli-cheddar soup, often made with heavy cream, has about 175 to 275 calories per cup; Au Bon Pain's has 215 calories (320 for 12 ounces). Try to avoid cream and cheese soups in general.

Chicken Noodle vs. Chicken Vegetable

While both are good choices, chicken vegetable is usually a bit lower in calories because it's missing the noodles.

- Campbell's Chunky Soup, Classic Chicken Noodle (1 cup): 110 calories, 2.5 g fat, 15 g carbs, 8 g protein, 890 mg sodium.
- Homemade chicken noodle soup, from scratch (1 cup): 300 calories, 7 g fat, 28 g carbs, 30 g protein, 1,430 mg sodium.
- Campbell's Chunky Soup, Hearty Chicken with Vegetables (1 cup): 90 calories, 1.5 g fat, 13 g carbs, 7 g protein, 790 mg sodium.

Black Bean vs. Lentil Soup

This one's a close call. The only thing that really makes lentil a better choice is the sour cream that's often served on top of the black bean soup (60 calories for 2 tablespoons). Both of these legumes offer health benefits, including significant folate, magnesium, antioxidants, fiber, and protein, with very low calories and fat. One additional benefit of black beans is the amount of iron they contain, because many Americans tend to lack iron in their diets.

- Panera Bread Low-fat Vegetarian Black Bean Soup (1 cup): 160 calories, 1 g fat, 31 g carbs (11 g fiber), 9 g protein, 820 mg sodium.
- Goya Black Bean Soup (1 cup): 210 calories, 1.5 g fat, 37 g carbs (20 g fiber), 11 g protein, 1,050 mg sodium.
- Amy's Organic Lentil Soup (1 cup): 150 calories, 4.5 g fat, 19 g carbs (9 g fiber), 8 g protein, 590 mg sodium.
- Coco Pazzo Tuscan Lentil Soup with Thyme (1 cup): 220 calories, 6 g fat, 30 g carbs (16 g fiber), 15 g protein, 610 mg sodium.

Minestrone vs. Split Pea Soup

Peas are an excellent source of fiber, folate, and potassium, but split pea soup is usually the loser caloriewise. It can be made a variety of ways, and when the peas are pureed, they're sometimes combined with butter and cream, which boosts the calorie and fat content. Minestrone, made with an assortment of vegetables, including leeks, carrots, onions, celery, potatoes, zucchini, tomatoes, and beans, is consistently the better choice. One cup is generally in the 100- to 180-calorie range, depending on the amount of beans and whether pasta is added.

- Campbell's Select, Minestrone Soup (1 cup): 100 calories, 0.5 g fat, 20 g carbs, 5 g protein, 950 mg sodium.

- Health Valley Organic Minestrone Soup (1 cup): 100 calories, 2 g fat, 17 g carbs, 4 g protein, 570 mg sodium.
- Progresso Vegetable Classics, Green Split Pea Soup (1 cup): 170 calories, 3 g fat, 25 g carbs, 10 g protein, 870 mg sodium.
- Amy's Organic Split Pea Soup (1 cup): 100 calories, 0 g fat, 19 g carbs, 7 g protein, 570 mg sodium.
- Au Bon Pain Split Pea with Ham (1 cup, but serving size is 12 ounces): 140 calories, 1 g fat, 28 g carbs, 12 g protein, 795 mg sodium.

Clam Chowder vs. Lobster Bisque

You might think that all clam chowders are equal, but the Manhattan version is tomato based, whereas New England clam chowder is made with milk or cream, which makes it higher in calories. But lobster bisque, typically made with heavy cream, can be the highest of all, coming in at 260 calories or more per cup, depending on the amount of butter, heavy cream, and lobster used in the preparation. Bisque, after all, means thick and creamy, so what would you expect?

- Progresso Traditional Soups, Manhattan Clam Chowder (1 cup): 110 calories, 2 g fat, 17 g carbs, 6 g protein, 880 mg sodium.
- Campbell's Chunky Soup, New England Clam Chowder (1 cup): 210 calories, 9 g fat, 25 g carbs, 7 g protein, 890 mg sodium.
- Boston Chowda Lobster Bisque (1 cup): 260 calories, 19 g fat, 12 g carbs, 9 g protein, 1,400 mg sodium.

Hot Dogs

Despite roots that go back to the wurst and sausages of Europe, hot dogs are a uniquely American phenomenon. Americans consume approximately twenty billion franks every year—that's seventy hot dogs per person.

Hot dogs are inexpensive, quick, filling, and taste great, but just one hot dog with a bun could have as many as 350 calories. Now add a few extras like baked beans, coleslaw, or mayo, have another dog or two, and you'll be eating upward of 1,500 to 2,000 calories (enough for an entire day), not to mention all the fat.

As with any great food, there are things you need to know to keep your calorie consumption to a minimum—even with a seemingly innocent hot dog.

What's Inside?

All hot dogs are cured and cooked sausages that consist mainly of pork, beef, chicken, and turkey, or a combination of meat and poultry. Other ingredients include water, curing agents, and spices such as garlic, salt, sugar, mustard, nutmeg, coriander, and white pepper.

By the way, the rumors—they're only partially true. Yes, nontraditional animal parts can be used to make hot dogs.

Variety meats or meat by-products such as hearts, kidneys, livers, and skeletal muscle may be included. But if by-products account for 15 percent or more of the mixture, the U.S. Department of Agriculture requires the manufacturer to declare those ingredients on the package with the statement "with variety meats" or "with meat by-products" and to specify which variety meat is included. Overall, most hot dogs are made from good quality meats.

It's Not Healthy

If a hot dog is made from all beef, turkey, or chicken, you may think it's a healthy choice—especially turkey. But be wary: Many of these dogs are full of fat. Also, make sure you consider the size of the frank in relation to the calories and fat; for example, Shelton's Turkey Franks are half the size of Oscar Mayer's XXL Deli Style Beef Franks.

Comparisons for one frank:

- Oscar Mayer XXL Deli Style Beef Franks (76 g): 230 calories, 22g fat, 1 g carbs.
- Oscar Mayer Beef Franks (45 g): 140 calories, 13 g fat, 1 g carbs.
- Hebrew National Beef Franks (49 g): 150 calories, 14 g fat, 1 g carbs.
- Nathan's Skinless Beef Franks (57 g): 170 calories, 15 g fat, 1 g carbs.
- Louis Rich Turkey Franks (45 g): 101 calories, 8 g fat, 1 g carbs.
- Shelton's Turkey Franks (34 g): 60 calories, 4.5 g fat, 1 g carbs.

Choose Reduced Fat or Fat Free

The calorie and fat savings are worth it—a real Calorie Bargain—and most people can't tell the difference, especially when the franks are barbecued and topped with all the extras. Try several brands to figure out which ones you like best.

- Ball Park Lite Beef Franks (50 g): 100 calories, 7 g fat, 3 g carbs.
- Ball Park Fat Free Beef Franks (50 g): 45 calories, 0 g fat, 5 g carbs.
- Ball Park Bun Size Smoked White Turkey Franks (50 g): 45 calories, 0 g fat, 5 g carbs.
- Healthy Choice Beef Franks (50 g): 70 calories, 2.5 g fat, 7 g carbs.
- Oscar Mayer 98% Fat Free Wieners (50 g): 40 calories, 0 g fat, 32 g carbs.
- Hebrew National 97% Fat Free Beef Franks (49 g): 45 calories, 1.5 g fat, 3 g carbs.

Watch Your Buns

The bun is what holds the frank and all the fixin's together, but the calories add up. Choose a brand that's lower in calories or wrap your hot dog in one piece of low-calorie toast (for instance, Arnold Bakery Light Wheat). If it's not a big deal to you, you could also try having your hot dog on a plate, with a knife and fork.

- Wonder Bread White Hot Dog Buns (1): 110 calories, 1.5 g fat, 21 g carbs.

- Pepperidge Farm Frankfurter Rolls (1): 140 calories, 2.5 g fat, 23 g carbs.

Vegetarian

Eating a meatless hot dog may save you calories and fat. That said, make sure you check the food label. Just because it says "vegetarian" or "meatless" doesn't guarantee that it will be low in calories.

- Morningstar Farms Veggie Dogs (57 g): 80 calories, 0.5 g fat, 6 g carbs.
- Yves The Good Dog Veggie Hotdogs (52 g): 100 calories, 5 g fat, 2 g carbs.
- Lightlife Smart Dogs Meatless Fat Free Franks (42 g): 45 calories, 0 g fat, 2 g carbs.

Trimmings

As always, mayo can be a problem. Coleslaw, potato, and macaroni salad all contain mayonnaise, which adds plenty of fat and calories. The trick with all of these extras is to have small portions, and if you can substitute reduced- or low-fat mayo for the regular, you'll be in good shape. But feel free to load up on the pickles!

- Bush's Original Baked Beans (1 cup): 300 calories, 2 g fat, 58 g carbs.
- Coleslaw (1 cup): 270 calories, 24 g fat, 13 g carbs.
- Potato salad (1 cup): 275 calories, 15 g fat, 33 g carbs.
- Macaroni salad (1 cup): 269 calories, 9 g fat, 43 g carbs.
- Pickles (1, 4-inch long): 24 calories, 0 g fat, 6 g carbs.

Calorie Bargain Spotlight

Calorie Bargain: Rick's Picks (Pickles)

The Why: If Peter Piper could have picked this peck of pickled peppers, he would have. He would also have enjoyed the pickled Mean (green) Beans, Spears of Influence, Phat Beets, Kool Gherks, and Windy City Wasabeans! Great pickles, great packaging, great names, and low calories. We'd even venture to say they'll be the most special pickles that you've ever tasted. They are a wonderful, flavorful addition to sandwiches, salads, or even just a fork—and with only 10 to 30 calories per serving, you can eat these to your heart's content.

The Health Bonus: Did you know that in addition to being low calorie, pickles are low fat or fat free and count toward your much-needed fruit and veggie quota?

What We Liked Best: So many fun types to try. They even come with suggestions for how to add them to favorite foods, in case you crave something other than straight from the jar.

What We Liked Least: If you're tempted by the idea of pickles, and then bite into one of these puppies thinking it's only gonna make you pucker—watch out! Some of the flavors were barely bitable to those with a low spice threshold on our tasting committee. (In other words, they're pretty hot.) The other slight problem is that they're not available everywhere.

The Price: Most of the varieties are $10.99 each.

Offerings: They are available in ten flavors: Windy City Wasabeans, GT 1000s, Phat Beets, Spears of Influence, Mean Beans, Smokra, Bee 'n' Beez, Kool Gherks, Pepi Pep Peps, and Slices of Life.

Website: www.rickspicksnyc.com.

Where to Buy: www.rickspicksnyc.com.

Ingredients: Each of the pickles has a little something different in the mix. Here's an example for Spears of Influence: cucumbers, vinegar, water, garlic, dill, salt, pickling spice, lime juice, cumin, dried chilies, peppercorns. For specific ingredients for each type of pickle, see the Rick's Picks website.

Nutritional Analysis per Serving: 1 Ounce (28 Grams)

Mean Beans	Spears of Influence
20 calories	10 calories
0 g fat	0 g fat
4 g carbs	2 g carbs
Less than 1 g protein	0 g protein
Less than 1 g fiber	0 g fiber
200 mg sodium	45 mg sodium

Toppings

All I can say is pack on the sauerkraut—it's your best bet. It has very few calories and no fat. Mustard, ketchup, and relish are also great deals in terms of calories. Steer clear of butter and mayo, which have a habit of turning up on almost everything we eat. Also, try to avoid cheese and chili whenever possible; they can add more than 250 calories and 15 grams of fat to your frank.

- Sauerkraut (1 cup): 27 calories, 0 g fat, 6 g carbs.
- Heinz Tomato Ketchup (2 tablespoons): 30 calories, 0 g fat, 8 g carbs.
- Gulden's Spicy Brown Mustard (2 tablespoons): 30 calories, 0 g fat, 0 g carbs.
- Sargento Fancy Mild Cheddar Shredded Cheese (¼ cup): 110 calories, 9 g fat, 1 g carbs.

- Hormel Chili with Beans (1 cup): 270 calories, 7 g fat, 34 g carbs.
- Heinz Sweet Relish (2 tablespoons): 40 calories, 0 g fat, 10 g carbs.
- Coney Island Style Hot Dog Sauce (1 cup): 303 calories, 20 g fat, 23 g carbs.

Cookies, Crackers, and Chips

Snacking sometimes gets a bad rap. A recent study in the *International Journal of Obesity* reported that people who are obese snack more frequently than nonobese individuals, and the more snacks people eat, the more calories they take in—specifically sweet and fatty foods. But snacking is not all bad. Healthy snacking is a good way to keep your hunger in check between meals so that you don't overeat, especially if you make healthy minimeals. Sometimes, though, the only snack options available are cookies, crackers, and chips, which really don't qualify as healthy, so you need to know how to make the best choices.

Oatmeal Cookies vs. Chocolate Chip Cookies vs. Fig Newtons vs. Graham Crackers vs. Animal Crackers

Almost any way you eat them, cookies are about 100 to 150 calories per ounce. No matter what kind of cookie, if it's made primarily of butter and sugar, it should be treated as an occasional dessert, not a healthy snack. Caloriewise, there's no difference between an oatmeal cookie and a chocolate chip cookie.

However, as far as health perks are concerned, while chocolate (at least dark chocolate) does have antioxidants, the better choice is the oatmeal cookies. They have fiber from the oats (a whole grain), which will fill you up more so you feel more satisfied.

There's a rumor going around that animal and graham crackers are healthy choices. Not true. Animal crackers have about 130 calories per ounce, and graham crackers are about 120 calories per ounce, although—because both cookies are smaller than the average oatmeal or chocolate chip—you feel like you're getting more, which is a good thing. For instance, you get about eight graham crackers for those 120 calories because each sheet weighs about ½ ounce.

Fig Newtons are lower in calories and make a better choice than the others, but, again, they're no health food at 55 calories per cookie (½ ounce).

- Chips Ahoy Chunky Chocolate (1 cookie, about ⅔ ounce): 80 calories.
- Keebler Country Style Oatmeal Cookies (1 cookie, about ½ ounce): 65 calories.

Fit Tip: Your best bet is to control your cookie portions. Don't eat directly from the bag or box. Take one at a time, put it on a plate or a napkin, and seal up the rest. As a rule, avoid low-fat or low-carb cookies, which often are just as high in calories as the regular versions. Your best bet: Go with those 100-calorie snack packs. Kraft currently has them for Chips Ahoy, Cheese Nips, Honey Maid Cinnamon Grahams, Ritz Crackers, Oreos, Planters Peanut Butter Cookie Crisps, and Wheat Thins. Other food companies make them too. Even if they're a bit more expensive, they will really help you control portions.

You can make your own 100-calorie packs using Ziploc bags. The only thing is, you might want to cut the cookies in quarters; otherwise you'll only have one or two cookies in each bag.

Beware of those giant cookies. One Pepperidge Farm Soft Baked Dark Chocolate Chunk Nantucket cookie (slightly more than 1 ounce) has 150 calories. Also, just one Double Stuf Oreo or Milano cookie contains about 70 calories—pretty high considering the size of what you get (and how many you end up eating).

Try to choose whole-grain alternatives if they're available. These are not health foods and may not even have fewer calories, but oftentimes they're still a better choice. For instance, 100% Whole Grain Fig Newtons are still 55 calories per cookie (same as regular Fig Newtons), but the first ingredient is whole-grain flour, which is more nutritious than refined flour. Even Chips Ahoy makes a 100 percent whole-grain cookie (but it does have 150 calories per 33 grams). Whole grains help you feel full longer, and they have certain benefits, including fiber and nutrients such as B vitamins, vitamin E, magnesium, and selenium.

Another choice: Bake your own and make them healthy. Oatmeal raisin cookies can be prepared using egg whites, skim milk, reduced-calorie margarine, and an artificial baking sweetener such as Baking Splenda.

Bagel Chips vs. Pita Chips vs. Potato Chips vs. Baked Potato Chips

Either baked or bread-based chips are a better bet than potato chips. Both bagel chips and pita chips typically have about 130 calories per ounce. Baked chips come in at around 110 to 120 per ounce, whereas potato chips fall in the 150- to-160-calorie range.

But while it's true that "baked" or "veggie" is usually code for healthy, it's best to read and compare the actual nutrition information. Not all foods that boast healthy sounding names are actually diet friendly. People seem to think they've earned a "health halo" when they buy a bag of Baked Lay's potato crisps, baked pita chips, or veggie chips (such as Terra chips, at about 11 calories per chip)—and then proceed to devour them as though they have calorie immunity. Unfortunately, the calorie difference isn't overwhelming.

Plus, you're not getting any notable health benefits. "Eating baked chips or veggie chips is not the same as eating a baked potato," reminds Bonnie Liebman, director of nutrition at the Center for Science in the Public Interest. "It's a big mistake to think a chip is a vegetable."

Fit Tip: Next time you get a craving for chips, try a 1-ounce bag. Prepackaged serving-size portions help on two levels: You can't eat more than one serving, and you can actually see how small those serving sizes really are—especially when you consider the number of calories they pack. Try other types of chips, such as Stacy's Soy Thin Crisps, which pack in 6.5 grams of protein at 110 calories per ounce, plus you get a lot more chips for slightly fewer calories per ounce.

But watch out, because there is no guarantee that making the switch from potato chips to soy crisps will save you calories. For instance, Glenny's Soy Crisps have 140 calories per 1.3-ounce bag, and since we always eat what's in the bag, that would be only 10 to 20 fewer calories than a 1-ounce serving of potato chips.

Buy soy chips in packages with 110 calories or less for the entire bag. And choose them only to replace higher-calorie chips already in your diet. Also, for 100 calories per ounce, there are Pretzel Crisps (www.pretzelcrisps.com), which are not bad and lower in calories than most other chips—so long as you remember to consume them responsibly.

You can also make your own whole wheat pita chips from Thomas' Sahara Whole Wheat Pita Bread, which is 140 calories for a 2-ounce pita. Give one a few squirts of margarine spray, add a bit of garlic powder and salt, cut into chips, and toast. You'll get double the amount of chips for half the calories.

Ritz Crackers vs. Saltines vs. Wheat Thins vs. Triscuits

Triscuits rack up 20 calories per cracker but could be your best bet because they're 100 percent whole grain—plus, you might eat a lot less because of all that fiber. Ritz crackers have about 16 calories each, whereas saltines have 12 calories per cracker. Wheat Thins come in at a bit more than 9 calories per cracker. It's important to note, however, that gram for gram, they all contain roughly the same number of calories. If you're thinking about going low fat, well, Health Valley Low Fat Whole Wheat Crackers have 15 calories per cracker, but you get a bit more cracker for your calories.

Fit Tip: Try to choose whole-grain crackers. Even if you don't save calories, at the very least you'll be getting the benefits of the whole grains. Kashi TLC Original 7 Grain crackers are about 8.5 calories per cracker, but they're whole grain and even have a seal of approval from the Whole Grains Council as a "good source" of whole grains. Or you can go with re-duced-fat Triscuits, which are 17 calories per cracker; a good bet if you practice portion control.

Condiments

There are many foods that I consider "free" foods, meaning that you can eat as much of them as you want, and it just doesn't count. But it's recently been reported that cutting just 100 calories from what you ordinarily eat each day can add up to significant weight loss over time—almost ten pounds a year. Wonder why you're not losing weight even though you've been making healthy food choices? It might just be the little things, such as the condiments you're using, that end up costing you big-time.

Ketchup

All those little ketchup packets can add up. They're still relatively low in calories, but *only* if you use them sparingly.

- Heinz Tomato Ketchup (2 tablespoons): 30 calories, 0 g fat, 8 g carbs.

Mustard

Plain old mustard is a great condiment, offering great taste for very few calories. But even mustard can be dangerous to your waist if you're not careful. Mustard mixed with honey is a relatively low-calorie condiment, but most honey mustard dressings are usually mixed with oil and sometimes cream.

- Burger King Honey Mustard Dipping Sauce (1-ounce packet—about 2 tablespoons): 90 calories, 6 g fat, 9 g carbs.
- French's Prepared Deli Mustard (2 tablespoons): 32 calories, 2 g fat, 3 g carbs.
- Grey Poupon Dijon Mustard (2 tablespoons): 36 calories, 2 g fat, 3 g carbs.

Horseradish

Famous as an ingredient in Bloody Marys, horseradish adds lots of flavor and no fat. One tablespoon of prepared horseradish has only 6 calories, 1 gram of carbohydrate, and no fat. But don't confuse horseradish with horseradish *sauce*. The addition of sour cream puts this condiment on the condemned list.

Oils

While it's true that oils such as olive, canola, or the popular flaxseed are heart-healthy choices, they are still high in calories and should be used sparingly. In fact, they all have the same number of calories.

- Olive oil (1 tablespoon): 119 calories, 13.5 g fat, 0 g carbs.

Spreads

Many sauces and spreads found on sandwiches or with appetizers are actually loaded with fat and calories.

- Starr Ridge Sun Dried Tomato Cracker Spread (2 tablespoons): 140 calories, 12 g fat, 6 g carbs.
- Pesto (2 tablespoons): 160 calories, 15 g fat, 2 g carbs.

Mayonnaise

This is by far the most condemnable of all the condiments! Just 2 tablespoons of Hellmann's has 180 calories, 20 grams of fat, and no carbs. Wow! It's used to make tuna salad, chicken salad, and Russian dressing, it's spread on top of hamburgers and sandwiches—mayo is everywhere. And, believe me, when it goes on as a condiment, people don't use it sparingly. Switching from 2 tablespoons of regular mayo to low-fat mayo on your daily sandwich would save you 36,500 calories and help you lose as much as 10 pounds after one year!

- Hellmann's Light Mayonnaise (2 tablespoons): 100 calories, 10 g fat, 2 g carbs.

Sour Cream

Sure, sour cream is great on Mexican food, in dips, and on a baked potato, but a serving of Breakstone's (2 tablespoons) has 60 calories, 5 grams of fat, and 1 gram of carbohydrate. Replace your full-fat sour cream with reduced-fat varieties, or better yet, use plain nonfat yogurt—it has only 7 calories per tablespoon!

Butter and Margarine

How much butter do you think you spread on your sandwich or toast? And do you think margarine is better? Check out these numbers:

- Land O'Lakes Butter (1 tablespoon): 100 calories, 11 g fat, 0 g carbs.
- Fleischmann's Original Margarine (1 tablespoon): 100 calories, 11 g fat, 0 g carbs.
- Parkay Original Stick margarine (1 tablespoon): 90 calories, 10 g fat, 0 g carbs.

Not much of a difference there. Also, keep in mind that many brands of margarine have trans fats, which may negate the health benefits of the decrease in saturated fat. Here are some healthier choices:

- Land O'Lakes Whipped Butter (1 tablespoon): 70 calories, 7 g fat, 0 g carbs.
- Parkay Light margarine (1 tablespoon): 50 calories, 5 g fat, 0 g carbs.
- Smart Beat Super Light Margarine (1 tablespoon): 20 calories, 2 g fat, 0 g carbs.

But if you do switch to a lighter version, keep in mind that even these calories can add up quickly; the fact that it's lower in calories still doesn't give you license to go wild. A good rule of thumb to remember is that a pat of butter or margarine is slightly more than one teaspoon.

Jams and Jellies

Although it's not as high calorie as peanut butter, jelly can still add significant calories to your day. Spread a thin layer on your bread or crackers, and opt for the sugar-free or no-sugar-added versions, which are better deals.

- Polaner All Fruit Strawberry Fruit Spread (1 tablespoon): 40 calories, 0 g fat, 10 g carbs.
- Smucker's Sugar Free Seedless Blackberry Jam (1 tablespoon): 10 calories, 0 g fat, 5 g carbs.

Diet Detective's What You Need to Know

True or false: Condiments like mayonnaise, ketchup, mustard, and barbecue sauce can last a long time in the fridge—almost forever?

True, but not forever. They'll last about six months, which to most of us sounds like a pretty short time considering that our condiments seem to be in there for years. They will eventually spoil, due to either chemical changes or bacterial growth. But keep in mind that these bacteria are not the ones that make us sick; they just spoil the taste, says Donald W. Schaffner, PhD, extension specialist in food science and professor at Rutgers, The State University of New Jersey. Also, "One of the reasons condiments last as long as they do is because they have an acidic environment (for example, the vinegar in ketchup), and bacteria don't do well in that situation," says Keith R. Schneider, PhD, a professor of food science at the University of Florida in Gainesville. As far as mayo is concerned, Dr. Schneider says it gets a bad rap and is not really as dangerous as its reputation for bacterial growth, but it is still bad in terms of calories. He also reminds us that rancid foods are not necessarily dangerous—they just taste bad.

Tartar Sauce

Tartar sauce goes best with fried fish—a combination that is deadly to the waistline. One ounce of Burger King's tartar sauce has a monstrous 160 calories and 16 grams of fat, with no carbohydrate. Kraft makes a fat-free tartar sauce that has 25 calories, 0 grams of fat, and 5 grams of carbohydrate per ounce (2 tablespoons). Use this, or switch to grilled fish with cocktail sauce or salsa for a delicious, lower-calorie alternative.

Barbecue Sauce

This sauce adds flavor to almost anything—it's sweet, tangy, and a must for any outdoor eating festival.

- Kraft Original Barbecue Sauce (2 tablespoons): 40 calories, 0 g fat, 11 g carbs.

Duck Sauce

Watch out for those seemingly harmless packs of duck sauce that come with your next order of Chinese food.

- Saucy Susan Duck Sauce (2 tablespoons): 80 calories, 0 g fat, 19 g carbs.

Steak Sauce

I was actually surprised at how few calories steak sauce contained.

- A.1. Steak Sauce (1 tablespoon): 15 calories, 0 g fat, 3 g carbs.

Salsa

Not only is salsa great on Mexican foods, it's also delicious on baked potatoes, grilled chicken, or seafood, and even sandwiches or burgers. Just two tablespoons are only 15 calories.

Calorie Bargain Spotlight

Calorie Bargain: Quaker Chewy 90 Calorie Granola Bars, Chocolate Chunk

The Why: These bars are tasty, low in calories, and low in fat.

The Health Bonus: They aren't whole grain, but they are *made* with whole grains, giving them some extra sustenance. And they provide 8 percent of your daily calcium needs.

What We Liked Best: These bars are an excellent and satisfying substitute for a candy bar or a bag of M&M's, either of which averages about 250 to 300 calories.

What We Liked Least: This is far from good wholesome ingredients. Fruit is always a bettter snack choice.

The Price: about $2.99 for a box of ten.

Offerings: Chewy 90 Calorie Granola Bar, Chocolate Chunk.

Website: www.quakersnackbars.com.

Where to Buy: local grocery store.

Ingredients: granola (whole-grain rolled oats, sugar, rice flour, whole-grain rolled wheat, partially hydrogenated soybean and cottonseed oils with TBHQ and citric acid added to preserve freshness and/or sunflower oil with natural tocopherol added to preserve freshness, whole wheat flour, molasses, sodium bicarbonate, soy lecithin, caramel color, barley malt, salt, nonfat dry milk), corn syrup, crisp rice (rice, sugar, salt, barley malt), semisweet chocolate chunks (sugar, chocolate liquor, cocoa butter, soy lecithin, vanillin [an artificial flavor]), sugar, corn syrup solids, glycerin, high fructose corn syrup, partially hydrogenated soybean and/or cottonseed oil, sorbitol, fructose, calcium carbonate, natural and artificial flavors, salt, soy lecithin, molasses, water, BHT (a preservative), citric acid.

Nutritional Analysis per Serving: 1 Bar
90 calories
2 g fat
19 g carbs
1 g protein
1 g fiber
80 mg sodium

Chocolate

Chocolate's getting a lot of attention these days, from its heart-healthy claims (which are only for dark chocolate) to its ability to reduce stress. So I was wondering if there was a way to make better chocolate choices and keep our waists trim. Test your knowledge and see if you're a chocolate expert.

M&M's vs. Raisinets

At first glance, there doesn't seem to be very much difference. While M&M's are slightly higher in calories (1.7 ounces, 240 calories), you also get a little more in the package. But beyond the straightforward calories per ounce, there are some important distinctions between the two. M&M's are 100 percent candy: bite-size pieces of milk chocolate covered in colored sugar. Raisinets (1.58 ounces, 185 calories), however, could be considered a chocolate-coated health food. Much like dark chocolate, raisins are packed with flavonols, the phytochemicals that give cocoa its health power. So while the calorie counts may be similar, the health benefits of Raisinets make them a much better option. Junior Mints (one 1.84-ounce box, 210 calories) can also be a decent choice.

Fit Tip: In terms of chocolate candy, individual bags with tiny pieces seem to last longer than a chocolate bar and might, therefore, be your best bet. Just be sure to eat those tiny chocolate pieces one at a time; don't empty the bag into your mouth all at once.

PowerBar vs. Hershey's Special Dark

Just because it comes in a sporty little wrapper with a slogan about strength, speed, endurance, and muscle mass doesn't mean a PowerBar isn't just a candy bar with extra protein, vitamins, and minerals. Yes, an energy bar has a few extra nutrients, but unless you're a serious athlete, you probably don't need one. And eating dark chocolate (Hershey's Special Dark Chocolate) has heart-healthy benefits, but you can get the same benefits from tea or wine. The bottom line is that it's fine to want a snack, but at least be honest with yourself: PowerBar or Hershey's Bar, it's still a snack.

- Hershey's Special Dark Chocolate (1.4 ounces): 220 calories, 12 g fat, 25 g carbs.
- Clif Builder's Chocolate Bar (2.4 ounces): 270 calories, 8 g fat, 30 g carbs.
- PowerBar Performance Bar, Chocolate (2.3 ounces): 230 calories, 1.5 g fat, 44 g carbs.
- Scharffen Berger 70% Bittersweet Gourmet Chocolate (1 ounce): 170 calories, 12 g fat, 14 g carbs.
- Snickers bar (2.07 ounces): 280 calories, 14 g fat, 35 g carbs.
- Hershey's Milk Chocolate (1.55 ounces): 230 calories, 13 g fat, 25 g carbs.
- Milky Way (2.05 ounces): 260 calories, 10 g fat, 41 g carbs.

Fit Tip: Watch out for some of those "health" bars; the calories can be as high as those in any candy bar. If you're looking for dark chocolate's antioxidant power, go for a Mars CocoaVia Chocolate Snack Bar (80 calories, www.cocoavia.com), which is tasty and has been scientifically designed to pack on the heart-healthy flavonols. (The Original Chocolate bar has 100 calories.) Or if it's simply a chocolate treat you're seeking, try a York Peppermint Pattie (1.4 ounces, 160 calories).

Godiva Chocolate Liqueur vs. Chocolate Martini

A chocolate martini, made with vodka, chocolate liqueur, cream, and dark crème de cacao, averages more than 60 calories per ounce, with an average of 4 to 6½ ounces per cocktail. On the other hand, Godiva Chocolate Liqueur is typically served over ice as a 1- to 2-ounce drink and averages 103 calories per ounce.

Fit Tip: Keep in mind that drinks have calories too, and they add up quickly. Alcohol also lowers your inhibitions, which makes you likely to eat more.

- Godiva Chocolate Liqueur (1 ounce): 103 calories, 7 g fat, 11 g carbs.
- Chocolate martini (6½ ounces): 438 calories, 20 g fat, 24 g carbs.

Chocolate-dipped Strawberries vs. Chocolate-covered Cherries

It's fairly close, but the strawberries are your best bet at about 45 calories each; plus you get the health benefits that are packaged with the dark chocolate and berries. While chocolate strawberries typically involve only strawberries and chocolate, the cherries (about 55 calories each) are made with a filling—the sugary sauce the cherries swim in—which adds extra calories.

Fit Tip: How about dipping your strawberries or fresh cherries into some delicious Jell-O Sugar Free/Reduced Calorie Chocolate Pudding? The entire container (almost 4 ounces) has 60 calories.

Oreo Chocolate Cookie Crumbs vs. Chocolate Sprinkles

The calories in ice cream toppings add up fast—so pay attention. Choosing chocolate sprinkles (1½ ounces, 38 calories) over Oreo crumbs (1½ ounces, 218 calories) saves you 180 calories. Think of it this way: At 145 calories per ounce, your Oreo topping adds the same amount of calories as another half serving of French vanilla ice cream.

Fit Tip: You can try dark Dolfin Belgian Chocolate Flakes at 75 calories for a ½ ounce—they are less sweet than other sprinkles, which helps curb the temptation to smother your ice cream in them, and you get the dark-chocolate health benefits. You can get them on the web at www.chocolatesource.com.

Scharffen Berger Dark Drinking Chocolate vs. Swiss Miss Hot Cocoa

Swiss Miss Milk Chocolate Hot Cocoa Mix has only 120 calories for a ¾-cup (one packet) serving, whereas the dark

Calorie Bargain Spotlight

Calorie Bargain: Swiss Miss Diet Hot Cocoa Mix with Calcium

The Why: How can you go wrong with only 25 calories—for hot chocolate?

The Health Bonus: When I first started losing weight, this was a comforting treat whenever my sweet tooth kicked in.

What We Liked Best: The product does not contain any aspartame.

What We Liked Least: The mix does contain Splenda.

The Price: $3.49.

Offerings: Diet Hot Cocoa Mix with Calcium, Hot Cocoa Mix, No Sugar Added.

Website: www.conagrafoods.com.

Where to Buy: grocery stores, supercenters, convenience stores, discount club centers, snack bars, entertainment venues, Amazon.com.

Ingredients: nonfat dry milk, cocoa (processed with alkali), calcium carbonate, modified whey, salt, less than 2 percent of: carrageenan, sucralose (Splenda brand), natural and artificial flavors, disodium phosphate, acesulfame potassium.

Nutritional Analysis per Serving
25 calories
0 g fat
4 g carbs
2 g protein
1 g fiber
150 mg sodium

chocolate, while having the health benefits of real chocolate, has 210 calories for ½ cup if made with 1 percent milk. What about other chocolate drinks? Nesquik contains 230 calories per 8 ounces, while Yoo-hoo has 130. A can of Creamy Milk Chocolate Slim-Fast (about 11 ounces) comes in at 190 calories; however, it's meant to be a meal replacement, not a drink.

Fit Tip: Hot chocolate made with nonfat milk has only 140 calories for an 8-ounce serving. Or you can make a low-calorie dark chocolate hot cocoa by mixing unsweetened cocoa powder with Splenda (or another sugar replacement, or even with a tablespoon of sugar is fine) and skim milk. You can also go with Yoo-hoo Lite, which has only 70 calories for 9 ounces. Or, go for the premixed Swiss Miss Diet Hot Chocolate (one envelope prepared with water, 25 calories). It may kill your nighttime chocolate cravings for fewer than 30 calories!

Chocolate Shake vs. Ben & Jerry's Chocolate Fudge Brownie Low Fat Frozen Yogurt

Of course, low-fat frozen yogurt has fewer calories and is your best bet. But the calories can be pretty close: One cup of Ben & Jerry's Chocolate Fudge Brownie Low Fat Frozen Yogurt has 380 calories. A 12-ounce McDonald's Chocolate Triple Thick Shake is only a little higher at 440 calories, but it has none of the possible health benefits of yogurt.

Fit Tip: There are many lower-calorie fat-free frozen yogurts. Look for those with fewer than 200 calories per cup. For instance, Edy's/Dreyers Chocolate Fat-Free Frozen Yogurt has only 180 calories per cup.

Calorie Bargain Spotlight

Calorie Bargain: Edy's No Sugar Added Fruit Bars

The Why: Not only do these fruit bars make excellent desserts (or summer afternoon snacks), they are also filled with real fruit juices and vitamin C.

The Health Bonus: Try substituting them for ice cream after dinner or sodas during the day—they are just as refreshing and satisfying, with a fraction of the calories.

What We Liked Best: Some of these bars have real fruit (for example: strawberry).

What We Liked Least: The ingredients. If you're not interested in having Splenda, the regular Edy's Fruit Bars are still only 80 calories.

The Price: $2.99 for a box of twelve.

Offerings: strawberry, tangerine, raspberry, black cherry, strawberry-kiwi, mixed berry.

Website: www.edys.com.

Where to Buy: Publix, Kroger, Meijer, Wal-Mart.

Ingredients: strawberry (water, strawberries, sorbitol, glycerin, white grape juice from concentrate [water, white grape juice concentrate], strawberry juice from concentrate [water, strawberry juice concentrate], polydextrose, maltodextrin, citric acid, ascorbic acid [vitamin C], natural flavors, sucralose [Splenda brand], acesulfame potassium, beet juice concentrate [color], guar gum, turmeric color, carob bean gum.

Nutritional Analysis per Serving
30 calories
0 g fat
8 g carbs
0 g protein
1 g fiber
0 mg sodium

Hershey's Kiss vs. Russell Stover Truffle

Although the truffles—or any kind of boxed candy—are tasty and rich, they are very high in calories, averaging around 70 to 90 calories each. In addition, all these bite-size candies come in large bags or boxes containing many, many mouthfuls. Given that most of us can't stop at just one, consider exactly how many it's going to take to satisfy your chocolate craving before you decide whether it's a bargain. Even if you have just two dark truffles, that's about 160 calories—equal to more than six Hershey's Kisses (25 calories each).

- Russell Stover Dark Chocolate Truffle: 80 calories, 4.5 g fat, 9 g carbs.
- Russell Stover Dark Chocolate Butter Cream: 70 calories, 3 g fat, 11 g carbs.
- Hershey's Milk Chocolate with Almond Kiss: 25 calories, 1.5 g fat, 3 g carbs.

Fit Tip: Tootsie Rolls (27 calories each) are a good bet because you have to chew them, which means they last longer, so you may be able to get away with just one. However, many sugar-free candies are just as high in calories as the regular versions. Hershey's Sugar Free Dark Chocolate Candy has about 35 calories per piece. And avoid those new Bites candies you can just pop in your mouth: Each one is about 10 to 14 calories, and they add up quickly. Also avoid mini Reese's Peanut Butter Cups, which have 42 calories apiece.

Chocolate-frosted Brownie vs. Double-dipped Chocolate Cupcake vs. Flourless Cake

The cupcake (2.5 ounces, 240 calories) actually comes in a bit ahead of the brownie (2.4 ounces, 280 calories). Despite the current carb scare, flourless doesn't mean healthy. In the case of flourless cake, it just means there's much more butter, chocolate, eggs, and sugar for about 390 calories per 3.2-ounce slice.

Fit Tip: While it's not exactly front and center on the food pyramid, stick to an old-fashioned cookie to satisfy your chocolate bakery craving. You can even get fancy with a double chocolate chunk cookie and still save about 70 calories over a cupcake. Or try meringue cookies—some are even made with Splenda, so they're fat free and sugar free. Miss Meringue Chocolate Cookies: thirteen cookies for 40 calories (www.missmeringue.com).

Calorie Bargain Spotlight

Calorie Bargain: Lightfull Satiety Smoothies

The Why: It's 8:13 a.m., and you're on the ball. You're dressed, you've packed your lunch and your gym bag, and even your teeth are brushed. As you fly out the door, you smile. Don't you just love days when you've got a little extra time? (Maybe you'll score that brownie point with your new boss?!?) Just then your stomach growls, and you realize what you missed: breakfast, the most important meal of the day.

You can have your breakfast and your brownie point too, thanks to Lightfull Satiety Smoothies. You dash back inside, grab one for the road, and arrive at work early *and* satisfied. These high-fiber and high-protein drinks are really great served nice and cold. They are also high in calcium and have a low glycemic index. They were designed as a healthy, quick, and affordable way to fill you up and keep you going. The great taste and low-calorie combo is achieved thanks to a zero-calorie sweetener found naturally in fruit.

The Health Bonus: Lightfull Smoothies are all natural, have 20 percent of the recommended daily value for calcium, and 5 grams of fiber.

What We Liked Best: The fruit-flavored ones were our taste testers' favorites—Strawberry Bliss, Peaches & Cream, and Mango Oasis are delicious. No high-fiber graininess here. If we didn't know better, it might even seem like dessert.

What We Liked Least: The Chocolate Satisfaction and Café Latte flavors. Also, this should not replace water or other low-calorie drinks. This should be a snack.

The Price: $2.19 to $2.49 per smoothie (the 8¼-ouncers are also available in a multipack, four for $7.99).

Offerings: Strawberries & Cream, Peaches & Cream, Café Latte, Chocolate Fudge.

Website: www.lightfullfoods.com.

Where to Buy: Amazon.com.

Ingredients: water, erythritol (natural sweetener), nonfat plain yogurt, mango puree, tangerine juice concentrate, contains 2 percent or less of the following: whey protein concentrate, dextrin, natural flavors, inulin (natural dietary fiber), crystallized cane juice, fruit and vegetable juice for color, calcium lactate, pectin, xanthan and guar gums, dipotassium phosphate, potassium citrate, gellan gum, salt, citric acid. Contains milk and soybeans.

Nutritional Analysis per Serving: 8¼ Fluid Ounces (Mango Oasis Flavor):
90 calories
0 g fat
38 g carbs
5 g protein
5 g fiber
70 mg sodium

Ice Cream

You might say that I have ice cream in my blood. My father started his career selling Good Humor ice cream and worked his way up to own one of the first Carvel franchise operations; he actually knew the founder, Tom Carvel. I wish I could say that eating all that ice cream while growing up left me sick of the stuff, but, unfortunately, that's just not the case. So I'm always looking for ways to indulge in ice cream treats without the calories. Here are a few tips I've picked up from my research that will help fellow ice cream lovers indulge without blowing their diets.

Juice Bar vs. Fudgsicle

They're both pretty good choices. You might think the fruit bar would be better for you because of the real fruit, but if you're craving chocolate, don't feel guilty about the very low-calorie Fudgsicle.

- Low Fat Fudgsicle: 60 calories, 1.5 g fat, 12 g carbs.
- Dreyer's Fruit Bar, strawberry: 80 calories, 0 g fat, 21 g carbs.

Italian Gelato vs. Sorbet vs. Italian Ices

I always thought that gelato was much lower in calories and fat than regular ice cream, but one cup of Ciao Bella gelato ranges from 360 to almost 500 calories, compared to 500 calories in a cup of Ben & Jerry's Cherry Garcia ice cream.

Sorbet or sherbet would be a better choice. For instance, Häagen-Dazs Strawberry Sorbet has 240 calories in a cup, and Edy's/Dreyer's Berry Rainbow Sherbet is only 260 calories per cup. Your best bet? Italian ices. Yes, that's right, Marino's Lemon Italian Ices are only 100 calories per cup—a real Calorie Bargain.

Wafer Cone vs. Sugar Cone vs. Waffle Cone

I was thrilled to find out that the wafer cone—which happens to be my favorite—is the best option of the three, at about 20 calories. Sugar cones have between 50 and 60 calories, while waffle cones are about 100 to 160. And watch out for the chocolate-covered waffle cones, which can pack on a whopping 320 calories—and that's before you even add the ice cream!

Ben & Jerry's Half Baked Low Fat Frozen Yogurt vs. Ben & Jerry's Half Baked Original Ice Cream

Any low-fat yogurt is typically a better deal than ice cream. Just make sure it's low fat or fat free.

- Ben & Jerry's Half Baked Low Fat Frozen Yogurt (½ cup): 190 calories, 3 g fat, 1.5 g saturated fat, 20 mg cholesterol, 35 g carbs, 5 g protein.

Calorie Bargain Spotlight

Calorie Bargain: The Skinny Cow Ice Cream Sandwiches, Vanilla

The Why: They call them sandwiches, but I refer to them as saucers (because they're round). Readers rave about these sandwiches.

The Health Bonus: They are filling (you will eat only one), tasty, and low in calories—what more can you ask?

What We Liked Best: I tasted them a number of times and thought they were pretty good, but everyone I gave samples to thought they were great.

What We Liked Least: the ingredients. In fact, the cookie part contains partially hydrogenated soybean oil (a sign of trans fat) and high-fructose corn syrup.

The Price: about $2.99 for a box of six.

Offerings: coffee, chocolate peanut butter, cookies 'n cream, mint, strawberry shortcake, vanilla, vanilla/chocolate.

Website: www.skinnycow.com.

Where to Buy: H-E-B, Randalls, Albertsons, Publix, Kroger, Meijer.

Ingredients: skim milk, wafer (bleached wheat flour, sugar, caramel color, dextrose, partially hydrogenated soybean oil, corn flour, high-fructose corn syrup, corn syrup, baking soda, modified cornstarch, salt, monoglycerides and diglycerides, soy lecithin, cocoa), sugar, corn syrup, water, polydextrose, cream, whey protein, fructan (dietary fiber), stabilizer (microcrystalline cellulose, cellulose gum, monoglycerides and diglycerides, locust bean gum, calcium sulfate, polysorbate 80, carrageenan), natural flavor, vitamin A palmitate.

Nutritional Analysis per Serving: 1 Sandwich
140 calories
1.5 g fat
30 g carbs
3 g protein
3 g fiber
90 mg sodium

- Ben & Jerry's Half Baked Original Ice Cream (½ cup): 280 calories, 14 g fat, 9 g saturated fat, 50 mg cholesterol, 34 g carbs, 5 g protein.

Organic vs. Regular Ice Cream

Just because the label says "organic" doesn't mean it has fewer calories. A ½-cup serving of Ben & Jerry's Vanilla Organic Ice Cream has 220 calories and 14 grams of fat, 10 of which are saturated. Ben & Jerry's Vanilla Original Ice Cream has 240 calories and 16 grams of fat (11 saturated) in a ½ cup. Organic cream and organic liquid sugars have no fewer calories than conventional cream and sugar.

- Ben & Jerry's Vanilla Organic Ice Cream (½ cup): 220 calories, 14 g fat, 10 g saturated fat, 65 mg cholesterol, 18 g carbs, 3 g protein.
- Ben & Jerry's Vanilla Original Ice Cream (½ cup): 240 calories, 16 g fat, 11 g saturated fat, 75 mg cholesterol, 19 g carbs, 4 g protein.

Sprinkles vs. Ground Walnuts

You'd think that sprinkles would be the clear winner because they're so small and seem so innocuous. But just one serving of either nuts or sprinkles has about 200 calories. If you really want one of these toppings, choose the nuts—at least they contain protein and more healthy fat.

- Walnuts (1 ounce): 190 calories, 17 g fat, 5 g carbs, 4 g protein.
- Sprinkles (4 tablespoons): 220 calories, 4 g fat, 46 g carbs.

Crushed Oreos vs. Hershey's Chocolate Syrup

There is no good choice here. Don't be fooled because the cookies are crushed; that just makes it easier to load two cookies' worth of crumbs onto your frozen yogurt for an additional 107 calories and 5 grams of fat. And don't let the "fat free" fool you: Just 4 tablespoons of Hershey's chocolate syrup has 200 calories! Also note that using peanut butter topping adds about 210 calories, and hot fudge about 140 calories. Best bet: fresh fruit (not in sugary syrup) or go bare!

- Oreo (2 cookies): 107 calories, 5 g fat, 16 g carbs.
- Hershey's chocolate syrup (4 tablespoons): 200 calories, 0 g fat, 50 g carbs.
- Smucker's Special Recipe Butterscotch Caramel Topping (4 tablespoons): 260 calories, 2 g fat, 60 g carbs.
- Smucker's Magic Shell Topping, chocolate (4 tablespoons): 420 calories, 34 g fat, 32 g carbs.

Calorie Bargain Spotlight

Calorie Bargain: PhillySwirl Fudge Swirl Stix and Sugar Free Swirl Pops

The Why: I've known about these great frozen treats for years, but they weren't available nationwide until now. The Stix are formulated just like ice cream, which improves the taste.

The Health Bonus: They're peanut/tree nut free, dairy free, egg free, soy free, and gluten free.

What We Liked Best: The Fudge Swirl Stix are my favorites. They're a bit higher in calories, but at 57 per serving, they're still low enough to be a Calorie Bargain.

What We Liked Least: Unfortunately, these are still a little hard to find. You can go to the company website and use the locator tool to find a store near you.

The Price: approximately $10 for a box of forty.

Offerings: Sugar Free Swirl Pops, Fudge Swirl Stix, Vanilla Cream, Raspberry, Strawberry, Orange Sorbet, Cherry Sorbet.

Website: www.phillyswirl.com.

Where to Buy: Sam's Club, Wal-Mart, local grocery store.

Ingredients

Sugar Free Swirl Pops
Water, sorbitol, erythritol, polydextrose, glycerine, natural and artificial flavorings, strawberry concentrate, lemon concentrate, orange concentrate, pectin, xanthan gum, guar gum, ascorbic acid (vitamin C), sucralose, acesulfame-K (sweeteners), Red 40, Yellow 5 and 6, Blue 1.

Fudge Swirl Stix

Water, sugar, milk fat, nonfat milk, buttermilk, whey, corn syrup, cocoa (processed with alkali), cellulose gum, disodium phosphate, guar gum, pectin, calcium phosphate, modified cornstarch, salt, locust bean gum, gelatin, vanilla, artificial flavor, caramel color, colors F, D, and C 5 & 6, Red 40, vitamin A palmitate.

Nutritional Analysis per Serving

Sugar Free Swirl Pops—(1 Bar)	Fudge Swirl Stix—(1 Bar)
10 calories	57 calories
0 g fat	0.5 g fat
4 g carbs	12 g carbs
0 g protein	1 g protein
1 g fiber	0 g fiber
0 mg sodium	15 mg sodium

Calorie Bargain Spotlight

Calorie Bargain: Klondike Slim a Bear 100 Calorie Bars

The Why: No more looking longingly through the frosty doors in the freezer aisle, marveling about what we would do for a Klondike Bar.

The Health Bonus: At only 100 calories each, you get to eat the whole thing and still feel like you're getting a good deal.

What We Liked Best: That nice, crunchy chocolate layer on the outside.

What We Liked Least: For the purists, these treats are not free from chemicals and preservatives. And they aren't great for the low-carb crowd.

The Price: about $4 for a six-pack.

Offerings: vanilla, vanilla-chocolate, fudge.

Website: http://www.icecreamusa.com/klondike.

Where to Buy: your local grocery store.

Ingredients: artificially flavored vanilla ice cream: nonfat milk, buttermilk, sugar, polydextrose, fructose, lactitol, milk fat, propylene glycol monoesters, monoglycerides and diglycerides, cellulose gum, locust bean gum, guar gum, natural and artificial flavor, carrageenan, vitamin A palmitate, annatto (for color), ice-structuring protein. Wafer: bleached wheat flour, sugar, caramel color, dextrose, partially hydrogenated soybean oil, corn flour, cocoa, high-fructose corn syrup, corn syrup, modified cornstarch, baking soda, salt, monoglycerides and diglycerides, soy lecithin.

Nutritional Analysis per Serving: 1 Sandwich
100 calories
1.5 g fat
21 g carbs
1 g protein
2 g fiber
20 mg sodium

Food Fads, Facts, and Fiction

There are a lot of marketing messages trying to get you to eat this or drink that, and while some are fact, many are fictions and fads. Here are a few of the fads, facts, and fictions on your supermarket shelves.

Special K Diet

Fad: By following the Special K plan, you will lose up to 6 pounds in just two weeks. The plan: Eat Kellogg's Special K cereal with ⅔ cup skim milk and fruit for two meals a day. Eat your third meal as usual. For snacks, choose from fresh fruits and vegetables or a Special K Cereal Bar.

Fact: One cup of Special K cereal has 110 calories. Add 60 calories for skim milk, 60 to 80 for the fruit, and you're about 230 calories per meal. Basically, you're lowering your overall calorie intake, so of course you're going to lose weight. However, you need to ask yourself if you can get by on just a bowl of cereal with a piece of fruit for breakfast *and* lunch.

Fiction: There's nothing about Special K that will cause you to lose more weight than if you were having a low-calorie, healthy, water-based soup twice a day. You could call that the

Soup Diet. Or how about the Carrot Stick Diet or the Oatmeal Diet? The question is: Can you stick with any of these diets? The answer is probably no.

Plus, Special K has added sugar and is one of the few remaining cereals that is not whole grain.

Bottom Line: You probably can lose weight eating just cereal for two meals a day. However, if you substitute any lower-calorie food for what you ordinarily eat, you will lose weight over time.

Low-fat/Low-carb Foods

Fad: The idea is that you will lose weight by consuming these foods as opposed to traditional versions.

Fact: Sometimes low-fat or low-carb foods really are better choices, but it depends. The best examples of great low-fat foods are dairy products like milk, cheese, and yogurt—all excellent sources of calcium. For instance, if you switch from 2 tablespoons of half-and-half in your coffee (39 calories) to skim milk (10 calories), you've just saved about 30 calories per cup. If you drink 3 cups per day, that's 90 calories, or about an 8-pound weight loss in a year. Other low-fat/low-carb options that probably make a difference include mayonnaise, certain soups, and sometimes even cakes, muffins, and chips.

Fiction: Many of these foods don't taste very good, and/or have added sugar (low-fat foods) or fat (low-carb foods), and end up having roughly the same number of calories as their traditional counterparts. Also, sometimes when we eat lower-carb or lower-fat foods, we think it's OK to overindulge because it's "diet food."

Bottom Line: Don't just go by what the label says. You also need to look at the calories, compare the taste, and watch your behavior—do you end up eating more?

Yogurt Cereal

Fad: If your cereal is made with yogurt, it must be healthy.

Fact: Low-fat and nonfat yogurts can be extremely low in calories and have many reported health benefits, including improved digestion, prevention of intestinal infection, and increased immune function.

Fiction: Unfortunately, you're really not getting all those yogurt-related health benefits when you grab a box of Yogurt Burst Cheerios Vanilla or Life Vanilla Yogurt Crunch. The assumption that the yogurt coating is somehow channeling the health perks of regular yogurt is not accurate.

Bottom Line: The coating appears to be nothing but a frosting. However, on the plus side, these cereals are made with whole grains, and the calories are not excessive: ¾ cup of Life's cereal has 126 calories, while ¾ cup of Cheerios has 120.

Whole Grains = Diet Food

Fad: Cereals, snacks, pasta—foods in all categories are becoming "whole grain" to convince you that eating them will make you healthier and trimmer.

Fact: When grains are refined, fiber and other nutrients, such as vitamin E, vitamin B_6, and magnesium, are removed. There

Diet Detective's What You Need to Know

Q: If the ingredient list says hydrogenated soybean or partially hydrogenated soybean oil, does that mean it's good for you?

A: Unfortunately, just because the label has the word *soybean* doesn't mean it's automatically healthy. If it has the word *hydrogenated,* it has trans fats; meaning the manufacturer has blasted corn, soybean, or other vegetable oils with hydrogen, which helps to keep them stable, makes them more solid, and lengthens their shelf life. This process turns good fats (unsaturated) into the unhealthiest fat: trans fat. Check the ingredient label of all processed food for the word *hydrogenated,* and avoid those foods when you can.

The good news is that if you see the words *nonhydrogenated* or *liquid soybean oil,* it means the product contains no trans fat.

has been evidence that whole grains reduce the risk of cardiovascular disease, diabetes, and certain cancers, whereas refined grains do not. Plus, fiber increases feelings of satiety, which may help you eat less—and lose weight.

Fiction: Most whole-grain products do not have fewer calories than products made with white flour. That's not to say you can't find a low-cal whole-grain food—you certainly can. But while switching from refined grains to whole grains is great, some of us are simply eating too much of them.

Bottom Line: They're better, but you can't give yourself carte blanche to eat more of anything that says "whole grain." The calories add up just as fast.

100-calorie Portion-controlled Snacks

Fad: Balance Bars, Oreo Thin Crisps, Wheat Thins, popcorn packs. Food companies are packaging 100-calorie snacks on the theory that by limiting your snacks, you will lose weight and be healthy.

Facts: Portion control is a huge issue. We eat what we see; therefore, packaging foods in smaller quantities helps. And seeing how little you get for 100 calories can also help you learn the true value of a calorie.

Fiction: "Know thyself." Will you really limit yourself to just one pack, or will you be going back for more?

Bottom Line: If you can avoid going for more than one pack, and it helps to limit your consumption, this is a great way to stay on track.

Part Four

AT HOME AND IN THE KITCHEN

Once you've found your Calorie Bargain foods in the supermarket, you'll need to know what to do with them once you bring them home to your kitchen. To help you do that, here are some great hints and tips for taking the calories out of your own favorites by substituting ingredients or reengineering the cooking method. I'll also provide you with suggestions for Calorie Bargain picnic foods and lunches you can pack. Before you start cooking, however, you need to know about some essential Calorie Bargain kitchen tools.

Kitchen Tools

There are many cooking techniques you can use to help control your weight and develop better food behaviors. Here are a few kitchen gadgets and appliances to get you on the path to healthier living.

Cooking Spray/Oil Mister

Since all oils contain about 120 calories and 14 grams of fat per tablespoon, using an oil mister or cooking spray can save you hundreds of calories per meal by significantly reducing the quantity of oil you are using.

Misters or cooking sprays can be used to flavor foods and to create a nonstick surface for sautéing, grilling, baking, or any form of cooking. Use olive or canola oil to fill your mister. Even though both still have calories, they're low in saturated fat and better for your heart. You can also fill your mister or a spray bottle with salad dressing to keep the calories down.

Expect to pay $10 to $20 for a good mister (example: Misto Sprayer), which you can find in any cookware or department store. If you'd rather use a ready-made version like Pam, keep in mind that although it appears to be calorie free, a one-second spray contains about 7 calories. Still, you would need about seventeen seconds to equal 1 tablespoon of oil, so you're still better off.

Steamer Basket

Steaming is a terrific way to keep calories low without losing valuable nutrients. You can steam chicken, fish, or vegetables—they're all delicious. For about $15, you can pick up an efficient, easy-to-use stainless steel steamer basket that you insert in a pot of boiling water. For extra flavor, add lemon juice, wine, soy sauce, or flavored vinegar to the cooking water, or add your favorite spices (thyme, rosemary, garlic, and so on). Or you can get an electric vegetable and rice steamer, which is a good investment.

Nonstick Pans

Everyone should have a set of nonstick pans in the kitchen. With a nonstick skillet and a quick blast of cooking spray, you have a recipe for success for any meal—from vegetable and meat dishes, to stir-fries and pasta sauces, or even egg-white omelets. A nonstick surface allows you to control the fat content by using less oil, without sacrificing flavor. Also, in a nonstick pan you can cook with low-sodium chicken broth or white wine for additional flavor and moisture without added fat.

A good nonstick frying pan (like Calphalon) will cost about $30 or so. Keep in mind that you will need to replace your pan as soon as it looks worn out. These pans don't last forever, and it's essential to keep the surface nonstick, or you will find yourself using more and more oil to get the job done.

Dishware

Believe it or not, when it comes to dishes, size matters. Experts have demonstrated that the smaller your plates, cups, or bowls, the less food you are likely to consume. I've seen this in my own kitchen. I used to have these oversized bowls that probably held about three cups of cereal. I replaced them with bowls that hold only about one cup and consequently cut back on my cereal consumption. It's a good idea to measure how much food your plates, bowls, and glassware hold. This will allow you to keep a closer watch on your portion sizes without stressing out.

Air Popper

Instead of making a batch of popcorn on the stove or buying microwave popcorn, invest in an air popper and a bag of kernels. You'll get more popcorn for less money, and you'll save plenty of calories and fat grams. Air-popped popcorn has about 30 calories per cup—not a bad treat. Or, as an alternative, Nordic Ware makes a microwave-safe container that you can use to pop your own microwave popcorn (about $9).

Rotisserie Ovens

You can use these ovens to cook chicken, turkey, ribs, Cornish hens, kebabs—just about anything you can grill. The concept of a rotisserie oven is to cook food using its natural fat so that no additional oil is necessary and the natural great taste of the food is maintained. If you don't want to spend the money on a rotisserie oven, try a roasting rack that suspends the meat above a roasting pan. For extra flavor, season the meat with your favorite herbs, such as rosemary or tarragon, before roasting.

Indoor Grills

Compact indoor grills allow you to enjoy grilled foods when outdoor grilling is just not possible. They use electric burners to provide smokeless, even heat and offer a nonstick surface that is much easier to clean than a standard outdoor grill. They work particularly well for vegetables, meat, fish, and chicken. Best of all, they are designed to drain away unnecessary fat and grease through special sloping grooves on the grilling surface.

One of the most famous indoor grills on the market is the George Foreman Grill, which starts at about $20. Alternatively, opt for one of the nonstick grills that sit on your stovetop and are designed to drip excess fat off the cooking surface into a pan filled with water. Le Creuset grill pans cost about $60 each, and the more affordable Chefmaster stovetop grills run about $15 to $20.

Plastic Storage Containers

If you're going to cook, you need somewhere to store leftovers. Invest in a durable set of lidded containers in various sizes and shapes. You can get the reusable ones by Ziploc or Glad, which are also dishwasher safe. That way you don't have to feel obligated to clear your plate or finish everything in the pot. These containers are also handy for taking your healthy leftovers to the office, saving you calories and money.

Kitchen Scales

How much are you eating? It's anyone's guess. Most people underestimate their portion sizes, which is why savvy dieters use kitchen scales to figure out exactly how much they're eating. Salter makes a variety of kitchen scales that typically sell for about $50 to $100, but less expensive scales are available too. There are also scales that give you nutrient information electronically—right on the scale—so you don't even have to look it up. Measuring cups, spoons, and ladles are also critical tools for the conscious eater. These are inexpensive and make it much easier to keep track of your portions.

Gravy Separator

Gravy is often the best part of the dish, but it's full of fattening grease. For about $15, you can purchase a gravy separator (such as the one sold by Sur La Table). This neat little device, with a spout that pours from the bottom rather than the top of the container, looks like something that belongs in a laboratory rather than a kitchen—and it actually removes the fat as you're pouring the gravy.

Other Kitchen Helpers

Food Processor, Mini Food Processor, Blender: The food processor slices, grinds, dices, chops, and shreds. "You can chop vegetables in the food processor by using the pulse button, although you have to be careful they don't turn to mush," says Nancy Mills, coauthor of *Faster! I'm Starving! 100 Dishes in 25 Minutes or Less* (Gibbs Smith, 2006). You can also turn your blender into a chopping device. Fill the blender halfway with water. Cut the vegetables into roughly 2-inch pieces, add them to the blender, and pulse until they are the size you want. Then drain the contents of the blender through a strainer, Mills adds.

Microwave: A microwave is invaluable for defrosting meat and reheating leftovers. It also bakes a potato in about seven minutes.

Knives: You need a good set of sharp knives for any preparation or cooking situation.

Preparation and Stocking the Kitchen

Although preparing your own meals can seem more complicated than eating out, here are a few tips that can help you to
streamline the process and make it simpler to create healthier
foods at home.

Prepare in Advance

If you think you're going to be able to wing it and prepare
quality foods quickly at home, you're mistaken. Planning
meals and shopping in advance ensure that you don't wind up
walking into your kitchen, opening the fridge, closing it in
frustration, and gathering the kids to go to McDonald's.

Cut It Up: Cut up vegetables such as onions, broccoli, peppers,
and asparagus in advance. Put them in pre-portioned baggies
or containers and store them in the fridge. "You can even
freeze them, so when you need chopped onions in a recipe,
you can just grab them out of the freezer," says Antoinette
Kuritz, a San Diego–based home-cooking expert and mom.
"Do the same with peppers and other vegetables, and cheeses
such as Parmesan, Romano, and Jarlsberg."

Buy Ingredients Partially Prepared: Although this can sometimes be more expensive, it still costs less than eating out—or

eating unhealthy meals. Get bags of prewashed lettuce, broccoli, and cauliflower florets or precut mixed vegetables. Check out the salad bar to stock up on other precut veggies. Buy jars of crushed fresh garlic. You can even get egg whites in containers so you don't have to crack any eggs—just pour the whites into a pan, add vegetables, and serve with whole wheat toast for a wonderful dinner omelet.

Cold Cuts: Low-calorie cold cuts such as sliced turkey and chicken are great to have on hand to create a quick and filling sandwich. They're presliced, so just slap a few slices onto a whole wheat wrap or piece of bread, add a little mustard, tomato, and lettuce, and voilà: a satisfying meal that's ready in minutes.

Precook Foods: Cook and freeze foods in advance. You can even prepare grains such as brown rice or quinoa and freeze them in serving-size portions in freezer bags. Simply take out a serving and thaw as needed for recipes for a main course or a side dish, suggests Janet Luhrs, author of *The Simple Living Guide*.

Plan before Shopping: Come up with general categories such as soups, stews, stir-fries, and grains. Within each category, have a recipe in mind, and write out your list of ingredients before you go food shopping, says Luhrs. Try to choose recipes for which all the ingredients are available at one location; you're more likely to give up if you have to shop at too many stores to get what you need.

Same Ingredients, Multiple Recipes: Pick a couple of recipe favorites and use them in different ways. For instance, use grilled chicken to top salads, pasta, and vegetables and to make sandwiches for lunch. A simple roasted chicken makes a fantastic and versatile entree that everyone loves, and the leftovers can be turned into a quick chicken salad, diced into curried rice or an omelet, or added to soup. It's easy to roast a couple of chickens at the same time and use one for Sunday dinner while reserving the other for turning into additional meals later that week, adds Chef Kirk Bachmann, vice president of Le Cordon Bleu Schools North America.

Buy It Smaller, Thinner, and Prepared: According to Nancy Mills, "The more surface area that is exposed to heat, the faster a food will cook, so buy your meats, poultry, and everything else cut into thinner and/or smaller pieces."

If you're parceling your meats yourself, Mills offers more tips to speed up the process. "It's easier to cut chicken and beef into thin slices or strips when the meat is partly frozen. Plus, you don't have to wait for the meat to completely thaw before cooking it. Steak or chicken cut into two-inch-long, half-inch-wide strips can be stir-fried in two to three minutes. Ground meat cooks much faster than whole pieces of meat. Thin slices of vegetables cook faster. For instance, very thin potato slices cook in less than ten minutes in soups, whereas a whole potato will take twenty to twenty-five minutes."

You can also pound boneless beef, pork, or chicken to help it cook quicker. Mills suggests pounding the meat between sheets of wax paper with a rolling pin or the side of a heavy can.

Get your hamburgers and turkey burgers in patty form, or package them yourself after buying ground meat and store them in the freezer in meal packs.

"Tired and Hungry" Recipes: Create three or four recipes that require very little thought and are ready to go. For instance, you might find it easy to cook frozen chicken strips or turkey burgers on the grill with some precut veggies. Come up with a few of these, and make sure that you always have the ingredients on hand.

Stock Up

Soups and Other Canned Foods: It is not cheating to open up a can of soup or tuna for a fast dinner. Stock up on these foods in abundance. They're filling, inexpensive, and right there when you don't feel like making a big deal out of dinner. To keep canned soups healthy, make sure the calories are below 120 per serving and the sodium under 750 milligrams.

Spices and Condiments: Creating healthier foods at home is also about having a well-stocked spice cabinet and lots of condiments in the refrigerator. Herbs and spices are a calorie-free way to add flavor to your meals. "If I could buy only five spices," says Chef John Greeley of the famed '21' Club in New York, "they would be black pepper, smoked paprika, curry powder, herbes de Provence, and coriander seed. I always have ketchup, mustard, vinegar, Worcestershire sauce, hot sauce, soy sauce, and honey on hand, as well as lemons and limes."

Other Healthful Helpers

- Fat-free cooking sprays are an easy way to eliminate fat from your favorite dishes.
- Fat-free, low-sodium chicken broth.
- Limes, lemons, and oranges add terrific flavor to any meal without added fat.
- Rice vinegar, apple cider vinegar, and balsamic vinegar add a lot of zing.
- Garlic and onions are another way to spice up whatever you're cooking.
- Barbecue sauce.
- Low-cal salad dressings (watch for sugar and sodium content).

- Canned beans.
- Bread crumbs.
- Flour.
- Carrots.
- Celery.
- Cornstarch.

Diet Detective's What You Need to Know

Avoiding the "Nibble Factor": A bite or two of a food never seems like it'll do much damage to your diet. But look back at your three-day food challenge—you'll be able to see how those little bites affect you over a whole day. Here are a few suggestions for getting away from the nibble factor:

- **When do you pick?** Stay conscious of your "picking times"; that is, when you're most likely to pick at food.
- **Leave the kitchen.** Stay away from key "picking areas," such as the kitchen or a buffet table.
- **Go ahead, waste it.** Don't finish the food your family or friends leave on their plates.
- **Elude the food.** Avoid leaving candy dishes or bowls of chips and other foods out and within easy reach.
- **Say no to freebies.** Skip free samples at stores, and don't feel you have to pick from other people's plates because you don't like wasting food.
- **Drink smarter.** Curb your urge to take a sip of someone else's beer or soda or to take a few swallows from the juice container when you open the door of the fridge.

How Those Nibbles Add Up: Whether it's unconscious eating in the kitchen or social eating at a party, those little bites can add up. Don't think it can be *that* bad?

The smallest nibble on the list—the Hershey's Kiss—can add up to almost three pounds if you eat it every day for a year.

The biggest nibble—the slice of cheese—can add up to almost 20 pounds!

And if you hate exercise, keep in mind that someone who weighs 150 pounds needs to walk for 15 minutes just to work off a 100-calorie snack. Remember that before you lick the peanut butter off the knife!

Passing through the Kitchen
- 4 spoonfuls of ice cream from the freezer: 150 calories
- 5 Lay's Classic Potato Chips: 40 calories
- 1 Double Stuf Oreo cookie: 70 calories
- 10 Rold Gold Classic Style Tiny Twists pretzels: 65 calories
- A handful of trail mix: 174 calories
- 1 Hershey's Kiss: 25 calories
- A handful of raisins: 86 calories

Cooking
- A slice of cheese: 189 calories
- Crumbs from the bottom of a bag of cookies: 140 calories
- A spoonful of cookie dough: 32 calories
- A spoonful of chocolate chips: 80 calories
- Licking peanut butter from a knife while making a sandwich: 95 calories

Out and About
- 4 wheat crackers: 76 calories
- 2 big handfuls of movie theater popcorn: 168 calories (and 13 grams of fat!)
- 1 bite of a hot dog at a baseball game: 48 calories

"Stealing" Food
- 2 bites of the chocolate cake your sister ordered for dessert: 117 calories
- 10 fries from your friend's plate: 53 calories
- A bite of a McDonald's cheeseburger: 40 calories

Leftovers
- 2 bites of cold pizza: 77 calories
- 3 bites of leftover Chinese food: about 70 calories

Drinks
- A gulp of OJ from the fridge: 28 calories
- A sip of soda: 25 calories

Secrets of Eating Healthy at Home

Buying healthy ingredients and cooking them at home gives you the best chance of controlling your weight. But even eating at home can have a negative effect on your waistline, depending on how you prepare the food. Here are a few tips for keeping your kitchen "light."

Stuff It with Vegetables

The next time you throw a burger on the grill, it doesn't have to wreak havoc with your diet. Just a few simple substitutions can save you a lot of calories and fat. To start, use lean ground beef instead of regular, or, for even less fat, try ground white-meat turkey. Next, give your burger some extra texture and flavor by mixing the meat with chopped mushrooms, peppers, and onions. You'll have the same size burger, but it will be much lower in calories—and you'll also be getting the health benefits of all those vegetables.

For variety, you can also experiment with chopped water chestnuts or sun-dried (not oil-packed) tomatoes. Vegetables are great as fillers for omelets and sandwiches, among other foods.

Try this when you're making meatloaf. To compensate for

the lack of fat in the beef, spray the pan with cooking spray to keep the meat from sticking.

- Hamburger with ground beef (6 ounces): 481 calories, 34 g fat, 0 g carbs, 40 g protein.
- Hamburger with lean beef and vegetables (6 ounces): 364 calories, 21 g fat, 14 g carbs, 30 g protein.
- Ground turkey breast, 99 percent fat free (6 ounces): 180 calories, 1.5 g fat, 42 g protein.

Replace Whole Dairy Products

You can replace almost any dairy product (cheese, milk, sour cream, to name a few) called for in a recipe with a low-fat or nonfat version, saving a significant number of calories. For instance, chef Terry Conlan, author of *Fresh* (Favorite Recipes Press, 2002) and executive chef at the Lake Austin Spa Resort in Austin, Texas, says his single favorite product for cooking is fat-free sweetened condensed milk. "It does everything that whole condensed milk will do for a lot less calories. We use it to make flan, cream pies, roasted tomato bisque, and much more." He also recommends melting reduced-fat or fat-free cream cheese to use in lieu of heavy cream or half-and-half. For example, he makes a quick and easy key lime pie using fat-free sweetened condensed milk with a combination of fat-free and reduced-fat cream cheese.

Pound It Out

One of the tricks I discovered when I owned a restaurant, and later used to help me lose weight, was to use a mallet to pound and tenderize chicken and other meats, making the portions appear larger. In fact, I now have the local supermarket pound out the boneless, skinless chicken breasts I buy so they are paper thin. This also allows for very rapid cooking using almost no oil.

Use Artificial or High-intensity Sweeteners

The word on the street is that Splenda (sucralose) can be used to replace sugar in almost all cooking, including baking, because it doesn't lose sweetness with high heat and because you substitute it in exactly the same measurements as sugar. So, if your recipe calls for a tablespoon of sugar, you can use a tablespoon of Splenda and get exactly the same results. Is it healthy? It's probably healthier to eat natural foods; however, the evidence seems to indicate that Splenda is not unhealthy or harmful.

Juice It

Using a juicer to make and create sauces is another way to cut hefty calorie costs while cooking at home. Scott Uehlein, executive chef at Canyon Ranch Resorts in Tucson, Arizona, finds that many vegetables and fruits can be juiced into a great sauce to replace the creamy, buttery sauces traditionally used to add flavor to foods. His favorite tip is to juice a golden, ripe pineapple, which makes a thick, tasty sauce with plenty of froth. The pineapple juice can be used as a sweet and sour dip and can also be brushed on steamed, grilled, baked, or broiled foods during the cooking process. He especially likes it with lobster tails.

Chef Uehlein also suggests juicing and then simmering sweet, ripe tomatoes or carrots in a pan until they reduce and thicken, then simply adding sea salt, lemon, and dill for a great-tasting, low-calorie sauce.

If you don't own a juicer, food processors and mixers often have juicing attachments available.

Make It Thick and Tasty

One of my favorite cooking tricks is to use cornstarch as an instant, fat-free thickener for sauces and gravies. "Just mix some cornstarch in cold water and add it to your stir fry," offers famed healthy-cooking expert Cary Neff, author of *Conscious Cuisine* (Sourcebooks Trade, October 2002) and culinary consultant to Jenny Craig. "Sauté vegetables with nonfat spray, seasoning, and lemon juice; add cornstarch, and then toss with pasta instead of making a cream-based pasta sauce. Or add cornstarch to meat juices to create a thick gravy without the added fat."

Pureed vegetables are another way to thicken sauces and stews. "Just a bit of cooked, pureed potato thickens 'cream' of asparagus soup so that no cream is needed. The same is true with pureed beans in veggie soup," says Jorj Morgan, author of *Fresh Traditions* (Cumberland House, August 2004).

Use Condiments, Herbs, and Spices

Whereas a bland "diet" meal can be pretty boring, highly flavored condiments help satisfy the senses. "Use a variety of vinegars such as raspberry, balsamic, and red wine," suggests Melanie R. Polk, MM Sc, RD, director of nutrition education at the American Institute for Cancer Research.

You can also use low-fat vinaigrette dressing for your cooking. "By coating vegetables, chicken, or other foods with a

Calorie Bargain Recipe

Guiltless Potato Fries
1 medium baking potato (3" diameter): 133 calories, 0 g fat, 31 g carbs.
Flavored bread crumbs (1 tablespoon): 28 calories, 0 g fat, 5 g carbs,
seasoning

OK, so they're not really fried, but they are just as good as fries, and
maybe even better because there's no dieter's remorse. I realize that the
carbs are a bit high for those on a low-carb program, but these fries are
so filling and low in calories that it's worth eating them to prevent other
cravings. (But remember, they should be considered a treat and eaten in
combination with other foods so that they don't cause a spike in your
blood sugar.) Here's how you make them:

Preheat oven to 450 degrees.

Scrub and wash one baking potato. Slice into eighths lengthwise.

Cover a baking sheet with aluminum foil and spray the foil lightly with
cooking spray.

Place potato wedges on the tray, and mist the potatoes with cooking
spray.

Sprinkle with onion powder, garlic powder, onion flakes, salt, pepper,
and paprika. Then sprinkle with 1 tablespoon of flavored bread crumbs.
Reapply a light coat of cooking spray and bake for approximately 40 to
45 minutes or to desired crispness. Spray with a light coating of I Can't
Believe It's Not Butter Spray before serving.

low-fat vinaigrette, you avoid the fattening oils [1 tablespoon
of oil has 120 calories], with flavorful results," reminds Neff.
In addition, culinary experts recommend cooking with fat-
free, low-sodium chicken or vegetable broth to avoid using
oil; it's a great way to bake, roast, simmer, or sauté.

You can also experiment with unusual condiments such as Liquid Smoke. "Liquid Smoke is a seasoning made from water and concentrated smoke that mimics the flavor of smoked meats," says Lawrence J. Cheskin, MD, professor of medicine and human nutrition at Johns Hopkins Bloomberg School of Public Health and author of *Recipes for Weight Loss* (Rebus, 2003). "It can be used to enhance almost anything, but especially split pea soup, braised greens, and baked beans, and it has virtually no calories." Buy Liquid Smoke online at www.colgin.com.

Melanie Polk also suggests using fresh herbs. "There's nothing like cutting fresh herbs such as thyme, cilantro, or rosemary from a pot on the patio and adding them to cooked grains, grilled chicken, or fresh green beans."

Fast and Healthy Home Cooking

Eating out is certainly convenient, especially with our busy lives. But there are ways to make cooking at home less time consuming and more feasible for even the busiest people. Here are a few tips for making faster food at home.

Batch Cooking and Other Ideas

Cook and Freeze: One of the most effective ways to ensure that you always have a healthy meal on hand is to cook several meals at once. Here's a recommendation from Antoinette Kuritz, a San Diego–based home cooking expert and mom: "Cook pork chops or chicken in huge batches, freeze on cookie sheets, and then store in the freezer in a sealed container with wax paper between the pieces. Take out only as many pieces as you need, spray both sides with no-stick spray, place them in a cold oven, set it to 425 degrees, and bake for twenty to twenty-five minutes, turning ten minutes before done."

Minimize Cleanup: Do all your major cooking the day before your regular housecleaning day. That way you won't have to clean the kitchen twice, adds Kuritz.

Form a Cooking Co-op: "Ask three friends if they'd like to form a cooking co-op," suggests Janet Peterson, author of *Family Dinners: Easy Ways to Feed Your Kids and Get Them Talking at the Table* (Gibbs Smith, 2006). "Each person prepares dinner one night a week for all four families. You get four great meals and only one night in the kitchen."

Have a Food Party: To make batch cooking a fun event and to share recipes to keep meals interesting, invite a friend or two over to cook batch meals together, or cook in your own kitchens and swap vacuum-sealed meals later, says Alicia Ross, coauthor of *Cheap. Fast. Good!* (Workman, 2005).

Make Theme Meals: To take the effort out of deciding what's for dinner, create a theme for each night of the week. For example, Monday can be soup night; Tuesday, taco night; Wednesday, salad bar, and so forth, suggests Carrie Hanna, the author of *Florida's Backyard* (Authorhouse, 2002).

Make Extra: As an alternative to cooking entire meals ahead, just double or triple up on some basic building blocks that will speed you through future meals. Browning batches of ground beef and onions, poaching or grilling chicken, and baking potatoes ahead of time are easy ways to cut down on meal prep time, says Alicia Ross.

Post the Menu: Plan weeknight meals in advance and post them, so there is no question of "What's for dinner?" when you get home. That way you shop once a week and get everyone on board, says Peggy Katalinich, food director for *Family Circle* magazine.

Cooking Out/Dining In: They're springing up all over the country, with names such as Dinner by Design (www.dinnerbydesignkitchen.com), Dream Dinners (www.dreamdinners.com), and Dinners Ready (www.dinnersready.com). These are basically storefront kitchens where you can prepare an entire week's worth of meals in one session. They do the planning, shopping, and chopping and provide everything you need to prepare healthy, delicious meals. Dinners Ready even has a chef and nutritionist on staff. People assemble their meals in the store, which is set up like a home economics class, then take them home, and freeze and cook as needed. That way you know you have all the ingredients, your meals are portion controlled, you can pick what's healthiest—and there isn't any cleanup.

Cookbooks

There are so many quick-and-easy cookbooks available that you would think nobody eats dinner out. Just take a peek on Amazon.com, and you'll find a host of books, including:

- *Rachael Ray's 30-minute Get Real Meals: Eat Healthy without Going to Extremes* by Rachael Ray (paperback, Clarkson Potter, 2005)
- *Weight Watchers Make It in Minutes: Easy Recipes in 15, 20, and 30 Minutes* by Weight Watchers (paperback, Wiley, 2001)
- *American Heart Association Quick & Easy Cookbook: More Than 200 Healthful Recipes You Can Make in Minutes* by the American Heart Association (paperback, Clarkson Potter, 2001)
- *Cooking Light Superfast Suppers: Speedy Solutions for Dinner Dilemmas* by *Cooking Light* magazine, Anne C. Cain and Anne C. Chappell, editors (hardcover, Oxmoor House, 2003)
- *Weight Watchers New Complete Cookbook* by Weight Watchers (ring-bound, Wiley, 2006)

Store It Right

Oxygen is not a friend to food, says Chef Kirk Bachmann, vice president of education for Le Cordon Bleu Schools North America, and freezing food that is not protected from oxygen will cause it to dry out. Refrigerators and freezers are actually

---

Calorie Bargain Recipe Spotlight

Calorie Bargain: Homemade Garlic or Herb Toast

The Why: You'll feel like you're cheating by eating great-tasting garlic bread.

The Health Bonus: Every time I make this for people, they're amazed at how delicious it tastes—and then they're blown away when I reveal that it's low in calories and fat.

Ingredients: 2 slices of low-calorie bread, preferably 100 percent whole grain (under 75 calories per slice), 5 to 10 quick sprays of margarine spray (for instance, I Can't Believe It's Not Butter Spray), garlic powder and/or herbs.

Preparation: Cover the bread with a few quick bursts of margarine spray, sprinkle with garlic powder, and cut up into strips. Toast the bread to desired crispiness.

Nutritional Analysis per Serving: 2 Slices of Arnold Bakery Light Wheat Bread
90 calories
1.5 g fat
17 g carbs
5 g protein
5 g fiber
150 mg sodium

cold dehumidifiers. One of the easiest ways to protect your food is to put it in a plastic bag with a zipper closing. Just make sure you get all the air out before you zip the bag shut. They come in a variety of sizes that you can use for different quantities.

You can also purchase storage containers in different sizes. Or, if you want to get fancy, you could invest in a sealing machine. "I use a vacuum sealer to freeze my food, but plastic wrap works just fine," says Chef John Greeley of the famed '21' Club in New York. "A vacuum sealer removes air and traps moisture in the product, avoiding freezer burn. When you're wrapping food to be frozen, do it tightly and avoid air pockets. Chicken, pork, and shrimp freeze well, but I avoid freezing fish," he adds, "although there are some exceptions to the rule."

Which foods don't freeze well? According to Chef Bachmann, "Foods with a low moisture content, such as baked goods, tend to get stale or become dry and brittle when they freeze. For example, frozen bread has a much shorter shelf life when it's defrosted. You can, however, freeze solid foods in broths or sauces relatively easily and still maintain the texture of the food. Stews, soups, chili, and spaghetti sauce freeze extremely well. Starchy foods like potatoes, turnips, pasta, dumplings, and rice tend to become mushy when frozen because the water crystals expand during the freezing process and tear apart the delicate, papery walls of the grains."

"Make sure to organize your freezer and keep a list of what's in there," says Antoinette Kuritz. "A full freezer is a wonderful thing, but not if you forget what you've prepared and leave it until it gets freezer burned." Also, keep in mind that the faster food freezes, the better chance you have of maintaining quality, adds Bachmann. And allow space between frozen items so that cold air can circulate around them.

Breakfast

It seems like at least once a month a new journal article touts the benefits of eating breakfast. One of the most persuasive statistics I've seen is that people who skip breakfast are four and a half times more likely to be overweight than those who don't. But just because it's important to eat breakfast doesn't mean that you don't have to watch *what* you eat. Here are a few tips to start your day with healthier choices.

Oatmeal vs. Granola vs. Farina (Cream of Wheat)

Most people assume that granola is a health food, but it's actually a snack food that originated in the late nineteenth century. Granola catapulted to fame in the 1960s, when the hippie movement made it its "all natural" cereal of choice as well as a popular and convenient treat at events like the 1969 Woodstock Music and Art Fair. Since the term *natural* is associated with *healthy*, granola "became" a health food. It had the right look: It's not frosted or brightly colored like high-calorie sweet cereals, and it looks like it should pack a lot of fiber, right? Unfortunately, granola fails to deliver as a healthy breakfast. With about 460 to 560 calories per cup, it's usually sweetened with sugar or honey and also comes with nuts and dried fruit, which significantly spike the calorie total. (To give you an idea, just 1 ounce of chopped walnuts has about 200 calories.)

Nearly all hot cereals—with the exception of farina and grits—are whole-grain dishes. Farina (cream of wheat) is made from the endosperm of the wheat kernel, which is milled to a fine consistency and then sifted to a texture similar to grits. The difference is that it's made from wheat instead of corn. One cup of farina has about 130 calories, not including any sugar you might add.

The clear winner from this group is the oatmeal, even though it could run a bit higher in calories. A ½ cup of dry quick oats—equal to about 1 cup cooked—has about 150 calories, but the instant oatmeal packets contain about 100 calories each. Oatmeal is packed with nutritional pluses, including protein, iron, magnesium, zinc, manganese, thiamin, and fiber. And you've probably seen food labels or TV commercials claiming that it lowers your cholesterol. That's because oats contain soluble fiber. According to research, soluble fiber (beta-glucan) may help lower blood cholesterol levels and reduce heart disease risk when included in a diet that is also low in saturated fat and cholesterol. The 3 grams per day of oat beta-glucan needed to lower cholesterol can be obtained by eating 1½ cups of cooked oatmeal (¾ cup of uncooked oatmeal), or roughly three packets of instant oatmeal. But be careful: Just as granola becomes a diet disaster as soon as it's sweetened and spruced up, oatmeal can deliver a higher-calorie punch if you add brown sugar, butter, honey, and/or whole milk.

Fit Tip: Stick to add-ons such as fresh fruit, cinnamon, and nutmeg to keep your oatmeal healthy.

Sausage vs. Bacon vs. Ham

Ham is the winner at only 25 to 30 calories per 1-ounce slice. In addition to being relatively low in calories, it's also low in saturated fat—the unhealthy fat that's linked to heart disease. Sausage and bacon, on the other hand, are not such good choices. If you were to pick between the two, sausage might just be the lesser evil. For instance, if you're frying up your own bacon, it's easy to start throwing strips in the pan, and before you know it, you'll have polished off a lot more than just two. At 70 or more calories per strip (not to mention 2 grams of saturated fat—about 10 percent of the daily recommendation), bacon is not a great choice. Caloriewise, things look a little better if you opt for Canadian bacon, which has 65 to 75 calories for 2 ounces. At least with the sausage, you probably won't eat more than two links, although they're no bargain either at 90 to 125 calories per link (and 3 grams of saturated fat). Sausage patties can be even worse, at almost 150 calories per patty.

Diet Detective's What You Need to Know

Q: Is butter better than margarine?

A: Even though margarine is often made with heart-healthy oil (for instance, canola), it fell out of favor for a while because it contained unhealthy partially hydrogenated oil, or trans fat. Plus, margarine has roughly the same amount of calories (about 100 calories per tablespoon) as butter. But now, especially since butter is loaded with unhealthy saturated fat, margarine has made a huge comeback because many manufacturers have eliminated trans fat from their products. Stick margarine still has trans fat, but the other types, including many tubs and sprays, have managed to do without. Check the label for saturated fat content and "trans fat free" claims.

Fit Tip: If you love bacon, try turkey bacon, which has half the calories (35 per strip) and saturated fat. Turkey sausage links are also better, at 67 calories each. But be wary of chicken apple sausage, which can be as bad as regular sausage. There are also some great meatless sausage links, such as Morningstar Farms Veggie Breakfast Sausage Links, which are only 40 calories each and also very low in saturated fat. Always check nutrition labels when available because calorie and fat content vary by brand.

Waffles vs. Pancakes vs. French Toast

Plain waffles and pancakes don't seem so bad caloriewise. And they're not if you just have one or two and are careful when applying the "extras" like butter, syrup, and sugar. A 6-inch homemade pancake has about 175 calories, whereas a waffle can be as high as 220 calories.

Fit Tip: Use whole wheat flour, whole wheat mixes, or whole wheat bread for your French toast. The calorie count doesn't always decrease noticeably, but at least you'll be getting whole-grain health perks. And try making your French toast or pancakes with egg whites. Also, add fresh fruit directly to the batter, and don't be shy about it. If you pack your pancakes with berries or bananas, each pancake will have fewer calories and more nutrients (the fruit displaces some calories from the pancake batter). Also, opt for light syrup, and don't pour it on—use a spoon and measure 2 tablespoons. Aunt Jemima Lite Syrup has 100 calories for ¼ cup (4 tablespoons) versus 210 calories for the regular version.

Butter is higher in calories and fat than syrup (100 calories per tablespoon). However, you can use a margarine spray (e.g. I Can't Believe It's Not Butter Spray), which has only a few

Calorie Bargain Spotlight

Calorie Bargain: I Can't Believe It's Not Butter Spray

The Why: You can spray it on toast, popcorn, vegetables. I use it on almost anything.

The Health Bonus: It's easy to control portions.

What We Liked Best: Even if you get up to 25 sprays (more than enough for a baked potato), it only has 20 calories and no trans fats. Compare that to 2 tablespoons of butter with 204 calories and 23 grams of fat.

What We Liked Least: The nutrition label is somewhat misleading; the product is not actually calorie free.

The Price: $2.39.

Offerings: original spray.

Website: www.tasteyoulove.com.

Where to Buy: local grocery store.

Ingredients: water, liquid soybean oil, salt, sweet cream buttermilk, xanthan gum, soy lecithin, polysorbate 60, lactic acid (potassium sorbate, calcium, disodium EDTA) used to protect quality, natural and artificial flavors, vitamin A (palmitate), beta-carotene (for color).

Nutritional Analysis per Serving: 1¼ Sprays
0 calories
0 g fat
0 g carbs
0 g protein
0 g fiber
0 g sodium

calories for 10 sprays. Also, don't confuse fruity syrup with fruit; they're not the same thing. Try a low-sugar or sugar-free jelly, which has about 10 to 25 calories per tablespoon (e.g. Smucker's Sugar Free, 10 calories).

Muffins vs. Scones vs. Croissants

Well, croissants are packed with loads of butter, and scones and muffins are typically large, individually baked pieces of cake. If you have to choose, a plain croissant is really your best bet. They generally range from 240 to 350 calories, and some may even be lower. Pillsbury Crescent Dinner Rolls, for example, are only 110 calories each, and you can buy them in advance and bake them at home. As for muffins and scones, they normally start in the 400-calorie range. A Panera Bread Cinnamon Chip Scone has 570 calories, and a Dunkin' Donuts Honey Bran Raisin Muffin has 480 calories. For a better muffin option, try making your own using a healthy recipe, or even a mix. One of my favorites is Vitalicious, a New York–based company that has come up with a great all-natural product that has fewer than half the calories of a regular muffin. Its mixes are available online at www.vitalicious .com.

Fit Tip: Split the muffin with another person; don't even tempt yourself by thinking you'll save the other half for later. Reduced-fat or fat-free muffins are not necessarily lower in calories either. For instance, Dunkin' Donuts Reduced Fat Blueberry Muffin has 400 calories, but at Panera, the Low Fat Tripleberry Muffin has 300 calories, and Starbucks's Low Fat Blueberry Muffin has 270 calories.

Calorie Bargain Spotlight

Oat Bran Blueberry Banana Muffins
Makes 12 muffins
Nutritional information per serving (1 muffin): 96.41 calories, 2.3 g fat, 13.57 g carbs, 1.77 g fiber, 3.42 g protein

2 cups Quaker Oat Bran
1¼ cups Splenda
2 teaspoons baking powder
½ teaspoon salt
1¼ cups skim milk
2 egg whites, slightly beaten
2 tablespoons vegetable oil
½ cup frozen or fresh blueberries
1 ripe banana, mashed

Heat oven to 425 degrees. Spray muffin tins with nonstick cooking spray. Combine dry ingredients. Mix well. Add milk, egg whites, and oil. Mix just until dry ingredients are moistened. Gently incorporate fruit. Fill muffin cups about ¾ full. Bake 15 to 17 minutes or until golden brown.

Bagel vs. Toast vs. English Muffin

As a rule, bagels are the worst choice. They're oversized and very dense, plus they keep lousy company (like cream cheese). For a plain bagel with nothing on it, you're looking at about 300 to 450 calories. A freshly baked plain bagel from Dunkin' Donuts will run you about 320 calories, for example. Some store-bought brands, such as Lender's plain frozen bagels (140 calories) and frozen New York–style bagels (230 calories), aren't a bad deal.

Your best bet, however, is an English muffin. They are reasonably portioned and denser than your average piece of

Calorie Bargain Spotlight

Calorie Bargain: The Alternative Bagel by Western Bagel

The Why: It isn't a traditional bagel, but for what it is, it is pretty amazing.

The Health Bonus: To keep them low in calories, Western Bagel has replaced flour with a combination of oat fiber, inulin fiber/bulking agent, and wheat starch, which helps reduce the carbs and increase the dietary fiber.

What We Liked Best: My family loved all the flavors, but our favorite was Sweet Wheat, which actually has 1 more gram of both protein and fiber than the others.

What We Liked Least: They're not 100 percent whole grain, and they're a bit small. Also, you might have to buy them from the website because they're not available everywhere.

The Price: $3.50 per bag.

Offerings: Cinnamon Spice, Sweet Wheat, Country White, Roasted Onion, and Very Blueberry.

Website: www.westernbagel.com.

Where to Buy: Kroger, Publix, Albertsons, company website.

Ingredients: enriched unbleached flour (wheat flour, malted barley flour, niacin, reduced iron, thiamine mononitrate, riboflavin, folic acid), water, whole wheat flour, wheat gluten, cornstarch, inulin, oat fiber, wheat bran. May contain 2 percent or less of: calcium sulfate, enzymes, L-cysteine, yeast, salt, calcium propionate and sorbic acid (preservatives), artificial flavor, dextrose, sucralose.

Nutritional Analysis per Serving: 2-ounce Bagel
110 calories
0 g fat
25 g carbs
6 g protein
7 g fiber
200 mg sodium

toast, so they're a pretty good choice at 120 calories. Toast can also be calorie controlled, but you need to be wary of all the options out there. Your average piece of white, multigrain, or wheat bread has anywhere from 45 to 80 calories, and the average whole-grain slice has 60 to 110 calories. Check the ingredient list if you're not sure your bread is a good choice. If the first item isn't wheat or whole grains, you could be eating white bread darkened with caramel coloring. Whole-grain breads, made with the whole wheat kernel, are not always lower in calories, but they provide many health perks plus feelings of satiety.

Fit Tip: Go for a whole wheat English muffin (120 calories) or a light multigrain English muffin (only 100 calories). Use a margarine spray if you want some buttery flavor without the calories of actual butter. If you prefer

Diet Detective's What You Need to Know

Q: Is honey better than brown sugar, and is brown sugar better than white sugar?

A: There is really no nutritional advantage to using honey or brown sugar over other sweeteners. Ounce for ounce, the nutrient content of honey is similar to that of white sugar, raw sugar, and brown sugar. Although some less-refined, more "natural" sugars may contain minerals, you would need to eat unreasonable amounts for them to make any meaningful contribution to your diet.

toast, stick to just two slices, and look for a sugar-free whole wheat bread. Also watch out for toppings or schmeers no matter which bread you choose. The ultimate health value of your breakfast may depend on the toppings you choose:

- 1 pat of butter: 25 to 30 calories.
- 1 scrambled egg: 80 to 95 calories.
- 2 tablespoons of cream cheese: 90 to 100 calories.
- 2 tablespoons of apple butter: 60 calories.
- 2 tablespoons of strawberry jam: 60 calories.

Calorie Bargain Spotlight

Calorie Bargain: Kellogg's Special K Chocolatey Delight

The Why: Chocoholics rejoice. Here's a great idea for you. For those times, late at night, when the hunger is "a-pokin' at ya', pokin' at ya'. . ." When you wish you were thirteen again and could down a king-size Snickers without thinking twice. How about a bowl of Kellogg's Special K Chocolatey Delight instead? Grab a cup or bowl, and you'll be on your way to a crunchy and chocolaty dessert that has fewer than half the calories of a Snickers bar.

The Health Bonus: Each ¾ cup serving has only 120 calories when served without milk.

What We Liked Best: That's the best way to eat it—dry. We had our taste testers try this chocolate treat many different ways and found that as a dry snack, served in a cup, it nicks those chocolate cravings. Keep in mind, this is not the perfect treat, but it does the job. Not every one of our tasters loved it, but the majority thought it was scrumptious. Lastly, watch how much you eat. It's a bit addictive, just like chips. Before you know it, the whole box could be gone—defeating the "bargain" aspect of the Calorie Bargain.

What We Liked Least: Keep in mind, this is *not* an all-natural product; also, it contains high-fructose corn syrup, but no trans fats.

The Price: $4.49.

Offerings: Kellogg's Special K Chocolatey Delight.

Website: www.kelloggs.com.

Where to Buy: local grocery store.

Ingredients: rice, whole-grain wheat, sugar, chocolatey chunks (sugar, partially hydrogenated palm kernel oil, cocoa processed with alkali, cocoa, soy lecithin, artificial flavor, milk), high-fructose corn syrup, salt, malt extract, natural and artificial flavors, ascorbic acid (vitamin C), reduced iron, niacinamide, pyridoxine hydrochloride (vitamin B_6), riboflavin (vitamin B_2), thiamin hydrochloride (vitamin B_1), vitamin A palmitate, BHT (preservative), folic acid, vitamin B_{12}, vitamin D, less than 0.5g trans fat per serving.

Nutritional Analysis per Serving: ¾ Cup
120 calories
2 g fat
24 g carbs
2 g protein
1 g fiber
180 mg sodium

Calorie Bargain Spotlight

Calorie Bargain: Cheerios

The Why: I've worked around plenty of registered dietitians, and I always see them snacking on dry Cheerios. Don't laugh until you try it; either plain or with a bit of artificial sweetener, they're pretty tasty. Or you can try the Honey Nut and MultiGrain varieties, which have 120 calories per cup—the choice is yours.

The Health Bonus: Cheerios are packed with essential vitamins and minerals and were one of the first cereals to be certified by the American

Heart Association for heart-protective benefits, including lowering cholesterol.

What We Liked Best: They're 100 percent whole grains. To tell you the truth, I never eat Cheerios for breakfast. Typically, I have a bowl as a mid-afternoon snack when I'm starving. They are also great because they have a decent amount of fiber, so you feel full.

What We Liked Least: They add sugar.

The Price: About $4.99 for a 15-ounce box.

Offerings: plain, Honey Nut, MultiGrain.

Website: www.cheerios.com.

Where to Buy: local grocery store.

Ingredients: whole grain oats, modified cornstarch, cornstarch, sugar, salt, calcium carbonate, oat fiber, tripotassium phosphate, wheat starch, vitamin E mixed tocopherols—added to preserve freshness, vitamins and minerals, iron mineral nutrient, zinc mineral nutrient, vitamin C (sodium ascorbate), niacinamide (a B vitamin), vitamin B_6 (pyridoxine hydrochloride), vitamin B_2 (riboflavin), vitamin B_1 (thiamin mononitrate), vitamin A palmitate, folic acid (a B vitamin), vitamin B_{12}, vitamin D.

Nutritional Analysis per Serving: 2 Cups
220 calories
4 g fat
44 g carbs
3 g protein
3 g fiber
210 mg sodium

A ½ cup of skim milk adds 43 calories, 0 grams of fat, and 6 grams of carbohydrate. You can eat 2 cups for only 220 calories.

Calorie Bargain Recipe Spotlight

Calorie Bargain: Egg-white Omelet with Veggies

The Why: You will not be hungry after eating this huge omelet—that's if you can even eat the entire thing. This is a real meal. It fills you up, it's packed with protein, it can be made in a matter of minutes, and it's perfect for anyone who wants to stay in shape.

The Health Bonus: If you think egg whites won't taste like eggs, you're wrong. They taste every bit as good as whole eggs, without any fat.

Ingredients: 8 egg whites, ½ cup frozen spinach, ½ medium green or red bell pepper, ½ cup mushrooms.

Preparation: Did you know you can microwave eggs? Just combine the egg whites and vegetables in a bowl, pop them in the microwave, and cook through (times vary).

Nutritional Analysis per Serving
176 calories
0 g fat
11 g carbs

Burgers

Here's how to make your burger healthier and tastier.

Traditional

Unfortunately, burgers are not exactly diet food, although research has demonstrated that a diet high in protein helps you feel full longer. A 6-ounce burger has more than 400 calories, but when you count the bun and all the toppings (mayo, cheese, bacon, ketchup, and so forth), you can hit 700 or even 800 calories.

And all those different types and cuts of meat—ground round, ground chuck, ground sirloin—can be quite confusing. Which do you choose? The less fat (especially the bad saturated fat) in a piece of meat, the healthier it is, and also the fewer calories it contains. For instance, ground sirloin has 300 calories and 15 grams of fat for 6 ounces, while the same amount of ground round has 360 calories and 26 grams of fat, and ground chuck, 435 calories and almost 35 grams (plus more than a half day's worth of saturated fat). Keep in mind, your home-barbecued burgers are generally much bigger than those you get in a restaurant—plus, many people typically eat more than one. So why not just go with the lowest-calorie meat? The problem is that leaner meats tend to have less flavor and dry out more during cooking. But it doesn't have to be like that.

BURGER FIXES

How do you make the healthy burger tastier?

Use vegetables and other fillers. Give your burger additional texture and flavor by mixing the meat with chopped mushrooms, peppers, and onions. You'll have the same size burger, but it will be lower in calories—and you'll also be getting the health benefits of all those vegetables.

Mix the meat with egg whites (two per pound), bread crumbs, water, salt, pepper, and onion and garlic powder.

Add herbs and spices. To make leaner cuts of meat tastier, try a blend of fresh herbs (such as thyme, marjoram, chives, and parsley) or dry ground spices (black pepper, smoked paprika, cumin, and cayenne), says John Greeley, chef at the '21' Club in New York. Herbs and spices add a lot of taste with practically no calories. Whether you use fresh or dried herbs, always crush them first to release their full aroma.

Marinate the meat overnight in a low-calorie marinade such as Lawry's Herb & Garlic, which has only 30 calories in 3 tablespoons.

Use cooking spray instead of oil. If you're grilling your burgers, spray the grill *before you light the flame* or the burger itself, with cooking spray to prevent sticking. If you're cooking in a pan, add 1 to 2 tablespoons of defatted broth, water, juice, or wine to the pan to compensate for the lower fat content of the beef.

Style matters. According to Paul Gayler, author of *The Gourmet Burger* (Gibbs Smith, 2005), "Meat should be coarsely ground. If it's too finely ground, the burger is more likely to fall apart, and the texture will be less satisfying." Also, keep the meat loose. Burgers will be less juicy if you over-pack the patties. Good burgers should be about an inch thick and have a slightly thinner center.

Once burgers are shaped, chill them again to firm up the meat before cooking, recommends Gayler.

Charbroiled burgers are best cooked over medium-high heat; in other words, when the red-hot coals are covered with a layer of white ash. "And don't press down on them with a spatula to speed up cooking. It dries out the burger, and precious flavor is lost," reminds Gayler. Also, make sure you cook them slowly, so they don't dry out.

Alternatives

Using other meats, poultry, or vegetables rather than beef for your burgers could reduce the calorie and saturated-fat content. But be wary—you still have to make smart choices.

- **Turkey and chicken burgers:** If they're not made from ground white meat, you might be better off with beef. A 6-ounce white-meat turkey burger has about 195 calories and almost 1 gram of fat (0 grams saturated). But when your turkey burger contains other, fattier parts of the turkey, a 6-ounce burger can run as high as 400 calories and 22 grams of fat. The same goes for chicken burgers; ground chicken breast is a better bet.
- **Pork burgers:** Try to find lean ground loin pork (10 percent or less fat), which has 300 calories and 16 grams of fat (5 grams saturated) for 6 ounces. However, if you get regular ground pork (20 percent or more fat), watch out: You're looking at 450 calories and 36 grams fat (9 grams saturated).
- **Salmon burgers:** These are pretty low in both calories and fat, plus you get the heart-healthy benefits of

omega-3s. A 6-ounce patty has 240 calories and 10 grams of fat (1.5 grams saturated). According to Chef Greeley, "Asian flavors such as soy, teriyaki, lime, wasabi, and sesame seeds work well with salmon burgers. Fresh herbs such as cilantro, scallion, and dill add good flavors. Also, you can brush your burger with a tamarind paste or barbecue sauce and a squeeze of lemon. Serve medium rare to medium with sliced avocado and pickled cucumber."

- **Veggie burgers:** They're lower in calories and fat than any other choice. For example, a Boca Burger has only 80 calories and 1 gram of fat. You can try different meat substitutes, above and beyond even the veggie burger. Try soy burgers, seitan patties, and other protein substitutes.

  Chef Greeley says that veggie burgers are the most difficult to make at home because without the correct blend of moisture and binder, they tend to crumble or fall apart. He uses ground smoked tofu, blending it with ground cooked mushrooms, tahini and hummus, and binding it with a little wheat flour. "Form into balls and coat with a light dusting of the wheat flour, then form into patties," suggests Greeley. "Flavors such as minced onion, garlic, black pepper, cumin, and tomato powder are fantastic. Almost any soft, fresh herb will work, including basil, oregano, chervil, tarragon, and chive. Brush the patties with olive oil and cook under a broiler, or lightly grill just enough to sear the outside and get the inside hot."

  Also, Chef Cary Neff's recipe for Black-Bean Griddle Patties from *Conscious Cuisine* is a delicious low-calorie treat. The recipe is available at www.dietdetective.com/articles/food/recipe_light.html.

- **Bison burgers:** These offer some savings in terms of

calories and fat compared to traditional beef burgers. A 4-ounce TenderBison Bison Burger (frozen) has 220 calories and 11 grams of fat (5 saturated).

- **More exotic alternatives:** According to Paul Gayler, "Other game meats make excellent burgers. Pheasant and ostrich are well flavored and nutritious. Because they are so lean, add a little fat to the mixture in the form of pork."

The Bun

Buns can add anywhere from 110 to 180 calories. A regular 1½-ounce white hamburger bun has about 110 calories, but kaiser rolls are normally higher, at 180 calories. For more fiber, try to get 100 percent whole-grain buns. But just because the package says wheat doesn't mean it's 100 percent whole grain. Make sure whole grains are the first ingredient. Your best bet is a whole wheat English muffin (120 calories) or a light multigrain English muffin (only 100 calories). Also, try no-sugar-added, low-calorie 100 percent whole wheat toast.

Burger Company

Watch out for the obvious: fries, potato chips (150 calories per handful), coleslaw (more than 250 calories per cup), pasta salad (depending on ingredients, you're looking at 400 to 500 calories per cup), and so on. All these sides are typically very high in calories and can turn your burger into a diet disaster. Instead of chips or fries, make your own grilled potatoes.

Toppings and Condiments

Instead of cheese (70 to 120 calories a deli slice; plus, cheese is high in saturated fat), add lettuce, tomatoes, onions, pickles, or even celery to your burgers. Or try reduced-fat cheese (Kraft Cracker Barrel Reduced Fat Cheddar Cheese, Jarlsberg Lite, Cabot Reduced Fat cheeses, Kraft Fat Free Singles, or Borden Low-Fat). Fat-free single-serving slices have about 30 calories each. Also look for cheeses that are not only reduced fat but that are thinly sliced; they're typically less than an ounce, with only about 40 to 60 calories.

For great flavor and virtually no extra calories, top your burger with tomatoes marinated in red wine vinegar, fresh basil, a drop of olive oil, salt, and cracked black pepper. And add some pickled red onions or pickled peppers, says Greeley.

Avoid mayo (100 calories per tablespoon) and stick to ketchup, mustard, or even steak sauce. At 30 calories per tablespoon, barbecue sauce has double the calories of ketchup or steak sauce (15 calories). That can add up fast if you're not paying attention; just ½ cup on your burger and fries adds 240 extra calories.

Mad Cow and *E. Coli*

Most food safety experts agree that mad cow disease poses a minuscule risk to U.S. consumers. However, food poisoning is another story. You can get food poisoning if you don't handle your meats carefully. Here are a few tips:

- Prevent cross-contamination—that is, don't let raw meat, fish, or poultry touch foods that won't be cooked, such as lettuce. Never use the same knife or cutting board without washing it first.

- Cook foods to the proper internal temperature (160 degrees for ground meats and pork; 170 for poultry breasts; 165 for leftovers, casseroles, and ground poultry).
- Wash your hands with soap and warm water for twenty seconds after handling raw meat.

(For more about food risk and *E. coli*, check out: http://www .dietdetective.com.)

Salads

What could possibly be fattening about a salad? Well, according to the USDA, the average woman, ages nineteen to fifty, gets more fat from salad dressing than from any other food source, and that's not including the various other toppings we pile on our salads. I don't know about you, but I used to think that if I ate nothing but salad, the weight would just drop from my body. In truth, however, with just a few wrong steps, a salad can end up in the food hall of shame alongside french fries and chocolate cake!

Salad consumption is at an all-time high, with 73 percent of American households serving salad as a regular part of their meals. We start out with great intentions: green, leafy lettuce, fresh peppers, onions, beets, cucumbers, and other healthy foods. However, the problems begin when we start dressing up the salad. We add dressing, croutons, cheese, oil-drenched sweet peppers, bacon bits, egg, ham, and anything else we can think of that packs on the calories and fat. People are looking for texture and—most of all—taste in everything they eat today, right down to the salad toppings. So what can we do to keep up the flavor and keep off the pounds?

Dressing on the Side

Regular dressing can be high in calories and fat, and very often salads are drenched in it, so use 1 to 1½ tablespoons. Choice of dressing is also important. Here's what can be found in 3 tablespoons (a standard restaurant serving) of some popular dressings:

- Blue cheese: 225 calories, 24 g fat, 3 g carbs.
- Ranch: 220 calories, 24 g fat, 3 g carbs.
- Thousand Island: 180 calories, 18 g fat, 6 g carbs.
- Italian: 130 calories, 12 g fat, 6 g carbs.
- Olive oil and vinegar: 225 calories, 24 g fat, 3 g carbs.

Switch Things Up a Bit

Try switching to a low-fat or fat-free dressing. Some of them actually taste good! Fat-free dressings, by law, contain fewer than 0.5 grams of fat per 2 tablespoons, and low-fat dressing must contain no more than 3 grams of fat per serving. Also, try balsamic vinegar, Dijon mustard, or fat-free yogurt as healthier alternatives.

Avoid the Crunch

Avoid crunchy additions such as croutons (½ cup = 86 calories and 3.5 grams of fat) and fried noodles. They add extra calories, with little or no nutritional value.

Calorie Bargain Spotlight

Calorie Bargain: Wish-Bone Salad Spritzers Vinaigrette Dressings

The Why: These dressings are quite the discovery for those who normally dump dressing onto salads, thinking that they're making a healthful choice.

The Health Bonus: The new spray bottle lets you monitor the amount of dressing you put on.

What We Liked Best: This is not just Wish-Bone's regular dressing; it's a lower-calorie version. One tablespoon (about 20 sprays) contains 20 calories, while 1 tablespoon of regular dressing has about 35 to 40 calories.

What We Liked Least: The sprays are made with high-fructose corn syrup.

The Price: $3.49.

Offerings: Asian Silk, Balsamic Breeze, Caesar Delight, French Flair, Italian Raspberry Bliss, Red Wine Mist.

Website: www.wish-bone.com.

Where to Buy: local grocery store.

Ingredients: (Balsamic Breeze) water, balsamic vinegar, high-fructose corn syrup, soybean oil, salt, distilled vinegar, extra virgin olive oil, onion juice, garlic juice, xanthan gum, natural flavors, sorbic acid and calcium disodium EDTA, wine, soybean lecithin. Contains sulfites.

Nutritional Analysis per Serving: 10 Sprays
10 calories
1 g fat
1 g carbs
0 g protein
0 g fiber
130 mg sodium

Don't Say Cheese

Try to avoid whole-milk cheeses. Even cottage cheese can be a source of unwanted fat. Many supermarkets carry prepackaged shredded low-fat cheese, ready to sprinkle right on.

Bacon

We all know that bacon is full of fat, so if you must have it, try cooking it on a paper towel in the microwave to absorb the fat and save some calories.

Potato, Tuna, and Egg Salads

In delis and markets watch out for premade salads such as pasta salad, potato salad, and coleslaw. Many of these contain mayonnaise. One cup can contain close to 30 grams of fat. Try for salads made from low-fat mayo, mustard, and/or vinaigrette. Or, better yet, make your own.

Mix It Up

Make your salad more exciting by switching from iceberg lettuce to a combination of greens. Not only will this improve the color and texture of the salad, but it also increases the nutritional value without adding too many calories (about 25 calories per ½ cup). Using greens like romaine lettuce, spinach, herbal greens, arugula, radicchio, and cabbage adds extra beta-carotene, potassium, and vitamin K. You can also try cherry tomatoes and baby carrots, which are nutritious additions that require little effort. Speaking of which, if putting all these ingredients together yourself seems like too much trouble, you can buy prepackaged mixed greens and bags of veggies (make sure to wash them, unless they're pre-washed) in almost any local supermarket.

Sauces

Sauce comes from a French word meaning to enhance the flavor of our meals. And while sauces are now an integral part of many popular dishes, they weren't always. In fact, before refrigeration, sauces were used to disguise the less-than-scrumptious flavor of meat, poultry, and fish that had aged a little longer than one would like. But even though they're no longer needed to cover up something that would otherwise taste really bad, sauces still improve the taste of a lot of different foods. They can, however, make or break your meal caloriewise. Take a look at these popular flavor enhancers and see where they rank on the weight-loss scale.

Pesto vs. White Clam Sauce vs. Red Clam Sauce

Pesto is delicious, but it's made with a lot more than chopped basil. It also traditionally contains ground pine nuts, olive oil, and Parmesan cheese, which is why a ½-cup serving has about 300 calories. Pesto packs more of a calorie punch than either of the clam sauces, but you might use less of it because it is denser. Between the two clam sauces, red sauce is better because its base is tomato, not butter and wine like the white sauce. Per ½-cup serving, red clam sauce has about 60 calories, and white clam sauce has 110 to 160. Also, remember that if you're ordering these sauces in restaurants, you're going to get significantly larger portions than you might use at home. For example, spaghetti with white clam sauce at the Old Spaghetti Factory has nearly 700 calories, and pasta with pesto basil cream sauce comes in even higher at about 800 calories.

Fit Tip: Some recipes cut down on the oil and add spinach to make up the difference. Pureed vegetables are another way to thicken sauces. You can reduce the oil by using lemon. Also, you can use reduced-fat Parmesan cheese.

Marinara vs. Meat or Bolognese Sauce vs. Vegetable Sauce

Most red pasta sauces have added sugar and oil or some other fat, but if used sparingly, they can all be OK. Not surprisingly, meat sauce (130 to 170 calories per ½ cup) is the one you probably want to stay away from. Marinara and vegetable sauces both have about 60 to 80 calories per ½ cup, but bear in mind that if you choose the vegetable sauce, you're getting a lot of variety, not to mention the health perks of the low-cal veggies in the sauce.

Another thing to watch out for is portion control. While 80 calories is certainly reasonable, if you use more than a ½ cup, you'll be getting additional calories with the additional sauce.

Fit Tip: There are many healthy ready-made marinara and meat sauces that are delicious and lower in calories. Look for sauces with 50 to 60 calories per ½ cup. And if you really love meat sauce, try lower-cal alternatives—they aren't that hard to find. Healthy Choice makes a number of low-calorie pasta sauces, including Garlic & Herb, which has 60 calories per ½ cup. Or try adding vegetables to regular tomato sauces. You'll get more quantity for fewer calories and feel full longer.

Coconut vs. Curry vs. Peanut Sauce

This gets a little tricky. Coconut sauce (50 to 70 calories in 2 tablespoons), which is made from coconut milk (extremely high in fat and calories; just 2 ounces have roughly 140 calories and 14 grams of fat), has slightly fewer calories than the others. But the bulk of the fat in the coconut is unhealthy saturated fat, so I'd prefer the peanut sauce, even though it does have more calories (80 calories in 2 tablespoons). Curry sauce is typically made with ginger and other spices, as well as onion, garlic, fried chilies, oil, and tomatoes, and it can be high in calories (2 tablespoons, 120 calories).

Fit Tip: Watch out for the sodium levels in the curry you purchase. And if you really love coconut sauce, make your own, starting with a low-fat coconut milk.

Sweet-and-Sour Sauce vs. Peking (Hoisin) Sauce vs. Duck Sauce

Looking at straight calorie counts, sweet-and-sour sauce (40 calories for 2 tablespoons) is the lowest. Peking sauce has 70 calories, and duck sauce has 60. But with these sauces, you've got to look beyond the sauce itself. Also think about what you'll be putting it on. If your duck sauce goes on cubed chicken that's been breaded and fried, as it often does in Chinese restaurants, you may be looking at up to 800 calories and 31 grams of fat for the meal. And if you're dipping fried noodles or a fried egg roll in the duck sauce, that can also be a Calorie Rip-off.

Fit Tip: The bottom line is that you have to watch not only your sauces but what's under them as well. If you're consuming fried, greasy, or fatty foods slathered with mammoth portions of any sauce, well, the calories are going to add up quickly. Try using the juice of a golden, ripe pineapple for a thick, sweet sauce with plenty of froth to replace a sweet-and-sour dip, or brush it on baked chicken for a low-cal sweet-and-sour dish.

Teriyaki vs. Soy Sauce

OK, before you start recommending soy as the best sauce, make sure you're reading the entire nutrition label. It may be an excellent option caloriewise, but soy sauce (10 calories per tablespoon) packs 920 milligrams of sodium. Teriyaki is a smarter option (1 tablespoon, 15 calories). Although it's still high in sodium at about 610 milligrams, it's not quite as high as soy sauce.

Fit Tip: If you're attempting to keep your sodium intake down, the light versions of both soy and teriyaki sauce can save you almost 50 percent.

Hollandaise vs. Béarnaise vs. White Sauce

While drenching your food in any of these sauces can be a calorie catastrophe, a béchamel (white sauce) at least has the fewest calories per ounce—about 60. White sauce is cream or milk mixed into a white roux (a combination of butter and flour that is cooked but not browned). Hollandaise (about 160 calories per ounce) is made with vinegar, egg yolks, and butter, and flavored with lemon. Béarnaise (100 calories per ounce) is actually similar to hollandaise but with the addition of wine, tarragon, and shallots.

Fit Tip: Start with broths, vegetables, or vegetable purees instead of butter as a base for your sauces. Using a juicer is another way to cut calories. Also, experiment with spices and fresh herbs to add flavor. Finally, there are ingredients that simulate the texture of fat without the fat. Try using cornstarch as an instant fat-free thickener for sauces and gravies. Just mix some cornstarch in cold water and add it to your stir-fry. Or, instead of a cream-based pasta sauce, sauté vegetables with nonfat spray, seasoning, and lemon juice, add cornstarch, and then toss with pasta.

For hollandaise sauce, begin with 1 percent milk, cornstarch, and a little lemon juice, and reduce the quantity of butter and eggs. I'm not sure how far you want to go with this, but there are recipes that use tofu and lecithin granules, and others that call for nonfat yogurt and/or nonfat mayo with a little mustard and lemon. I would probably just keep the sauce on the side.

Barbecue Sauce vs. Steak Sauce vs. Ketchup

A tablespoon of any of these sauces doesn't really do any damage to a diet; however, the steak sauce and the ketchup have half the calories (15 per tablespoon) of the barbecue sauce (30 calories). But this is another instance when it's important to remember that you're probably not eating the sauce by itself—and the stuff you're slathering it on might just do some serious diet damage.

Fit Tip: Although the calories per tablespoon are all low, if you become a heavy user, they add up. For instance, if you pour a ½ cup of barbecue sauce on your burger and fries, you've just eaten an additional 240 calories. To keep track, use a tablespoon to add sauces to your food, and avoid pouring them directly from the bottle. For barbecues, instead of coating your ribs, chicken, wings, or meat with an excessive amount of sauce beforehand, cook it first with lots of seasonings, then spoon on your sauce sparingly. That way you won't end up having eight servings of sauce with every few bites.

Brown Gravy vs. Sausage Gravy vs. Mushroom Gravy

Typical brown gravy has only 30 calories in a ½ cup. The problems start with the country-style, beef, mushroom, and pork varieties. These gravies are made with high-calorie ingredients like oil, fat skimmed from cooking, and whole milk. For instance, country-style sausage gravy (about 200 calories per ½ cup) has almost ten times the calories of turkey gravy.

Diet Detective's What You Need to Know

Q. True or false: Buttermilk is the most fattening milk of all.

A. False. In fact, buttermilk is usually made from skim milk, so it's actually lower in calories than whole milk, at 100 calories per cup compared with 150 in whole milk. Buttermilk is also low in cholesterol and fat. At one time, buttermilk was what was left after butter had been churned from cream. It was a way of using up the leftovers in the interest of conservation. Now, however, it is fermented (with cultures) from skim milk.

And it isn't going to fill you up significantly more or give you any health perks. Canned mushroom gravy has about 60 calories for a ½ cup. Remember that eating your meat au jus is not the same as covering it with gravy. *Au jus* means the meat is cooked and served in its own juices, while gravy includes the juice of the meat combined with broth, wine, or milk, plus a thickening agent such as flour or cornstarch.

Fit Tip: To lower the calories in your gravy, remove the fat with a fat separator (a cup with a spout designed to pour the juices from the bottom and leave the fat on top). Or add ice cubes to the pan juices so that the fat hardens and clings to the ice. If you have enough time, refrigerate the pan drippings so that the fat rises to the top and hardens, allowing you to scrape it off before reheating the gravy. Oh, and if you're trying to cut down on calories, avoid using bread or biscuits to mop up extra gravy.

Alfredo vs. Marsala Sauce

Marsala wine sauce (160 to 180 calories for a ½ cup) is a better choice than Alfredo. Wine itself contains 140 calories per ½ cup; however the sauce is traditionally prepared with mushrooms and olive oil, so the calories climb a bit higher, depending on how much oil is added. Alfredo sauce, on the other hand, is problematic because its primary ingredients are cheese, heavy cream, and butter, all of which can add up to 300 to 400 calories for a ½ cup.

Fit Tip: To keep down the calories in Marsala sauce, use a minimal amount of oil. And there are light versions of Alfredo sauce available that can cut calories in half.

Calorie Bargain Spotlight

Calorie Bargain: Quaker Quakes Rice Snacks—Chocolate

The Why: Rice cakes may conjure up images of Styrofoam, but these little snacks are packed full of flavor.

The Health Bonus: You get seven minicakes for only 60 calories. The best part about these rice cakes is that you don't feel deprived, and they don't taste like you're eating something low calorie.

What We Liked Best: I love both the chocolate and caramel corn flavors. They taste amazing and are a much better deal than chips.

What We Liked Least: They're very artificial, and they have high-fructose corn syrup. Also, it's easy to get carried away and eat too many—keep an eye on your portion size!

The Price: $2.59.

Offerings: Apple Cinnamon, BBQ, Caramel Corn, Cheddar Cheese, Chocolate, Kettle Corn, Nacho Cheese, Ranch, Sour Cream.

Website: www.quakerricesnacks.com.

Where to Buy: local grocery store.

Ingredients: rice flour, corn (with germ removed), sugar, maltodextrin, milk chocolate chips (sugar, chocolate liquor, milk, cocoa butter, soy lecithin, vanillin), high-fructose corn syrup, sunflower oil with natural tocopherols added to preserve freshness, natural and artificial flavors, cocoa, salt, soy lecithin, caramel color, sucralose, acesulfame potassium, citric acid, sodium citrate. Contains milk and soy ingredients.

Nutritional Analysis per Serving: 7 minicakes
60 calories
1 g fat
13 g carbs
1 g protein
0 g fiber
45 g sodium

Tartar Sauce vs. Cocktail Sauce

Tartar sauce (74 calories per tablespoon) is made with mayonnaise, which has about 100 calories per tablespoon. Cocktail sauce (15 calories per tablespoon) is the clear winner.

Fit Tip: Try making your own tartar sauce with reduced-fat or nonfat mayo.

Barbecues and Picnics

Sure, we all know everyone eats a lot at a barbecue or picnic, but how much we really eat is astonishing. The average barbecue or picnic meal contains well over 3,500 calories! That's 1,500 calories more than a full day's worth of meals. Yet it's not always easy to make healthy decisions. Here's a quiz to help you get on the right track:

Which are the better choices and why?

Hamburger or Frankfurter?

Hot dogs seem like a better choice, but nobody eats just one. And nobody eats them plain. The best toppings to use are sauerkraut, good old ketchup, mustard, and relish. Stay away from cheesy sauces and chili. Two low-calorie hot dogs (for example, Healthy Choice Beef Franks) with sauerkraut and mustard but without the buns add up to fewer than 200 calories.

Burgers aren't so innocent either. Do you know anyone who eats a plain burger? Mayo will add 100 calories per tablespoon! Stick to ketchup, mustard, pickles, and veggies for extra flavor. Make your burgers with the leanest beef you can find and toss in veggies like mushrooms, onions, and peppers to increase nutrients and lower the calorie content without reducing the volume. Go bunless to save yourself even more calories and carbs. Eating your burger with a knife and fork will also prevent you from scarfing it down and then wanting another one a minute later. Save even more calories with a 4-ounce turkey burger (130 calories, 0.5g fat, 0 g carbs, 28 g protein) or a Gardenburger veggie pattie (100 calories, 3.5 g fat, 14 g carbs, 5 g protein).

- Plain hamburger (¼ pound) on bun: 447 calories, 22 g fat, 32 g carbs, 27 g protein.
- Plain frankfurter on bun: 260 calories, 16 g fat, 20 g carbs, 9 g protein.
- Healthy Choice Beef Frank: 70 calories, 2.5 g fat, 7 g carbs, 6 g protein.
- Ball Park Bun Size Smoked White Turkey Frank: 45 calories, 0 g fat, 5 g carbs, 6 g protein.
- Sauerkraut (1 cup): 27 calories, 0 g fat, 6 g carbs, 1 g protein.
- Heinz Tomato Ketchup (2 tablespoons): 30 calories, 0 g fat, 8 g carbs, 0 g protein.
- Gulden's Spicy Brown Mustard (2 tablespoons): 30 calories, 0 g fat, 0 g carbs, 0 g protein.
- Sargento Fancy Mild Cheddar Shredded Cheese (¼ cup): 110 calories, 9 g fat, 1 g carbs, 7 g protein.
- Sweet relish (2 tablespoons): 30 calories, 0 g fat, 6 g carbs, 0 g protein.

Coleslaw or Baked Beans?

Baked beans might be slightly higher in calories, but they're lower in fat and higher in protein and fiber. The problem is, the baked beans you buy in the supermarket are made with sugar or molasses. Instead, make your own bean salad.

Choose your favorite beans, chop up an onion and some peppers, add a little lemon juice and vinegar for flavor, and you've got a nutrient-packed side dish!

- Coleslaw (½ cup): 135 calories, 12 g fat, 7 g carbs, 1 g protein.
- Baked beans (½ cup): 150 calories, 1 g fat, 29 g carbs, 7 g protein.
- Bean salad (½ cup): 73 calories, 0 g fat, 14 g carbs, 4 g protein.

Caesar Salad or Macaroni Salad?

Veggies versus pasta sounds like a no-brainer. But even though macaroni salad is usually made with mayo, Caesar salad typically has egg, cheese, and sometimes mayo or oil. The Caesar dressing alone has 25 grams of fat! Your best option is to avoid both and stick with a regular garden salad and nonfat dressing.

Pasta or macaroni salad generally has, in addition to the pasta itself, some type of creamy or fattening dressing made with mayonnaise or olive oil, plus cheese, nuts, vegetables, ham, eggs, chicken, tuna, and even pepperoni. For 1 cup, depending on ingredients, you're looking at 500 to 650 calories.

- Caesar salad (1 cup): 302 calories, 28 g fat, 3 g carbs, 10 g protein.
- Macaroni salad (⅔ cup): 420 calories, 28 g fat, 28 g carbs, 5 g protein.

Try making your macaroni salad with 100 percent whole wheat pasta (not semolina or 100 percent pure durum semolina). This will increase the fiber content and help you fill up faster. Another way to increase your portion size without adding calories is to use lots of vegetables. Isn't that the idea of a salad anyway? But the most important fix is the dressing. Most salad dressings, including those made with olive oil, are packed with calories. Your best bet is a light vinaigrette or low-calorie Italian dressing, or one made from a light mayonnaise base. You can also go very light by using an olive oil mister and seasoning the salad with spices such as pepper, garlic, oregano, or basil to liven things up without extra calories. One cup of vegetable pasta salad made with light vinaigrette has 206 calories. Or skip the pasta altogether and go for a cucumber salad made with sliced onion, vinegar, salt, pepper, and a pinch of sugar or Splenda, or a cucumber and tomato salad made with vinegar, no oil. Both have 48 calories per cup.

Cornbread, Biscuits, or Corn on the Cob?

Corn on the cob is the clear winner if you avoid butter and use a margarine spray instead (1 ear with 10 sprays: 69 calories). Biscuits are typically made with tons of butter or shortening, so if you're looking for something doughy, stick with cornbread.

- Corn with butter (1 ear with 2 tablespoons of butter): 263 calories, 24 g fat, 14 g carbs, 2 g protein.
- Homemade cornbread (1 piece, 65 g): 184 calories, 6 g fat, 28 g carbs, 4 g protein.
- Homemade buttermilk biscuit (63 g): 224 calories, 10 g fat, 28 g carbs, 4 g protein.

Minestrone or Chili?

No contest here. Bring your minestrone soup in a thermos, and don't forget bowls and spoons! Even if you add a tablespoon of Parmesan cheese (20 calories), minestrone still has fewer calories than chili.

- Minestrone (1 cup): 233 calories, 13 g fat, 22 g carbs, 9 g protein.
- Chili (1 cup): 321 calories, 14 g fat, 27 g carbs, 22 g protein.

PB&J or Ham and Cheese?

Your basic peanut butter and jelly is usually the better choice. If you keep it down to just two slices of ham and one slice of cheese, the ham and cheese wins in terms of calories (314 calories, 14 grams of fat, 28 grams of carbs, 21 grams of protein). But don't forget that peanut butter is a great source of heart-healthy unsaturated fat, while ham and cheese both contain unhealthy saturated fat.

- PB&J sandwich (2 tablespoons peanut butter, 1 tablespoon jelly): 381 calories, 19 g fat, 45 g carbs, 14 g protein.
- Ham and cheese sandwich (4 slices ham, 3 slices cheese): 576 calories, 31 g fat, 32 g carbs, 42 g protein.

Wine or Light Beer?

Ounce for ounce, light beer is lower in calories. But most people will drink the whole 12-ounce bottle, whereas they might drink only a few ounces of wine. Plus, with wine you get the purported benefits of protection against heart disease and cancer.

- Bud Light (12 ounces): 110 calories, 6.6 g carbs.
- Red wine (5 ounces): 106 calories, 3 g carbs.

Brownie or Apple Pie

You might think that apple pie sounds better for you (and your waistline) than a delectable fat-drenched brownie. Think again. They both can pack on the pounds. Try No Pudge! Fudge Brownie mixes (www.nopudge.com), made with yogurt, and cut your calories by more than half. Or how about a baked apple made with Splenda and cinnamon (80 calories) or a fruit salad (174 calories for 2 cups)?

- Brownie (142 g): 580 calories, 23 g fat, 88 g carbs, 9 g protein.
- Apple pie (169 g): 550 calories, 31 g fat, 66 g carbs, 4 g protein.

Barbecued Spareribs

Ribs are typically made with sugar, barbecue sauce (which also contains sugar), honey, and other assorted fattening extras, adding up to more than 1,000 calories for six medium ribs. The sauce itself wouldn't be so bad if it were applied lightly, but it's usually slathered on. Since just 2 tablespoons of barbecue sauce have 50 calories, you can see how the damage adds up quickly.

Nutrition Fix: First of all, use babyback ribs. They're the smallest, which helps with portion control. Place them on the grill without any barbecue sauce; just season with kosher salt, fresh pepper, and garlic powder, and cook for thirty to forty minutes. Watch carefully so that they don't burn. Serve with barbecue sauce or hot sauce on the side.

If you feel you must have regular ribs, be sure to trim off the visible fat; that will save close to 250 calories. Also, skip repeated coatings of heavy barbecue sauce during cooking: Use one coating and serve extra sauce on the side.

Fried Chicken

Deep-fried chicken with the skin can be very costly caloriewise. Just one 3½-ounce fried breast has about 250 calories, and one drumstick with skin has about 200 calories.

Nutrition Fix: Remove the skin from the chicken. Put two beaten egg whites in one bowl and bread crumbs in another. Dunk the skinless chicken into the egg whites and then into the bread crumbs. Coat the pieces lightly with a cooking spray such as Pam and bake in the oven at 350 to 400 degrees for about thirty to forty-five minutes. This saves more than 75 calories per piece of chicken.

Potato Chips

Chips are a natural part of summer barbecues, picnics, or poolside snacking. But at 150 calories an ounce (or handful), they can do a lot of damage.

Nutrition Fix: Make your own chips by thinly slicing a medium baked potato, microwaving it on high for about six minutes, and then grilling the slices or baking them in the oven until they're crisp. Salt them and coat them lightly with a bit of margarine spray. Each potato is 100 calories, and it's pretty filling. Plus the work it takes to make them allows you to enjoy them much more.

Coleslaw

Coleslaw is basically cabbage, mayonnaise, sugar, and vinegar, but some recipes also add olive oil and other ingredients. The end result can be more than 350 calories per cup.

Nutrition Fix: Buy a coleslaw mix in the vegetable section at the grocery store and make your own slaw with light or nonfat mayonnaise and Splenda, and add some julienned green and red peppers to increase the yield while cutting calories per cup.

Ice Cream

Ice cream is pretty much synonymous with summer—and it's also one of the premier diet busters. One cup of premium ice cream can have more than 500 calories, and we typically eat 2 cups plus toppings.

Nutrition Fix: Use a cup, not a cone, and save anywhere from 20 calories (for a wafer cone) to more than 300 calories (for a waffle cone with chocolate). Avoid nut toppings and sprinkles (2 tablespoons have 100 calories). Try to go with an ice cream bar—the low-cal versions, such as Fudgsicle, have only 40 calories—or a frozen fruit bar (70 calories). They're portion controlled, and you can't add toppings. Avoid gelato and stick

Calorie Bargain Spotlight

Calorie Bargain: Jell-O Sugar Free/Reduced Calorie Pudding Snacks

The Why: I've always been fond of these treats, but until now they were available only in vanilla and chocolate. Kraft finally came out with a few new flavors, the most notable of which is Double Chocolate.

The Health Bonus: It's sugar free and has only 60 calories per cup.

What We Liked Best: It's not ice cream, but the creamy, smooth flavor will satisfy your sweet tooth when you're craving something cold and delicious.

What We Liked Least: lots of chemicals.

The Price: $3.69.

Offerings: Chocolate, Chocolate Vanilla Swirl, Double Chocolate, Vanilla.

Website: www.kraftfoods.com.jello.

Where to Buy: local grocery store.

Ingredients: water, xylitol, modified food starch, cocoa processed with alkali, milk protein concentrate, contains less than 1.5 percent of hydrogenated vegetable oil (coconut and palm kernel oils), salt, sodium stearoyl lactylate (for smooth texture), sodium alginate, calcium phosphate, sucralose, acesulfame potassium, natural and artificial flavor, artificial color.

Nutritional Analysis Per Serving: 1 Container
60 calories
1 g fat
1 g saturated fat
13 g carbs
1 g protein

to sorbet: You'll save a couple hundred calories. Or try Italian ices at only 100 calories per cup. And don't be fooled by frozen yogurt (either regular or soft serve). It can be just as high in calories as regular ice cream, so always choose fat-free versions and watch portions to save calories.

Lemonade

On a relaxing summer day, a pitcher of lemonade on the front porch sounds good, but if it's made with sugar, it can also be very high in calories, especially when it's hot outside and we drink a lot. Just a few glasses could cost about 600 calories.

Nutrition Fix: Make it yourself and squeeze real lemons. Three ounces of lemon juice have about 30 calories. Use about one-third juice and two-thirds water and add Splenda to taste.

Brown-bag Lunches

What can you bring for lunch on the go? Sounds like a simple question, but finding the answers turned out to be more difficult than I thought, requiring a trip to the supermarket and some serious brainstorming. When we're on the move, and all we can do is pack a brown paper bag or a lunch box, it's tough to find tasty, portable options. Here are a few suggestions:

Pack It Cold

It seems that—with just a few exceptions—almost all foods have to be kept cool to remain safe to eat. Get a well-insulated lunch bag and use an ice pack or freeze a water bottle, which can double as something to drink after it thaws.

eBags (www.ebags.com) has great insulated coolers that are both stylish and convenient. The Lunch Cooler ($19.95) keeps food cold for four to six hours with proper ice packs, and profits from the pink version are donated to breast cancer research. Aladdin (www.aladdin-pmi.com) makes a series that has insulation to keep salads, fruit, and other foods crisp and chilled.

Test your bag's insulation with a refrigerator thermometer. The temperature should stay below 40 degrees until lunch. Also, chill foods thoroughly before packing them.

Sandwiches and Wraps

Chicken, turkey, lean cold cuts, or low-fat cheese on 100 percent whole-wheat bread (whole grain must be the first ingredient) are all great options. Wraps, whole wheat pita bread, and tortillas (not fried) are also good, but always check the calories. A 1-ounce corn tortilla has about 70 calories. Avoid mayo, tartar sauce, creamy dressings, and cheese. Use mustard, ketchup, salt, pepper, or vinegar as condiments.

Pasta

Use whole wheat pasta, and add vegetables and a low-calorie sauce (50 to 60 calories per ½ cup). Pack it in a plastic container like GladWare or Tupperware. One cup of cooked whole wheat spaghetti has 170 calories.

Salads

Buy prepackaged bags of salad and keep them in your cooler, then add your low-calorie dressing at lunchtime. Or get McDonald's Newman's Own Low-fat Balsamic Vinaigrette at only 40 calories per packet—you can buy packets of them there for about 30 cents each (they're not sold in stores). Avoid nuts, croutons, noodles, and creamy salad dressings.

Chicken, Turkey, and Sushi

All of these can be eaten cold. With chicken and turkey, opt for white meat and remove the skin, which has most of the fat. Sushi is sold in many supermarkets in plastic containers perfect for taking "to go." Choose vegetable rolls (such as California or cucumber) to get fiber and flavor for fewer calories.

No Cooling Necessary

GO FISH
If a cool pack isn't an option, buy low-calorie single-serving cans or vacuum-packed pouches of tuna. Three ounces of white tuna packed in water (110 calories), with two pieces of whole wheat bread (220 calories) and one packet of mayonnaise from a deli (100 calories), totals 430 calories. Chicken of the Sea also sells a 3-ounce vacuum-packed Smoked Pacific Salmon, which has only 120 calories.

PB&J
Peanut butter and jelly are among the few foods that require no cooling or heating. Though peanut butter is high in calories, using a moderate amount can keep your meal low calorie and nutritious. Two tablespoons of natural peanut butter (190 calories), sugar-free jelly, such as Smucker's (20 calories for 2 tablespoons), and two pieces of low-calorie, whole wheat bread (120 calories) totals just 330 calories.

MEAL REPLACEMENT SHAKES
They're fine if you have one with a salad or soup and a piece of fruit. Just make sure it's satisfying, so that you don't feel hungry too soon. Low-carb Slim-Fast has about 180 calories—taste-test and find the ones you enjoy.

SOME LIKE IT HOT
To keep almost any food hot—especially soups, stews, or chilis—Aladdin's Heat & Go series has a double wall of foam

insulation that's activated in the microwave and can keep food hot for more than four hours. Thermos (www.thermos.com) and other companies also make insulated vacuum containers to keep liquids hot.

MICROWAVE, BUT NO FRIDGE

A few companies make low-calorie microwavable meals (although many are high in sodium). Some from Simply Asia (www.simplyasia.net) taste great, especially the Soy Ginger Noodle Bowl at just 420 calories for the entire 8-ounce meal. The meals from Fantastic Foods (www.fantasticfoods.com) are organic and lower in sodium. They use an innovative cooking technology developed by NASA to preserve the flavor and nutrition. Try the Spanish Paella at only 280 calories for the entire 8-ounce meal.

SOUPS

Hot in an insulated container or cold soups are great, especially since research shows that low-calorie soups (fewer than 120 calories for 8 ounces) are very filling and help you eat less. But soups can have a lot of sodium. Your best bets are those with less than 600 milligrams per serving, such as Healthy Choice and the low-sodium versions of Progresso and Campbell's. Also look for Moosewood's excellent line of low-calorie organic soups (www.fairfieldfarmkitchens.com).

Even if you have just hot water, there are low-calorie soups from Fantastic Foods and Health Valley to which you only need to add hot water. Make sure to follow the directions, and don't add too much.

There are also microwavable "soups to go"; both Campbell's and Progresso make them.

SNACKS AND SIDES

Fruits and vegetables are low-cal, nutritious, filling, and don't have to be refrigerated or reheated. Apples, pears, grapes, and

Calorie Bargain Spotlight

Calorie Bargain: FruitaBü Fruit Twirls

The Why: You know that grocery aisle with all the junky, high-calorie sweet snacks? The one that's usually frequented by moms, snatching up boxes of fruit-flavored, sugary packets to throw in their kids' lunch bags? Well, this calorie bargain will give you a feel-good reason to go down that aisle. Kids will love 'em, and even adults can look forward to this fun, tangy snack. The twirls are long, thin strips of dried fruit puree, pressed onto wax paper and all rolled up. These are a great, portion-controled snack, and since there are about eighteen inches of fruit to enjoy, it lasts a long time. Part of the fun is picking your twirl-eating style. Some of our tasters unrolled the whole thing first. Others went the silly route, and ate and unrolled as they went along.

The Health Bonus: Each twirl has 1 serving of organic fruit. In fact, they say the extra *O* in *smoooshed* is for Organic.

What We Liked Best: The all-natural ingredient list, grabability, and tangy fruit kick.

What We Liked Least: Not much bad to say here, except that maybe that you have to deal with a piece of sticky paper . . .

The Price: $3.69 to $3.99 for a box of six.

Offerings: available in Smoooshed Fruit Strawberry, Smoooshed Fruit Apple, and Smoooshed Fruit Grape.

Website: www.fruitabu.com.

Where to Buy: Fruit Twirls are available nationwide in health food stores and major grocery chains. You can also visit the FruitaBü site to purchase online, or look up a store near you.

Ingredients: organic apple puree concentrate, organic apple juice concentrate, organic white grape juice concentrate, organic strawberry puree concentrate, organic apple, organic palm fruit oil, citrus pectin, natural strawberry flavor, fruit juice for color, citric acid, sodium citrate, acerola cherry extract (natural vitamin C), soy lecithin.

Nutritional Analysis per Serving: 1 Twirl
80 calories
1.5 g fat
16 g carb
0 g protein

cut-up melon are durable and portable. Enjoy unsweetened all-natural applesauce packs or a small box of raisins. Other good choices:

- Nonfat yogurt is a great portable snack, but it's perishable, so pack it in an insulated bag or freeze it the night before.
- Low-calorie cereals (for instance, Kashi Seven Whole Grain Puffs Cereal, at only 70 calories per cup) work well in a sealable bag. Choose cereals with no more than 160 calories per cup, and avoid added sugar and partially hydrogenated oil.
- Hard-boiled eggs pack well, and you can either eat only the whites or go for the entire egg for about 80 calories.
- Whole-grain rice cakes vary widely in calorie and fat content. Quaker Lightly Salted Rice Cakes are only 35 calories each.
- Energy bars tend to be high in calories and fat but are an acceptable alternative to candy bars. One bar shouldn't exceed 200 calories.
- Soy chips or baked chips come packed in 1-ounce portions. Look for brands with fewer than 120 calories per ounce (potato chips are about 160).

- Jell-O Sugar Free Reduced Calorie Pudding Snacks are 60 calories and can be kept in a cooler until lunch.
- Jell-O Smoothie Snacks are 100 calories and great if you're not a yogurt fan.
- Nabisco makes 100-calorie portion-controlled snack packs (Oreo Thin Crisps, Wheat Thins Minis, to name two) that have no trans fat. They're a decent snack once in awhile, but don't start choosing them instead of fruit.

A Campout for Lunch

A lot of interesting (but often high-sodium) on-the-go foods come from the camping and/or military crowd, who need tasty yet convenient chow. AlpineAire Foods (www.aa-foods .com) sells self-heating food packages: Pull a tab, and in just fifteen minutes the package actually cooks itself. The Chicken Pasta Parmesan (280 calories per 12-ounce portion, but more than 1,000 milligrams of sodium) and the meatless Mountain Chili (280 calories per 12 ounces, but more than 1,500 milligrams of sodium) are both very tasty and low in fat. They're about $8 per meal, plus shipping.

Beverages

Choose unsweetened iced tea, bottled water, or other low- or no-calorie drinks. Try Crystal Light On the Go. Pour a packet into any 16.9-ounce (0.5-liter) bottled water and shake. Avoid high-calorie sodas, fruit juices, teas, or anything else with more than 30 calories per 8 ounces.

Combination Brown-bag Lunches

4-ounce white-meat turkey breast sandwich on 100 percent whole wheat bread with 1 slice low-fat provolone, mustard, lettuce, tomato, onion: 360 calories.
1 Jell-O Sugar Free Reduced Calorie Pudding: 60 calories.
1 banana: 120 calories.
Total calorie count: 540 calories.

4 ounces smoked salmon on 100 percent whole wheat bread with 2 tablespoons of low-fat cream cheese and dill: 420 calories.
Low Fat Hickory Barbeque Kettle Chips (1-ounce bag): 110 calories.
Nonfat, sugar-free vanilla yogurt (6 ounces): 90 calories.
Total calorie count: 620 calories.

2 ounces hummus on 100 percent whole wheat pita with lettuce, tomato, and onion: 250 calories.
2 dill pickles: 5 calories.
Kashi 7 Whole Grain Puffs Cereal (1 cup): 70 calories.
Progresso Vegetable Classics Vegetable Soup (1 cup): 80 calories.
Apple: 80 calories.
Total calorie count: 485 calories.

1 medium grilled chicken breast on 100 percent whole wheat bread with roasted red pepper, lettuce, and mustard: 390 calories.
3-ounce side salad with packet of Newman's Own Low Fat Balsamic Vinaigrette: 55 calories.
1 orange: 60 calories.
Total calorie count: 505 calories.

Calorie Bargain Spotlight

Calorie Bargain: Snack Factory's Pretzel Crisps—Everything Flavor

The Why: Pretzel Crisps are a very tasty alternative to potato chips (150 calories per ounce) when you're in need of a good salt fix.

The Health Bonus: They're low calorie and also low in fat—no trans or saturated fats.

What We Liked Best: My favorite flavor is Everything.

What We Liked Least: Make sure you portion them, because they're addictive. Though Pretzel Crisps are lower in calories than potato chips, it's only slightly. (So you can't eat the whole bag.)

The Price: $2.99

Offerings: Original, Buffalo Wing, Chipotle Cheddar, Garlic, Honey Mustard & Onion, Everything.

Website: www.pretzelcrisps.com.

Where to Buy: www.snackaisle.com.

Ingredients: wheat flour, seasoning (salt, sesame seeds, poppy seeds, dehydrated garlic, dehydrated onion, caraway seeds), sugar, barley malt.

Nutritional Analysis per Serving: 1 Ounce
100 calories
0 g fat
21 g carbs
3 g protein
1 g fiber
350 mg sodium

4 ounces (2 to 3 slices) deli ham on 100 percent whole wheat bread with 1 slice low-fat Swiss cheese, lettuce, tomato, and mustard: 420 calories.

½ cup grapes: 60 calories.

Campbell's Kitchen Classics Chicken Noodle Soup (1 cup): 90 calories.

Total calorie count: 570 calories.

Part Five

HOLIDAYS AND OTHER SPECIAL OCCASIONS

Holiday celebrations aren't the only potential diet busters. Meals on the road or in the air, business lunches, and romantic dinners—even the foods you eat in front of the tube while watching the big game—can all turn into diet disasters. To avoid the calorie overload that can sneak up on you when you're most vulnerable, the Diet Detective has searched out the best alternatives for keeping you on track.

Halloween Choices

According to the National Confectioners Association, more than 93 percent of children go trick-or-treating each year. But it's not just kids. Ninety percent of parents admit to sneaking goodies from their kids' trick-or-treat bags. Don't worry, I'm not going to take the fun out of one of the great "treat" holidays of all time. While I do believe that small things make a difference, and I strongly advocate dietary consistency for long-term weight control (no one-day breaks), I'm not going to spoil your Halloween. However, I do have a few healthier choices to share.

Candy Corn vs. Mini Chocolate Candy

Based simply on calories and fat, candy corn is the better bet. Because it's so sweet, it's hard to eat more than a couple of 1-ounce packages (220 calories for two packages), and it's virtually fat free. On the other hand, you can eat a lot of chocolate very quickly, and each one of those mini candy bars has about 45 to 80 calories. But while chocolate has more saturated fat, on the positive side it also has some antioxidants and calcium (keep in mind it is still not a health food). So choose the chocolate minis—but only two or three.

- Reese's minis (5 pieces): 210 calories (about 45 calories for 1).
- Mini Nestlé Crunch bars (1 bar): 30 calories, 1.5 g fat, 4 g carbs.
- Mini mix (5 bite-size pieces, including Snickers, Milky Way, 3 Musketeers, and Twix): 200 calories, 9 g fat, 29 g carbs.

Fit Tip: If you want a chocolate taste with fewer calories, opt for mini York Peppermint Patties—only 50 calories and 1 gram of fat for more than a ½-ounce portion.

Pumpkin Seeds vs. Gummi Bears

Gummi bears have fewer calories—140 for 16 bears (1½ ounces)—and because they're so chewy and sticky, you may eat a lot less. But they offer no nutritional value, whereas pumpkin seeds are loaded with nutrients such as protein, healthy fat, iron, magnesium, manganese, phosphorous, and other minerals. Unfortunately, they also pack on the calories: 180 to 200 for a ¼ cup. I'd still vote for them, but be sure to watch how many you eat.

Chocolate Covered Raisins vs. Hershey's Kisses

The key here is knowing how many it's going to take to satisfy your chocolate craving. If you have six Hershey's Kisses (25 calories each), that's 150 calories, whereas 1 ounce of chocolate-covered raisins has about 120 calories—not too bad if you buy 1-ounce bags—plus you get the health benefits of the raisins. And if you eat them one at a time, they'll last longer then a few Kisses.

Fit Tip: Why not have plain old raisins? They have iron, potassium, and fiber, are low in sodium, fat free, and loaded with antioxidants. While not a calorie bargain, they're still healthier than either of the candy choices. A very small box (½ ounce) can pack 45 calories—about 1 calorie per raisin.

- Hershey's Kiss: 25 calories, 1.5 g fat, 3 g carbs.
- Raisins (¼ cup, or 1 box): 130 calories, 0 g fat, 31 g carbs.
- Raisinets (3 mini bags): 200 calories, 8 g fat, 34 g carbs.

Rice Krispies Treats vs. Halloween Sugar Cookies

It's a pretty close call: A Rice Krispies Treat (90 calories, 2 g fat, 18 g carbs) contains 10 fewer calories than a 1-ounce cookie (100 calories, 6 g fat, 12 g carbs). It's also lower in fat and individually wrapped to help control overeating, all of which makes it the better option. Not only that, but how many of us can really eat just one cookie?

Fit Tip: For a cookielike taste with fewer calories, try Miss Meringue. The sugar-free and fat-free free Vanilla Mini has 35 calories per 13 cookies; sugar-free Chocolate Minis have 40 calories per 13 cookies; Chocolate, Vanilla, and Rainbow Vanilla Minis all have 110 calories per 13 cookies.

Smarties vs. Skittles

Smarties, like their name, are the smarter choice. You can have two rolls of Smarties (total: thirty candies) for just 50 calories. Skittles, on the other hand, have 170 calories per 1½-ounce bag.

Halloween Cupcakes vs. Pumpkin Pie vs. Halloween Chocolate Layer Cake

Layer cake is by far the worst choice, at more than 400 calories. The cupcake and the pumpkin pie are close when it comes to calories, but since portion sizes are usually bigger for pie, a cupcake is typically your better bet. Definitely skip the whipped cream if you choose pumpkin pie—it adds 80 to 100 calories per serving. Oh, and a scoop of vanilla ice cream to make it à la mode tacks on another 270 calories.

- Entenmann's Halloween cupcake: 290 calories, 14 g fat, 40 g carbs.
- Entenmann's pumpkin pie (one slice, or one-fifth of the pie, 120 grams): 300 calories, 13 g fat, 41 g carbs.

Apple vs. Candy Apple

OK, this is a giveaway, but the point is the huge difference in calories: 60 to 80 for a plain old apple compared with 330 calories or more for a candy apple.

Tootsie Roll Midgee vs. Tootsie Pop

Tootsie Pops—about 60 calories each—last a lot longer than a single Tootsie Roll Midgee, which is about 25 calories. It might do more to satisfy your candy cravings.

Halloween Tips

Perhaps you went overboard last Halloween, and it spiraled into a Thanksgiving feeding frenzy that became a Christmas

Calorie Bargain Spotlight

Calorie Bargain: York Mints

The Why: What a beautfiul evening. Perfect weather. Great food and conversation—the energy between you made you feel like you were floating on a cloud. A good hair day. Even the heels you're wearing turned out to be comfortable. After dinner, the check arrived with a handful of just what you needed: a little bit of chocolate and a nice minty crunch. Wonder if those just blew the diet??

Well, now you can carry a tin of York mints with you in your bag at all times. At only 10 calories for three mints, they'll end the perfect evening (or lunch, or boring meeting) without blowing the diet.

The Health Bonus: You'll get a nice bite-size dark-chocolate fix without packing on the pounds.

What We Liked Best: the taste, the calories (that there aren't many), and the tin. Plus, there are health benefits to chocolate.

What We Liked Least: no real nutritional value here, and not exactly all-natural ingredients.

The Price: $1.85 per tin.

Website: www.hersheys.com/products/details/york.asp?id=4757-2615.

Where to Buy: Amazon.com.

Ingredients: sugar, dextrose, semisweet chocolate (chocolate, sugar, lactose, cocoa, cocoa butter, milk fat, soy lecithin, PGPR, emulsifiers, vanillin, artificial flavor); corn syrup, contains 2 percent or less of glycerin, artificial color, gum acacia, natural flavors, resinous glaze, carnauba wax, invertase.

Nutritional Analysis per Serving: 3 Mints
10 calories
0 g fat
3 g carbs
0 g protein

binge, which turned into a 5-pound weight gain. Sound familiar? Well, this year will be different. Here are a few unusual and not-so-unusual tactics for treating your friends, foes, and family instead of treating yourself.

Keep It High: Place the candy for trick-or-treaters upstairs so you have to run up and down the stairs to get it. Do this ten times, and you've burned about 68 calories.

Walk It Off: Take your children trick-or-treating and keep up with them! Three hours can burn 300 to 500 calories.

Don't Go Far Out: Don't buy Halloween candy too far in advance; you'll have less time to eat it!

Don't Enjoy: When buying candy for trick-or-treaters, choose kinds *you* don't really like.

Work It: Make your child's costume. Sewing burns about 100 calories per hour.

Get Full: Have a satisfying and nutritious lunch or dinner before trick-or-treating; you'll be less likely to pick at the candy bag if you're full!

Keep It at 100: Today there are a number of 100-calorie snack packages that are perfect for Halloween. They include: Planters Peanut Butter Cookie Crisps, Oreos, Chips Ahoy, Pringles, Cheese Nips, Wheat Thins, and Jolly Time Healthy Pop popcorn.

Thanksgiving Dinner

Is overeating on Thanksgiving really so bad? In spite of all the hype about excessive consumption—eating more than 2,000 calories in a single meal—you can rest easy. One day is just not that terrible.

However, don't jump for that shovelful of stuffing just yet. There are a few reasons you might want to be concerned. The first is that Thanksgiving is the start of a six-week downward spiral for dieters that ends with a few extra pounds added to your waistline. The other is that it sets the tone for the way you eat throughout the new year. Research shows that those who maintain the same diet regimen throughout the year are more likely to maintain their weight loss than those who take "breaks" for special occasions.

I'm not going to bore you with more stories about how fattening a Thanksgiving meal can be. Nor do I want to take the thrill out of your meal on one of the most important eating days of the year. However, I do believe that picking the right foods doesn't mean you're going to starve or that you won't enjoy your dinner.

Candied Sweet Potatoes vs. Mashed Potatoes

I was hoping that the candied sweet potatoes would somehow turn out to be less fattening, but no such luck. A cup of mashed potatoes has about 240 to 300 calories, depending on how much butter (each tablespoon is 100 calories) and what type of milk or cream you use. Candied sweet potatoes, however, also contain butter—as well as brown sugar and sometimes even marmalade, honey, maple syrup, marshmallows, and/or pecans, which can add up to more than 450 calories for a 1-cup portion.

Your best bet? Stick the sweet potato in the microwave until it's soft, then mash it up with some margarine spray and salt; you'll probably be more than satisfied at about one-third the calories. You can also cut the sweet potato into six pieces, put it in the toaster oven, and then coat the cooked potato with margarine spray for "guiltless" sweet potato fries. Or, to reduce the calories in regular mashed potatoes, prepare them with skim milk, low-fat plain yogurt, or poultry broth, and fat-free sour cream instead of whole milk and butter.

Apple Cider vs. Beer vs. Wine

Apple cider has about 120 calories per 8-ounce serving, which is similar to many beers and wines. Just watch how many glasses you're having because the calories can add up quickly, especially when you're eating a lot of salty food. Alternatives: unsweetened iced tea with mint, water with lemon, or diet soda.

Sausage Stuffing vs. Wild Rice

Regular wild rice (about 160 to 220 calories per cup) is not so bad, but when you start dressing it up for Thanksgiving with loads of olive oil, pecans, and cranberries, it can add up to 550 or 600 calories per cup. However, the same amount of stuffing made with eggs, butter, and sausage is in that same high-calorie range. (By the way, you don't have to use butter in stuffing at all unless you're cooking it in a pan outside the bird, in which case you have a choice of basting it with the turkey drippings or dotting it with butter.) Stick with the rice; at least it offers some health benefits because of the nuts and cranberries. Or try preparing the stuffing with croutons, chopped apple, celery, and onion, and moistening it with chicken broth.

Traditional Turkey Gravy vs. Cranberry Sauce

Funny, I thought cranberry sauce would be the winner, but gravy is the right choice. Per ½ cup, cranberry sauce has 180 calories compared with only 80 calories for traditional turkey gravy.

If you want to make the gravy lower in calories, you can remove the fat with a gravy separator (a cup with a spout designed to pour the juices from the bottom and leave the fat on top), or you can add ice cubes to the pan juices so that the fat hardens and clings to the ice. If you have enough time, you can also refrigerate the pan drippings so that the fat rises to the top and hardens, allowing you to scrape it off before reheating the gravy.

Turkey: White Meat vs. Dark Meat

The dark meat has about 15 percent more calories. A 3½-ounce serving of turkey breast with skin has about 153 calories; dark meat with skin has about 182 calories. If you really want to save, you need to remove the skin, but not until after the turkey is cooked; otherwise the meat will dry out during the long cooking time. Removing the skin saves another 10 percent in calories. White meat without skin: 135 calories; dark meat without skin: 162 calories.

Other healthy suggestions include roasting your turkey on a rack so that it is not sitting in its own juices. The rack does not have to be metal. A bed of chopped onions and carrots, or quartered apples, or a medley of lemon, orange, and lime quarters not only acts as a rack, it also adds wonderful flavor and fragrance to the holiday bird. You can also baste the turkey with apple juice or low-fat chicken broth instead of its own juices.

Butternut Squash vs. Pumpkin Soup

In this case, they're both pretty good bargains. Creamy butternut squash soup has about 90 to 140 calories a cup. Pumpkin soup is also very low in calories, coming in at about 100 to 140 calories per cup. But either one can quickly turn into a diet disaster, depending on how much butter, oil, or cream is used in the preparation. Try nonfat yogurt rather than sour cream or heavy cream as your thickener if you don't want the calories per cup to shoot up to as much as 400.

Creamed Pearl Onions vs. Creamed Sweet Corn vs. Sautéed Spinach with Garlic

I guess with *creamed* in the name, you would immediately assume that the onions and corn weren't fat free or calorie free. And you'd be correct. Creamed pearl onions are traditionally made with milk, butter, flour, and sometimes nuts and have about 225 calories per 1 cup serving. The spinach with garlic is your best bet at about 175 calories per cup. And the big loser is the creamed corn, at a whopping 325 calories per cup.

Pumpkin Pie vs. Apple Pie vs. Pecan Pie

The pumpkin pie is actually the best of the three, coming in at 270 calories per slice, but the apple pie is a close second at about 350. Pecan pie, however, is a dietary mess at more than 700 calories. Whichever one you choose, definitely skip the whipped cream—it adds an extra 80 to 100 calories per serving. Oh, and if you add a scoop of vanilla Häagen-Dazs ice cream to make it à la mode, tack on another 270 calories.

Christmas and Other Holiday Parties

OK, so a few years ago the *New England Journal of Medicine* reported that holiday weight gain isn't so bad after all: only 1 pound per year on average. The problem is, you never lose that 1 pound you gained. I know that if I let go every holiday season and didn't make at least a few healthy choices, well, let's just say I'd be back to shopping for my clothing in the husky department. So here are a few pickier choices you can make, whether you're at a holiday party, a family dinner, or even deciding what to eat from that holiday gift basket.

Chocolate Martini vs. Eggnog vs. Champagne vs. Hot Buttered Rum

The hands-down winner is champagne. A 4-ounce glass contains about 85 calories. A chocolate martini, made with vodka, chocolate liqueur, cream, and dark creme de cacao, has about 440 calories. Eggnog has 340 to 460 calories per 8-ounce glass, depending on the ingredients used (typically egg, heavy cream, and cognac). You can, however, make your eggnog lower in calories by using nonfat milk, egg whites, and artificial sweetener, which would drop it down to about 100 to 110 calories per 8 ounces. Oh, and if you think hot-buttered rum is much better, think again. It's made with butter (just 1 tablespoon has 100 calories) and sugar, and it weighs in at about 220 calories per 8 ounces.

Candy Cane vs. Chocolate-covered Marshmallow Santa vs. Hollow Milk Chocolate Santa

The candy cane wins at 55 calories (for a ½-ounce cane). What surprised me is that the chocolate-covered marshmallow Santa (180 calories for 1½ ounces) by Russell Stover has fewer calories than the hollow milk chocolate Santa (280 calories for 1¾ ounces). The main reason: Although it contains sugar, the marshmallow is fat free, and fat has more calories per gram than sugar (9 calories per gram for fat versus 4 for sugar). However, if you're looking to save even more calories, Russell Stover has a sugar-free Santa that's only 90 calories, but it's only 1 ounce. Yes, it's smaller, but it will probably satisfy you—that's the beauty of portion control.

Mixed Nuts vs. Sugar-coated Pecans

Nuts may have health benefits, but they also have a whole lot of calories. Even so, the mixed nuts have fewer than the sugared pecans. Mixed nuts have 170 calories per ounce, while the pecans, which are coated with egg whites and sugar, have 220 calories per ounce. Here are a few other stomach stuffers: a handful of honey-roasted peanuts: 152 calories; 10 veggie sticks and a bit of dip: 76 calories; one handful of potato chips: 198 calories.

Diet Detective's What You Need to Know

Holiday Fit Tips

Eat First

It may sound absurd, but if you are going to a holiday party, eat ahead of time. I know plenty of people who starve themselves before going to a party so they'll have room for all the great food. They arrive—stomachs rumbling—and make a beeline for the high-calorie, high-fat appetizers and finger foods, easily eating more than a day's worth of calories. Instead, try eating enough healthy food beforehand so you're full before you arrive. You'll have much more self-control around those tempting party treats.

All or Nothing

I don't know how many times I've heard someone say "I've already ruined my diet, so it doesn't matter what I eat now." I'm not sure how that myth got started, but it can be hazardous to your waistline. The bottom line is, an extra calorie is an extra calorie—so eating a slice of pie shouldn't give you an excuse to eat two more. And after a bowl of ice cream, you don't have to eat whatever is left in the container. Have you ever heard of cutting your losses? Well, the same rule applies to cutting your gains. It's never too late to stop.

Strategize

You might think that planning what you're going to eat beforehand takes all the fun and spontaneity out of the occasion, but that's just not so. You're probably thinking about what you're going to eat anyway, so why not make it work for you instead of against you? In fact, practicing good eating behavior at special events could actually make you feel more relaxed and empowered, not frustrated or disappointed. It gives you the sense of being in control of your environment instead of being lured into the dark world of overindulgence. So plan what and how much you're going to eat at the event before you even get there. Set limits, and you'll feel better.

For instance, if you know there's going to be cake and ice cream, and you typically have two or sometimes three servings, mentally rehearse having only one serving of each. And if you know you're going to want dessert, cut back on your main course or make sure to have a low-calorie option ready, such as fruit.

Watch Out for Food Pushers

How many times has a family member or friend told you that you'll spoil the party if you don't partake in the food festivities, or that it's bad luck not to have at least one slice of cake? Have your answer ready for those diet saboteurs. Mentally rehearse a few key phrases like, "Oh, no thanks. I couldn't eat another thing." Or try the truth: "I'm dieting, and that piece of cake will throw me completely off track."

Recruit Your Friends

Getting the support of your friends and family is not always easy, but it's worth a try. Talk to them about the healthy changes you're making and enlist their help. The idea is not to have them police your behavior but for them to empower you by being encouraging and enthusiastic about your new way of life.

Balance It Out

Looking for a guilt-free way to enjoy your favorite holiday treat? Try consuming fewer calories the day before and after the holiday. It's basically a matter of calorie balance. By consuming 500 fewer calories on either side, you're leaving room for 1,000 extra calories. So a rich holiday dinner or party can be balanced by a lighter meal the day after.

Trade-Off

Do a trade-off. Eating more during the holidays can be offset, at least in part, by a moderate increase in daily exercise. Keep in mind that every 100 calories is equal to about twenty-five minutes of walking. Here's an example of a Thanksgiving meal:

- 5 crackers with 1 ounce of cheese: 140 calories
- 4 thick turkey slices with gravy: 375 calories
- A mound of stuffing: 530 calories (1½ cups)
- ½ cup cranberry relish: 245 calories

- Sweet potato casserole: 285 calories (6 ounces)
- A mound of mashed potatoes: 240 calories (1½ cups)
- 1 slice of pumpkin pie: 240 calories
- 1 slice of apple pie: 290 calories
- Cider with rum: 160 calories (8 ounces)

That's approximately 2,500 calories; if you normally eat 1,500 calories per day, you'd have to walk for about four hours to compensate for the additional 1,000.

Bring Your Own Food

Offer to bring a dish to the next party. By supplying your own food, you can eat without abandoning your healthy diet, bypass the foods high in fat or sodium, and still feel a part of the crowd.

Take Control

Host a holiday event or party yourself. Believe me, with all that constant moving, planning, cooking, and preparing, you are bound to lose weight (as long as you give away the leftovers). Or, if you don't want to be the host, try helping out. If you're constantly on your feet, setting up, serving, and cleaning, you'll have less free time for nibbling.

Enjoy It

We often eat without thinking. We're so engaged in conversation and socializing that we stuff our faces without even realizing what or how much we're eating. Remember what your mom always told you: Don't talk with your mouth full. And make a conscious effort to pay attention to what you're eating—you might even enjoy it more.

It Pays to Be Picky

During the holidays, foods you wouldn't normally eat suddenly become more appealing (especially with a "you only live once" attitude), so be selective. Eat the things you really love—maybe a small serving of mashed sweet potatoes, a sliver of pecan pie—and ignore the not-so-thrilling stuff.

Easy on the Alcohol

Alcohol decreases inhibitions—potentially causing you to eat more—plus it's loaded with calories. If you're going to drink, stick with wine or beer and stay away from exotic fruity cocktails or fancy coffee drinks.

Feeling Full

Most people miss the physical cues signaling that they have eaten enough. Instead of waiting until you're bursting out of your clothes, try eating whatever you want, but stop once you are full. How will you know you're full? Wait fifteen to twenty minutes after you've finished what's on your plate before requesting seconds or dessert. By delaying, you may find that your appetite for a second helping decreases.

Dumplings vs. Mini Egg Rolls vs. Mini Pizzas

Waiters are roaming the room, passing out delicious appetizers. Which ones should you choose? Don't let those mini pizzas go by; they might be your best bet among these three: about 35 to 55 calories each. Whether the dumplings are filled with pork, vegetables, chicken, or beef, the calories still add up. You're looking at about 50 to 200 calories for each dumpling, depending on the size and the ingredients, whereas one mini egg roll has about 40 to 50 calories. Some other appetizers to keep in mind: mozzarella sticks: 431 calories; six Buffalo wings with blue cheese dressing: 316 calories; large chicken fingers: 634 calories.

Stuffed Brie vs. Port Wine Cheddar Log

Stuffed brie is by far the worse choice here, at about 420 calories per 3 ounces. It's made with butter, brie, and phyllo dough (puff pastry) and is often stuffed with some type of chutney or filling. A cheddar log, believe it or not, is a much better deal. For instance, Hickory Farms Cheese Celebration (a port and cheddar log covered in fresh nuts) has 240 calories for 3 ounces.

Baked Country Ham vs. Turkey vs. Prime Rib

You're at the carving station of the buffet at your holiday party (or the dinner table at your friend's or relative's house) and you want to make the best choice. If you guessed that the turkey is the best deal, you're right: White-meat turkey without the skin has about 193 calories for 5 ounces. A country ham is made with brown sugar, apple cider, and red wine vinegar and has about 340 calories for 5 ounces. And forget the prime rib—it's the worst of the three, at 450 calories for a 5-ounce portion.

Roasted Potatoes vs. Asparagus with Parmesan Cheese

Three pieces of roasted potato (half a medium potato) have about 80 calories. Compare that to five medium asparagus spears cooked with oil or butter and topped with grated Parmesan cheese at about 105 to 120 calories (depending on how much cheese is used). The potatoes look like the winner here in terms of calories—assuming you don't eat more than three pieces. But both have vitamins and minerals that make them nutrient-dense foods.

One Genoa Salami Slice on a Cracker with Cheese = Wrapping Presents for 55 Minutes

Those tiny little slices of salami may seem harmless, but take a closer look. See those little white flecks, the ones that take up a good 25 percent to 50 percent of the slice? Those are little bits of calorie-laden lard. So if you plan to go to town on the salami appetizer, I hope you've also gone to town on your present buying.

Fit Tip: If you have a salami weakness, at least make sure to skip its best friends—the crackers and cheddar cheese. One cracker adds 16 calories, and just a ½ ounce of cheddar tacks on another 55. So if you really want the salami, enjoy it by itself.

Two Christmas Cookies = 27 Minutes Shoveling Snow

Holiday cookies vary in size and shape, but what with the butter or shortening, sugar, frosting, and sprinkles, expect the calories for a typical sugar cookie to be in the range of 50 to 120. And a gingerbread cookie, also made with butter or shortening with the addition of molasses, can be even worse, at up to 190 calories. That may not sound so bad, but be honest with yourself—can you really stop at just one? We're talking almost a half hour of nonstop hardcore snow shoveling for just two cookies. So check out the snowdrifts in your driveway before you grab that second cookie.

Fit Tip: Don't keep cookies in a dish or bowl where you can see them, especially while you're talking on the phone or sitting in front of the television. Instead, store them in an airtight container on a very high shelf.

One Slice of Fruitcake = Building a Snowman for 80 Minutes

At 325 calories for a 3½-ounce slice, traditional fruitcake, made with walnuts, cherries, raisins, pineapple, and molasses and spiced with cinnamon and cloves, will add up to a long stretch of snowman building—eighty minutes, to be exact. At that rate, you may have to borrow snow from your neighbor to use up the last few calories.

Fit Tip: According to the *Wall Street Journal,* fruitcake bakers believe the serving size should be only 1½ ounces, or about 160 calories. And maybe they have a point. The redeeming quality of fruitcake is that it's incredibly dense— so dense, in fact, that you probably don't need a 3½-ounce serving to feel satisfied.

Four Bite-size Mini Pizzas (3.1 Ounces) = Waiting to See Santa with Three Rambunctious Kids (Mild Calisthenics) for 40 Minutes

Those little pizzas with lots of cheese (and sometimes pepperoni) disappear so fast that it seems they were never there, but your waistline knows the truth. And even chasing your kids around the mall won't burn enough calories to keep you trim.

Fit Tip: Make 'em yourself. Toast pita bread with a sprinkle of Parmesan or part-skim mozzarella and some low-calorie tomato sauce. Then throw on veggies and enjoy a low-cal, easy-to-make snack.

One Large Scoop of Bread Stuffing with Sausage = Performing *The Nutcracker* for 65 Minutes

A scoop of stuffing made with eggs, butter, and sausage can be in the range of 350 to 500 calories, which means you'll be doing pirouettes, spins, jumps, and pliés for sixty-five minutes nonstop. Don't kid yourself: Stepping in for the sugar plum fairy doesn't mean bopping to "Rockin' around the Christmas Tree"—ballet is a high-end aerobic workout.

Fit Tip: Prepare the stuffing with croutons, chopped apple, celery, and onion, and moisten it with chicken broth. By the way, you don't have to use any butter at all unless you're cooking the stuffing in a pan outside the bird, in which case you have a choice of basting it with the turkey drippings or dotting it with butter.

One Cup of Eggnog (8 Ounces) = Decorating the Tree for 97 Minutes

Eggnog is a diet catastrophe. It packs about 340 to 460 calories, depending on the ingredients and proportions. Typically it includes raw egg, heavy cream, and a shot or two of brandy. Exercisewise, you're looking at ninety-seven minutes of continuous tree decorating—up and down the ladder, finding the ornaments, and reaching up to the top.

Fit Tip: Make your eggnog with skim milk. At least you'll deduct the heavy cream from this diet disaster equation.

One Candy Cane (½ Ounce) = Writing Holiday Greeting Cards for 60 Minutes

Have you fallen a bit behind on your winter correspondence? Well, now is the time to get back in the game of shooting those family portraits and signing your name on the back. And if you're trimming the tree with candy canes, you'd better have a lot of friends and family to send cards to this season. A full hour of addressing and signing greeting cards burns the 60 calories in a single cane.

Fit Tip: Lick, don't bite; it will last longer. And don't start popping those red and green M&M's while you're practicing your penmanship.

Three Mini Spring Rolls with Dipping Sauce = 19 Minutes Dancing as a Rockette at Radio City Music Hall

At only 45 calories per 1-ounce roll, these might not seem like a bad deal. After all, a Rockette burns those calories in just six minutes on stage. But before you dig into the appetizer plate, give this a try: Kick your leg up to your nose. If you're still standing up, do it again. In fact, do it for six minutes without taking a single break. How'd that work out for you?

The problem with those mini rolls is that they're relatively insubstantial, and they're often fried. So while one may not seem like a lot of calories, it becomes a lot when you're on your seventh.

Fit Tip: First off, steam or bake—don't fry—them. And at your holiday party, work hard to escape the "have to eat it all now" mentality. You know what I mean: You see the buffet table and make a beeline for it, piling three of anything that looks good onto a napkin to make sure you get enough of the good stuff. We all do it. But it means that we end up with a lot of greasy, calorie-packed food in our hands—and in our stomachs.

Four Pitted Olives in Extra-virgin Olive Oil (1 Ounce) = Preparing for and Serving at the Holiday Party for 51 minutes

They're little, and they seem pretty healthy, right? Unfortunately, even soaking olives in their own heart-healthy oil leaves them dripping with excess calories—150 for 1 ounce, or four olives, to be precise. That's the equivalent of fifty-one minutes of cooking, prepping, timing, slicing, arranging, and serving at your annual holiday gala.

Fit Tip: There are some good olive choices. Cracked green olives have only 8 calories apiece, so if you like the oil-soaked variety, at least mix them up. That way you can eat a few more without overdoing the calories. And while getting things ready in the kitchen, snack on baby carrots. If you opt for olives, you'll OD on calories before the party even gets started.

The following are typical holiday foods and the number of minutes required to burn them off after you've exhausted your daily caloric budget.

HOLIDAY FOOD	AMOUNT	CALORIES	WALK	BIKE	RUN	SWIM	YOGA	DANCE
Prime rib	½ pound	675	174	96	72	82	230	115
Cheese lasagna with meat sauce	9-ounce slice	490	126	70	52	60	167	83
Honey-glazed ham	6 ounces	210	54	30	22	26	71	36
Bite-size mini pizza	4 minis	163	42	23	17	20	55	28
Cracker with cheese	1 cracker	71	18	10	8	9	24	12
Christmas cookies	2 cookies	120	31	17	13	15	41	20
Fruitcake	3½-ounce slice	325	84	46	35	40	111	55
Pecan pie	1 slice (⅛ of a pie)	503	130	71	54	61	171	86
Cocktail peanuts	3 ounces (90 nuts)	510	131	72	54	62	173	87
Candy cane	1½-ounce cane	55	14	8	6	7	19	9
Homemade pumpkin pie	1 slice (⅛ of a pie)	316	81	45	34	38	107	54
Beef franks in a blanket	5 pieces (2¾ ounces)	290	75	41	31	35	99	49
Mini crab cakes	4 pieces (57 grams)	70	18	10	7	9	24	12
Chicken fingers	2 pieces (1½ ounces)	240	62	34	26	29	82	41
Cheddar cheese	2 cubes (1 ounce)	110	28	16	12	13	37	19
Dinner roll	1 large (3½-inch diameter)	136	35	19	14	17	46	23
Ritz crackers	5 crackers	80	21	11	9	10	27	14
Deviled egg	1 egg / 2 halves	145	37	21	15	18	49	25
Gingerbread cookie	1 cookie	145	37	21	15	18	49	25
Regular beer	12 ounces	153	39	22	16	19	52	26
Martini	4 ounces	274	71	39	29	33	93	47
White wine	4 ounces	98	25	14	10	12	33	17
Eggnog	1 cup	343	88	49	37	42	117	58
Hot buttered rum	8 ounces	220	57	31	23	27	75	37

At the Mall

During the holiday season, my family generally spends many hours in our local mall. We walk, browse, buy gifts, go to the movies—and eat. And that's where the potential problems begin. With more than 1,130 shopping malls in the United States and the majority of us eating something whenever we visit one, there's potential for doing some serious diet damage during the already difficult holiday eating season. With a few key strategies, however, you can steer clear of Calorie Rip-offs while you're bargain hunting for the holidays.

Don't Starve

Resist the urge to starve yourself until you feel compelled to run to the food court and eat the first thing you can get your hands on. Ideally, eat before shopping. Or, if it's going to be a full day at the mall, schedule a meal break somewhere in the middle.

Avoid Variety

When you're strolling through the food court, watch where you're going. Research from the University of Pennsylvania has demonstrated that an increase in variety only adds to the amount we end up eating. The more choices there are, the worse it is. Decide what you're going to have before you get to the food court. Many malls have listings of all their food establishments on their websites, or you can look on the many mall directories that list them. Don't just walk in there without any preparation and be tempted by all the choices.

Mix and Match

Remember, there's no law that says you can't mix and match foods from different vendors, as long as you've planned ahead. For example, get the chicken teriyaki at the Japanese restaurant, a vegetable soup at the Italian place, and a low-fat frozen yogurt from the ice cream shop.

Eat for Real

You may think you just want something to "hold you over," but most times you'd be better off having a full-blown meal. Snacks can easily add up to the same amount of calories and fat as a meal. Then you end up eating twice, with double the calories. Just take a look at these classic mall treats: Cinnabon—more than 800 calories; Mrs. Fields chocolate chip cookies—more than 200 calories per cookie; Auntie Anne's Sesame Pretzel with butter—more than 400 calories. And avoid muffins; they often have well over 500 calories.

Diet Detective's What You Need to Know

Food Court Quick Tips

- Say no to butter, mayo, tartar sauce, creamy dressings, or extra cheese.
- Get Chinese food steamed with the sauce on the side; try the mixed vegetables or chicken and broccoli. Avoid egg rolls, fried rice, and deep-fried dishes like sweet-and-sour chicken, sesame chicken, or General Tso's chicken (more than 1,000 calories). And skip the duck sauce—just 2 tablespoons have 80 calories.
- Use mustard, ketchup, salt, pepper, or vinegar as fat-free ways to season your food.
- Even nonfat frozen yogurt can be a no-no if you get a large serving with toppings.
- Instead of cheese, opt for lettuce, tomato, and onion on your sandwich or burger; taking off one slice of cheese can save you about 100 calories.
- Top your pizza with vegetables instead of meat, and ask for half the cheese. Skip the stuffed pizza and the baked ziti or lasagna.
- Potatoes sound healthy, but the calories in the toppings can add up. Skip the butter, bacon, and sour cream. Try vegetables, and sprinkle with a light coating of cheese.

Drinking Hazards

Keep in mind that smoothies sold at places like Smoothie King, Orange Julius, and Jamba Juice are food, and they have as many calories as most meals. For example, a 20-ounce Smoothie King Banana Boat has 520 calories. Decide if you're having the smoothie as a meal replacement or simply as a drink with your burger and fries. Also watch out for specialty coffee drinks at Starbucks or Dunkin' Donuts; they too can be in the 350- to 500-calorie range.

Watch Your Steps

The average shopper spends more than eighty minutes per visit at the mall during the regular season, and that number probably doubles during the holidays. And since the typical mall is more than 850,000 square feet, there's plenty of room for walking. Bring a pedometer and see if you can get to 5,000 steps, which is about 2.5 miles. Make it your goal to walk the entire mall before you even start shopping or eating and again afterward—it might even help you find the best bargains. And don't park too close to the entrance; every step counts!

Free Equals Fat

Holidays bring about many "giveaways," including the free samples at the food court and in the stores. But remember, just because it's free doesn't mean it's calorie free. In fact, I was just in Williams-Sonoma, where they were offering some tasty samples, but when I stopped and looked at the packaging, I was amazed to find that a few of those little samples contained almost 300 calories. That's at least half a meal.

Bring Your Own

We pack lunches, drinks, and snacks for our younger kids when we go out with them—why not do it for ourselves? Since most malls have an open seating policy, you can bring your own sandwiches or other food to enjoy in the food court. You'll be eating healthier and saving money too.

Some Suggestions

Fruit: Apples, pears, and grapes are durable. Cut-up melon or other fruits become portable in a small container with a lid.

Nonfat yogurt: Yogurt is a great portable snack, but it is perishable, so pack it in an insulated bag or thermos.

Sandwiches: Precut them into portion-controlled sections so you can pull them out at different times without making a mess. Peanut butter, chicken, turkey, cold cuts, and cheese (on 100 percent whole wheat bread) are all great options for sandwiches on the go.

Sports and TV Watching

Throughout the year, many of us spend a lot of time in front of the TV watching football, basketball, baseball—and stuffing our faces. The problem is, we tend to forget the high-calorie snacks we munch on mindlessly as we watch. Overeating by 1,200 calories per game can pack on an extra 5 pounds during the football season alone. But with a few careful choices, you can reduce a potential food disaster to something like a controlled frenzy.

Guinness Draft vs. Sam Adams Light vs. Michelob Light

Amazingly, Guinness (only 125 calories per 12 ounces), which has been brewed using the same formula since 1759, has about the same number of calories as either Sam Adams Light (124 calories) or Michelob Light (134 calories). Michelob ULTRA is actually the lowest, with only 95 calories, but if you want a "regular" beer, Guinness is the answer.

Ham and Cheese vs. Turkey Sandwich

- Schlotzsky's Ham & Cheese—The Original-Style: 512 calories, 19 g fat, 85 g carbs, 30 g protein.

- Schlotzsky's Turkey—The Original-Style: 583 calories, 24 g fat, 54 g carbs, 36 g protein.

You'd think the turkey would be the clear winner, but not if you add mayo, which, with 100 calories per tablespoon, turns this seemingly healthy option into a diet debacle. Substitute mustard, a fat-free dressing, or ketchup to save calories and still enjoy great taste. White-meat turkey has about 50 calories in 1 ounce, and ham has about 70, so if you keep the cheese to one slice (100 calories and 8 grams of fat), the turkey is still better, but not by much.

When making any sandwich, the key is to start with leaner cold cuts like turkey, chicken, roast beef, and ham. On average, these contain no more than 110 calories and 5 grams of fat for a 2-ounce serving. Avoid higher-fat meats like bacon, bologna, salami, pimento loaf, and sausage. Cheese is a great source of calcium and protein, but it's also a source of excess calories and fat—primarily saturated fat. One ounce of regular cheese contains about 100 calories and 8 grams of fat, of which 5 grams are saturated. If you're bringing your food home from a deli, watch out: They typically add three to five slices per sandwich, which sends the calorie and fat content skyrocketing. For more flavor and to fill you up, add vegetable slices, sweet peppers, pickles, and plenty of lettuce.

Chicken Wings vs. Pepperoni Pizza

- 5 chicken wings with hot sauce and 3 tablespoons blue cheese dressing: 599 calories, 50 g fat, 3 g carbs, 33 g protein.
- 1 slice stuffed-crust pepperoni pizza: 370 calories, 15 g fat, 42 g carbs, 17 g protein.

Here again, you might think to yourself, "How harmful can wings be? They're small, and it's chicken, after all!" But the reality is, those chicken wings are deep fried with their skin, making them a borderline health hazard, especially with the blue cheese dressing. So skip the dressing (without it, the wings and pizza are almost tied for calories), or, better yet, go for a thin-crust veggie pizza.

Veggies and Dip vs. Chips and Salsa

- 15 carrot sticks and ¼ cup French onion dip: 146 calories, 9 g fat, 12 g carbs, 3 g protein.
- 1 cup tortilla chips with ½ cup salsa: 165 calories, 7 g fat, 24 g carbs, 4 g protein.

Believe it or not, it's close. Vegetables are typically a low-calorie choice, but it depends on what you do with them. Just as french fries start out with fiber- and nutrient-rich potatoes but end up high in calories and fat, carrot sticks dunked in a mayo- or sour cream–based dip aren't exactly a health food. Try using a low-calorie dip (4 tablespoons reduced-calorie dip: 88 calories, 7 grams of fat, 5 grams of carbs, 2 grams of protein) or make your own with nonfat yogurt or mayo. Oh, and just in case you don't think it matters what you dip with, compare 15 potato chips (150 calories) with 15 baked tortilla chips (81 calories). Why not skip the dip altogether and have some air-popped popcorn (3 cups: 92 calories, 1 gram of fat, 19 grams of carbs, 3 grams of protein) instead?

Chicken Nuggets vs. Pigs in a Blanket

- 5 chicken nuggets: 271 calories, 17 g fat, 13 g carbs, 15 g protein.

- 5 cocktail-size pigs in a blanket: 332 calories, 25 g fat, 17 g carbs, 9 g protein.

Because the chicken nuggets are fried, I was sure they'd be higher in calories. But the fat in the pigs and the dough in the blankets more than make up for the breaded and fried nuggets. Make grilled chicken breast strips, and you'll save serious calories. Also, be sure to use mustard, barbecue sauce, or ketchup instead of mayo or other high-calorie condiments.

Peanuts vs. M&M's

- ½ cup M&M's: 480 calories, 20 g fat, 68 g carbs, 4 g protein.
- ½ cup roasted peanuts: 424 calories, 36 g fat, 14 g carbs, 19 g protein.
- ½ cup pistachios in their shells: 164 calories, 13 g fat, 8 g carbs, 6 g protein.
- ½ cup roasted chestnuts: 175 calories, 2 g fat, 38 g carbs, 2 g protein.

The surprising thing is how similar M&M's and peanuts are in terms of calories. Yes, nuts are the better choice. They have more protein, which has been shown to make you feel full and more satisfied. Plus, nuts have unsaturated "good" fat, fiber, and plenty of other healthy nutrients. But they're also high in calories, and you can down a cup of nuts in no time. If you plan on eating peanuts, choose ones still in their shells— or go for pistachios. They take longer to eat, and it also looks like you're eating more because the shells pile up. You might want to try roasted chestnuts: They're big and bulky, low in fat, and very flavorful. And if they're in their shells, it will take you a while to peel them.

Honey Mustard Pretzels vs. Cooler Ranch Doritos

- 1 ounce Snyder's Honey Mustard & Onion Pieces: 140 calories, 7 g fat, 18 g carbs, 2 g protein.
- 1 ounce Cooler Ranch Doritos: 140 calories, 7 g fat, 18 g carbs, 2 g protein.

Neither choice has very much nutritional value. But if you must eat pretzels or Doritos, at least buy single-serving bags rather than the huge family size. They might cost a little more, but they'll save you from eating a lot more without thinking.

Other Tips and Suggestions

- Instead of snacking, eat your regular meals as you watch the game. This is food you'd be eating anyway, and if it's portion controlled, you'll be satisfied without over-eating.
- If you're going to overeat anyway, try picking foods that are low in calories to compensate. Air-popped popcorn, watermelon, baby carrots, or other vegetables without fattening dips let you eat a lot more for a lot fewer calories.
- Go for a walk at halftime.
- Don't serve all the snacks at once. Try putting something new out each quarter of a football or basketball game, or during the seventh-inning stretch if you're watching baseball.
- Keep the extra food in the kitchen. Out of sight, out of mind.
- Use small plates and bowls to encourage smaller serving sizes.

The Big Game

Let's all get together and huddle around the buffet: It's the Super Bowl. The Super Bowl has become much more than a football game. It's an eating event, just like Thanksgiving. Super Bowl Sunday with friends and family is now the second biggest day for food consumption in the United States after Thanksgiving. Discover the true costs of those game-day treats by learning how much time a 155-pound person would have to spend in his or her favorite Super Bowl activities to burn them off. What follows is not meant to ruin your day—just to give you a few tips for choosing the most splurge-worthy foods. And keep in mind that we all have a daily caloric budget, so it is only after you exhaust your daily budget that these exercise equivalents kick in.

Single Tortilla Chip Topped with Seven-Layer Dip = 9½ Minutes of Climbing the Stadium Stairs

To make seven-layer dip—perfect for dipping tortilla chips—refried beans are layered with guacamole, seasoned sour cream, veggies, and cheese. That's some serious calorie damage! Every time you dip into this combination, you're looking at about ten minutes of climbing the stadium stairs (based on 60 to 70 calories per ounce, depending on the recipe, plus one restaurant-style chip, which has about 22 calories, for a grand total of almost 90 calories).

Fit Tip: Use light or baked chips to reduce the per-chip calories to about 15, and switch to salsa—2 tablespoons have only about 15 calories. For seven-layer dip, use reduced-fat or nonfat cheese, baked chips, nonfat refried black beans, and nonfat sour cream.

Single Ritz Cracker with Cheez Whiz = 13 Minutes of Performing in a Marching Band

Yes, that's right. A simple Ritz Cracker has 16 calories, and just a tablespoon of Kraft Cheez Whiz contains 45 calories, for a grand total of 61 calories in a single bite.

Fit Tip: Avoid the cracker altogether and cut up small squares of low-fat cheese; you really won't notice the difference. In fact, you would probably eat cardboard if someone put it in front of you during the game.

"Nice Size" Helping of Meat Lasagna = Running 89 Football Fields

You're looking at pasta, mozzarella, creamy ricotta, meat, and other assorted high-calorie goodies. A 9-ounce portion (which is pretty large) has about 500 to 700 calories, again depending on the ingredients used.

Fit Tip: If you need pasta, skip the meat, cut back on the cheese, and bulk up your portion by filling your bowl at least halfway with vegetables.

Two Handfuls of Potato Chips = Running 45 Football Fields

Two handfuls of chips—about 2 ounces—have about 300 calories. Oh, and if you add just 2 tablespoons of onion dip (about 60 calories), you'll be running another nine football fields.

Fit Tip: Make homemade pita chips with margarine spray, or try Low Fat Kettle Chips and save more than a few football fields. Use plain nonfat yogurt instead of sour cream to mix up the dip.

Two Slices of Cheese Pizza = Doing the Wave 1,182 Times

Yes, pizza is a delicious snack food, but with the cheese and dough (forget about additional toppings, which would require additional waves), a typical slice has at least 260 calories.

Fit Tip: Try cheeseless pizza topped with plenty of veggies—broccoli, spinach, tomatoes, zucchini, mushrooms, or even artichoke hearts. Or go for thin-crust pizza with vegetable toppings instead of meat and extra cheese. Also, avoid personal pan pizza and stuffed-crust pizza: The thick, oily crust equals added fat and calories.

Handful/Gulp of Beer Nuts = 21 Minutes of Cheerleading

Don't kid yourself—cheerleading is not easy. Beer nuts have about 170 calories per ounce, which is just about a handful.

Nuts are a good source of "healthy" fat and protein, but they are packed with calories. Macadamia nuts, for example, contain 200 calories per ounce.

Fit Tip: Munch your heart out on Kashi Good Friends Cinna-Raisin Crunch or some other delicious low-cal cereal.

One Oreo Double Stuf Cookie = Pro Football Coaching for 15 Minutes

You think it's easy? With the stress, pacing up and down the sidelines, waving your hands and screaming, coaching pro football takes its toll. But in the end, you're still burning only one 70-calorie Oreo Double Stuf for fifteen minutes of coaching.

Fit Tip: Have a few chocolate meringue cookies instead. Try Miss Meringue's sugar-free, fat-free cookies; they're amazing (www.missmeringue.com).

A Handful of Doritos Chips = 43 Touchdown Dances in the End Zone

Chips, in general, are pretty expensive calorically. A handful of Cooler Ranch Doritos: 140 calories.

Fit Tip: Eat one at a time, and don't put out huge bowls of them—make it so that you have to get up each time you want more than six chips.

Two Slices of Stuffed Pizza with the Works = 197 Minutes Cleaning the Stadium after the Game

Having two slices of Pizza Hut's 14-inch (large) Stuffed Crust Pizza means that you're looking at more than 800 calories. It's the word *stuffed* that should give you a clue.

Fit Tip: Get thin-crust pizza with veggies, and eat it for lunch or dinner instead of a halftime snack.

Five pretzels = 15 Minutes Walking Around Looking for Your Car after the Game

Yes, I'm talking about five regular pretzels out of a bag (for example, Rold Gold Classic Style Pretzel Thins). They add up to about 60 calories. For some reason, people think pretzels are healthful. Well, they don't have fat, but they also have no nutritional value.

Fit Tip: Make sure you avoid those pretzels that are loaded with cheese—wow, are they high in calories.

Four Beers = 64 Minutes of Climbing the Stadium Stairs

Who would've thunk it? Beer has calories: about 150 calories per 12 ounces. And no, I'm not going to tell you not to have a few beers.

Fit Tip: There are some great light beers out there. Do a taste test before the game. See if you can make the event more special with some fancy low-cal beers.

Part of a Giant Italian Sub = 138½ Minutes Performing in a Marching Band

This is for a 6-inch sub with salami, pepperoni, ham, lettuce, tomato, and mayonnaise. It's about 650 calories.

Fit Tip: Go for low-fat cheese and skip the mayo.

Five Buffalo Chicken Wings = 102 Minutes of Refereeing the Game

The wings are fried and high in calories, and that blue cheese dressing can be caloric suicide. Just five chicken wings with hot sauce and 3 tablespoons of blue cheese dressing: 599 calories.

Fit Tip: Use the hot sauce and skip the blue cheese. Make the wings yourself. Go skinless, and bake them instead of frying. With all that football action to distract you, you probably won't even notice the difference.

Half Order of Baby Back Ribs = 73 Minutes of Cheerleading

Ribs are good, but they're packed with calories—as if you didn't know. They're fatty, and the sauce is sugary.

Fit Tip: Trim all visible fat from the ribs before and after cooking. Also, instead of coating your ribs with an excessive amount of sauce beforehand, partially cook them loaded with seasonings, brush them lightly with the sauce, and then finish cooking.

One Quesadilla with Cheese (5½ Ounces) = 176 Minutes of Standing Up and Cheering While Waving Your Hands

A 5-ounce mozzarella cheese quesadilla has 516 calories.

Fit Tip: Make your quesadillas with low-cal mozzarella, and try baking, not frying them. Skip the sour cream.

Two Handfuls of Chex Mix = 30 Minutes Jumping Up and Down after Your Team Scores

At 280 calories, 1 ounce of this mix is still calorically expensive even though it's lower in fat than chips.

Fit Tip: Don't eat it by the handful, or skip it altogether and go for some low-cal microwave popcorn instead. Even better, make it air-popped and use a margarine spray.

A Nice Portion of Baked Ziti = Playing Pro Football for 39½ Minutes

Baked ziti is basically pasta with lots of cheese and sauce. It's the cheese that makes it so high in calories: 420 calories for 6 ounces.

Fit Tip: If you're going to have baked ziti, make it a meal, not just an after-dinner snack (or a predinner appetizer). Try making it with low-fat mozzarella and a lower-calorie sauce.

Two Pieces of Fried Chicken = Doing the Wave 3,220 Times

That's for one deep-fried chicken breast and one thigh— about 660 calories combined.

Fit Tip: Go skinless and bake your chicken instead of frying it.

A Bowl of Chili = Running 100 Football Fields

A 16-ounce bowl of chili packed with beef, beans, and assorted vegetables comes to about 500 calories. A few tablespoons of sour cream and some shredded cheese add 150 calories more, for a grand total of 650 calories.

Fit Tip: Use ground sirloin or white-meat turkey, or make it vegetarian. Skip the sour cream and cheese, or go for no-fat or low-fat versions.

Fueling for a Job Interview

These situations can be stressful simply because they're so unpredictable. Being prepared is important, but you also want to make sure you fuel your body for peak performance. You have to strike the right balance: You want to be organized, but you also want to be flexible and responsive to unforeseen questions or situations. The last thing you need to worry about is feeling queasy, hungry, overstuffed, or anything else the wrong meal might provoke.

Objective: Don't show up for an interview with your stomach making all kinds of feed-me, feed-me noises.

Pick These foods: Three to four ounces of lean protein such as fish, chicken, low-fat cottage cheese, or an egg-white omelet, one slice of whole-grain bread or brown rice, and 1 cup of fruit or vegetables. If you normally drink coffee, tea, or other caffeinated beverages with your meal, continue to do so, says Judith Wurtman, PhD, a research scientist at Massachusetts Institute of Technology.

Why? You are eating protein to make sure that your brain is manufacturing two chemicals (norepinephrine and dopamine, made from tyrosine) that control mental alertness.

Calorie Bargain Spotlight

Calorie Bargain: Fruit²O

The Why: Ideally, we would thirst for plain old water, drink plenty of it, and live in hydrated happiness. However, many of us just don't dig plain H_2O. And don't be fooled—some of the other clear liquids out there that look like viable water alternatives are wolves in sheep's clothing. Drinking multiple servings a day of a sugary drink could lead to a calorie budget disaster. Fruit²O, on the other hand, is a refreshing alternative that is calorie free, sugar free, and offers flavors with added healthy themes: Immunity, Energy, Hydration, and Relax.

The Health Bonus: Aside from counting toward your daily water requirement, some of the flavors have added vitamins and minerals.

What We Liked Best: The water smells good and tastes good. It's also slightly sweet (from the artificial sweetener Splenda).

What We Liked Least: It's a lot sweeter than water; you've really got to be in the mood for something sugary. Also, if you're a purist and don't go for artificial sweeteners, this isn't for you.

The Price: About 99 cents to $1.29 per bottle.

Offerings: Energy (raspberry flavor with caffeine), Immunity (berry pomegranate with antioxidants C and E and vitamin A), Hydration (electrolytes with vitamin B), and Relax (tropical fruit blend with chamomile and hibiscus).

Website: www.kraftfoods.com/fruit2o.

Where to Buy: They are available nationwide at select drug, convenience, and grocery stores, as well as club and mass-merchandise outlets.

Ingredients: Purified water, contains less than 2 percent of natural flavor, citric acid, malic acid, sucralose and acesulfame potassium (sweeteners), plus unique ingredients for each of the four varieties.

Nutritional Analysis per Serving: 8 Ounces.

Energy
0 calories
0 g fat
0 g carbs
0 g protein
10 mg sodium

Hydration
0 calories
0 g fat
0 g carbs
0 g protein
70 mg sodium
30 mg potassium

Immunity
0 calories
0 g fat
0 g carbs
0 g protein
10 mg sodium

Relax
0 calories
0 g fat
0 g carbs
0 g protein
10 mg sodium

"Ordinarily we eat enough protein, so this is not a problem, but after an overnight fast, not eating any protein for many hours—until dinner, for example—could limit the synthesis of these neurotransmitters," says Wurtman. "The carbohydrate, fruit, or vegetables are included to nourish you and make sure your body is getting enough calories and nutrients. The caffeinated beverage is important if you normally depend on it to make you awake and keep you that way. You don't want to fall asleep during your job interview."

When Should You Eat It? Eat your meal at least an hour or an hour and a half before the interview to make sure it is at least partially digested and its effects on your brain are in process.

How Much Should You Eat? Eat a moderate amount because you don't want to feel bloated or stuffed. Stay away from bulky vegetables because you don't want to feel uncomfortable.

Avoid These Foods: High-fat foods like butter, mayonnaise, cheese, and cream.

Why? Because they will make you feel muddleheaded and mentally fatigued. Avoid alcohol unless your interview is at a bachelor party.

At the Office

We spend almost 25 percent of our adult lives at work, and that in itself can easily become a diet trap for many of us who are trying to stay fit and trim. The workplace is a dieting minefield, with tremendous pressure and stress, food pushers everywhere, and bad foods lurking at every cubicle. It's a wonder that any of us can stay focused on our job, much less on our diet.

Declare a No Food Zone

Most of us tend to eat unconsciously at our desks, at the computer, or on the telephone. To combat these forces of diet destruction, set up a neutral territory where unhealthy food cannot be left out or stored. This safety zone might be no bigger than your own desk, but that's an ideal place to start.

Take It Off

Do you really think that keeping a bowl of candy on your desk is harmless? After all, a few pieces of candy that are 20 or 30 calories each couldn't really matter, could they? The problem is that those calories do add up. Research shows you eat more food when it's left out on your desk—more than twice as much as when it's kept behind closed doors. So keep all foods, including candy, out of sight. And keep apples, oranges, or other healthy snacks in your desk drawer for when a snack attack hits.

Make It Social

There's strength in numbers! Team up with a coworker determined to lose weight. An office diet buddy can provide you with emotional support and reminders. Walk together. Exchange recipes. Share information by taking turns looking up nutrition facts about a food you both like and help each other make better and more interesting choices.

Preapproved

Gather menus from all local restaurants, as well as convenient take-out and fast-food eateries. Then scan them for healthy foods. Narrow your choices to those that sound best. For instance, think grilled or baked chicken instead of chicken Parmigiana. Then call up to inquire how the dishes you've chosen are prepared. Don't be shy about finding out what you need to know. You might ask, "Will you make special orders? Is this dish fried? Is it cooked with oil or butter? Can you steam the vegetables or fish? What do you use to make the sauce? Can you prepare it without the cheese/sauce? Can you serve the sauce on the side? How many ounces is the serving of beef, chicken, or fish? Do you offer any other healthy choices that are not listed on the menu?"

Don't refrain from making special requests because you're embarrassed. You are the only one who will suffer. Just to make things simpler, I often tell the server that I'm allergic to certain foods. Remember, if you don't care for a particular food—say, Gorgonzola cheese on a Cobb salad—you wouldn't have a problem asking your server to leave that off. Once you compile your list of approved restaurants and your new healthy menu choices, you can be even more organized and create a phone or fax list of your top selections. Better yet, prearrange a delivery or pick-up time with a few places for certain days of the week. That way, you'll never find yourself so hungry that you scarf down a few slices of the stuffed-crust pizza your officemates just ordered.

Pack It Up

Because restaurant foods are usually higher in calories and fat, contain less fiber, and come in larger portions that encourage overeating, your best bet is to bring your own food to work. Plan and pack meals the night before. Make sure you also bring a few snacks to ward off hunger throughout the day. The hungrier you are, the more likely it is you'll lose control and make an "unhealthy" choice. Good lunch foods that are easy to prepare and travel well include sandwiches made with lean deli slices, peanut butter, or tuna on 100 percent whole wheat bread. Soups, nonfat yogurt, nonfat cheese, and cut-up vegetables are also great snack options. And don't forget plastic cutlery to keep you from wandering into the deli next door!

Chill Out

For $40 to $100, you can purchase a mini refrigerator to chill healthy foods, snacks, and drinks so that you're always prepared when hunger strikes. Fill it with fresh fruit, vegetables, whole-grain cereals, and/or breads, and nonfat dairy products to help "keep the adversities of the nutritional climate at bay." Store the fridge under your desk, right at your feet. Be careful not to overstock, because that could lead to overindulging.

Breathe Easy

Keeping your breath fresh can also help keep hunger at bay. This may not be great for everyone (frankly, it doesn't work for me), but I know people who dissolve a Listerine Breath Strip in their mouth or brush their teeth to help them overcome cravings and create a "just finished eating" feeling. It's worth a try! See if this helps you cut down on your desire to indulge in high-fat sweets. Invest in a spare toothbrush, paste, and holder to keep in your desk.

Set Rules

Many offices are breeding grounds for nibbling on foods just because they're available—from donuts and cookies, to pizza and homemade lasagna. But a nibble here and there can easily add up to more than a meal. To combat temptation and empower yourself, set some ground rules. If you give in just this once, and just that once, and just this once again, before you know it, you'll always be giving in. Instead, set strict limits. Tell yourself, "I will never eat foods others bring into the office." Or, "I will eat only foods others bring into the office on these days/occasions." Remember, an extra bagel and cream cheese on "bagel Fridays" can add an additional ½ pound per month!

If you are going to indulge, do *not* eat directly from the

bag, pan, or serving plate. That only makes it harder to keep track of how much you're eating.

Be cautious when participating in office lunches. They aren't always the healthiest foods, even if it's salad. Instead, bring your own lunch. That way, you'll have much more control over what you eat.

Vending Machines

Be wary of vending machines. They are designed to sell, and what sells most? Lots of calories, fat, and carbs. So if you have to choose something, pick nutrient-rich choices such as nuts or seeds, even though these options may be high in calories. In the end, you'll be much more satisfied and less likely to keep reaching for more.

Calorie Bargain Spotlight

Calorie Bargain: Balance 100 Calories Bars—Vanilla Caramel Crisp

The Why: If you enjoy energy bars, or you're looking to replace your daily candy bar, consider Balance Bar's new 100-calorie version.

The Health Bonus: There is the added bonus of calcium, protein, and 5 grams of fiber.

What We Liked Best: I was expecting it to be tiny but was surprised at the size—and the taste.

What We Liked Least: Look at the list of ingredients. Also, it's easy to eat too many.

The Price: $1.

Offerings: Chocolate Caramel Crisp, Vanilla Caramel Crisp, Peanut Butter Crisp.

Website: www.balance.com.

Where to Buy: drugstores, grocery stores, health food stores, www.balance.com.

Ingredients: soy protein crisps, soy protein isolate, tapioca starch, salt, maltitol syrup, inulin for fiber, brown rice syrup, oligofructose for fiber, fractionated palm kernel oil, maltitol, sugar, glycerin, butter, cream, salt, natural flavor. Less than 2 percent: nonfat milk, milk protein isolate, soy lecithin, reduced minerals whey, salt, erythritol, palm oil, milk, sodium phosphate, fish gelatin, carrageenan, beta-carotene, ascorbic acid (vitamin C), calcium phosphate, ferric orthophosphate (iron), vitamin E acetate, phytonadione (vitamin K), thiamin mononitrate (vitamin B_1), riboflavin (vitamin B_2), niacinamide (vitamin B_6), cyanocobalamin (vitamin B_{12}), biotin (vitamin H), calcium pantothenate (vitamin B_5), potassium iodide, zinc oxide, sodium selenite, chromium chloride, sodium molybdate.

Nutritional Analysis per Serving: 1 Bar
100 calories
4 g fat
16 g carbs
5 g protein
5 g fiber
180 mg sodium

Wedding Day

If you're the bride, you've probably spent the last six months starving yourself to fit into that expensive one-time-only dress, so, ideally, you'll need to eat something that will not send you into a tailspin and will help you feel calm and collected on your big day. You'll have plenty of time to hang out later with your husband and your good friends Ben & Jerry while sitting around watching *American Idol*. (Research shows that people gain an average of 6 to 8 pounds during the first two years of marriage.)

Objective: For the actual wedding day, you need to eat something that will be easy on your stomach. Lots of nervousness and emotion can build up when you're about to make that lifelong commitment.

Pick These Foods: Dr. Judith Wurtman suggests eating a substantial breakfast, such as scrambled eggs, toast, and juice; or yogurt and cereal; or fresh fruit, yogurt, and a low-fat muffin. Then, while you're getting ready, eat foods that are easily digested and bland: a banana or melon, plain crackers, cereal and milk, a nibble of some plain chicken, and maybe a small roll. Drink water so you will not be dehydrated.

Why? Breakfast may be the only meal you get to sit down and eat, and your body will appreciate having those calories. Once you start getting ready for the wedding, eat small snacks because you do not want to upset your stomach or feel bloated. The water is good because you may not have time to drink much once the wedding celebration begins.

When Should You Eat It? "Try to fit in your snacks during the preparation time, when your hair and makeup are being done," says Wurtman. Then have a member of your wedding party bring you something to eat after the ceremony while you are having your pictures taken. If you are too busy to eat, have some juice to get a few calories; you probably won't eat anything during the reception.

How Much Should You Eat? Only what feels comfortable, says Wurtman.

Avoid These Foods: Alcohol before you eat, or anything gassy.

Why? Alcohol on an empty stomach may make it even harder to control your emotions on this very emotional day.

Romantic Dinner for Two

If you're looking at a fifty-year anniversary dinner, you're probably fine, but if the romantic night is more along the lines of a first date, you might be a little nervous beforehand. Also, this is a time to impress your date, so you want to eat right (and properly).

Objective: to be calm and feeling good, debonair, funny, sexy, and not too hungry.

Pick These Foods: Eat a light meal, such as a small chicken sandwich or scrambled eggs and toast before you get dressed for your date. For your dinner, order foods that are easy to eat and don't require too much attention. Fish (so long as it doesn't have bones) is a good choice because you don't have to fuss with cutting tough meat or spending a lot of time chewing. You should be talking instead. Never order pasta; it's too messy. Same with salads—you risk dropping the lettuce on your lap. Nibble on some crackers or a piece of bread before the meal is served. Be careful about your alcohol consumption; drink water if your mouth is dry.

Why? Eating ahead of time will allow you to focus on your dinner partner and not on your hunger. Eating carbohydrates before the meal is served will calm you down, says Dr. Judith Wurtman.

When Should You Eat It? Eat your at-home meal about two hours before the date so you will be full. If you don't get to finish your entire meal at the restaurant because you're so busy talking, don't worry about it. You can eat a big breakfast the next morning.

How Much Should You eat? At the restaurant, eat about half of what is served; the portions are usually twice as large as anyone should be eating.

Avoid These Foods: Any high-fat foods like three-cheese pizza or nachos dipped in cheese sauce.

Why: They tend to make you feel sluggish.

Calorie Bargain Spotlight

Calorie Bargain: Kettle Bakes Potato Chips—Hickory Honey Barbeque

The Why: Kettle Foods is a company that takes pride in its ingredients and uses no artificial flavors or coloring or hydrogenated oils.

The Health Bonus: Compared with regular chips, Kettle Bakes Chips have 30 fewer calories. If you wouldn't ordinarily eat any chips, pretzels, or other snack foods, I wouldn't start eating these, but if you're looking for a substitution for chips, they are a good deal.

What We Liked Best: Although I'm not much of a chip lover, these really grew on me after awhile.

What We Liked Least: can be difficult to find in stores.

The Price: $2.99.

Offerings: Lightly Salted, Hickory Honey Barbeque, Aged White Cheddar.

Website: www.kettlebakes.com.

Where to Buy: Albertsons, Whole Foods Markets, Trader Joe's, Wild Oats Marketplace, Publix, Meijer, Kroger, H-E-B, Randalls, www.snackaisle.com, www.shopnatural.com.

Ingredients: select russet potatoes, expeller-pressed high monounsaturated safflower and/or sunflower oil, honey powder (evaporated cane juice, honey), salt, onion powder, tomato powder, paprika, yeast extract, torula yeast, chili peppers, garlic powder, citric acid, paprika extract, natural hickory smoke flavor (maltodextrin, natural hickory smoke flavor).

Nutritional Analysis per Serving: 1 Ounce
120 calories
3 g fat
21 g carbs
3 g protein
2 g fiber
160 mg sodium

Compare to similar products:
- Lay's KC Masterpiece Barbecue Flavor Potato Chips (1 ounce): 150 calories, 10 g fat, 15 g carbs.
- Stacy's Simply Naked Pita Chips (1 ounce): 130 calories, 4 g fat, 18 g carbs.
- Baked Lay's KC Masterpiece Barbecue Flavor Potato Crisps (1 ounce): 120 calories, 3 g fat, 22 g carbs.

Traveling

Whether you're traveling by car, plane, train, or boat, keep these tips in mind so you can stay on the road to wellness.

Plan Ahead

First, figure out what, where, and when you're going to eat on your trip. It may sound unromantic or tedious, but give it a try—it might actually enhance your dining and travel experience. Write a meal plan for yourself. Traveling is stressful enough, and you'll be amazed how liberating it is not to have to worry about food while you're on the road!

On the day you're traveling, be sure to eat a meal before you leave your home or hotel. Don't let yourself become ravenous; that's the quickest way to end up eating garbage foods. If you're on the road, pack nutritious snack foods such as individual servings of cereal, yogurt, raisins, fruits, or vegetables in resealable bags, or animal crackers. Wherever you're going, be sure to pack a water bottle. Traveling can be notoriously dehydrating, leading to a false feeling of hunger, dizziness, headache, or fatigue.

Dining Out

When you are in a new place, it's hard to know which restaurants to choose. Buy a travel guide to help you become familiar with some local eateries, or ask the concierge of your hotel what he or she recommends for healthy dining. Be prepared to be specific—there are varying degrees of what one might consider healthy. Don't be afraid to call ahead and ask the restaurant if it has healthy selections (look for menu items that are baked, grilled, steamed, or broiled). Even fast-food restaurants have healthy choices; take a look at their websites for nutritional information.

Another tip is to request a room with a kitchen when you book your hotel. This way you can actually make meals for yourself if you can't find any restaurants that suit your tastes or your healthy lifestyle. In fact, there are many hotels, such as Residence Inn, Extended Stay America, and Homestead Studio Suite hotels, where rooms with kitchens are standard, and they're reasonably priced.

Exercising without Your Gym

While a large number of hotels have workout facilities, there are many that do not. Call the hotel to find out if it has a relationship with any fitness clubs. If not, or if it can't recommend a nearby club, contact the local chamber of commerce. Additionally, the International Health, Racquet & Sportsclub Association (IHRSA) has established the IHRSA Passport Program to give members of participating IHRSA facilities (approximately 20 percent of all fitness clubs in the U.S. are members) guest privileges in more than 3,600 clubs worldwide, so ask your current fitness facility if it participates in

Calorie Bargain Spotlight

Calorie Bargain: Sensible Foods Crunch Dried Fruit and Vegetable Snacks—100% Organic Apple Harvest and 100% Organic Supersweet Corn

The Why: With just 70 calories per package, the salty Supersweet Corn is an excellent substitute for potato chips. If you're in the mood for something sweet, try the Apple Harvest.

The Health Bonus: These crunchy, dried treats by Sensible Foods are fat free and 100 percent natural.

What We Liked Best: One package is equal to a ½ cup of fruit, or one serving. Each bag contains only one serving, which will help you keep an eye on portion control.

What We Liked Least: a bit pricey.

The Price: $40.56 for twenty-four ¾-ounce bags.

Offerings: Orchard Blend, Tropical Blend, Cherry Berry, 100% Organic Apple Harvest, 100% Organic Supersweet Corn, 100% Organic Cherry Berry, Organic Crunch Dried Roasted Soy Nuts.

Website: www.sensiblefoods.com.

Where to Buy: company website.

Ingredients

Supersweet Corn
100 percent organic sweet corn, sea salt.

Apple Harvest
100 percent organic apples.

Nutritional Analysis per Serving

Supersweet Corn—1 Bag	**Apple Harvest—1 Bag**
70 calories	80 calories
1 g fat	0 g fat
17 g carbs	19 g carbs
0 g protein	0 g protein
3 g fiber	1 g fiber
190 mg sodium	115 mg sodium

this program. You can search for participating clubs at www.healthclubs.com.

If there are no gyms available, there are many exercises you can do in your hotel room, such as crunches, push-ups, wall sits, squats, and lunges. Pack a jump rope, resistance bands, water-inflatable weights, or workout tapes—these are easy to carry and provide a good workout without any professional equipment. For water-inflatable weights, visit: www.aquabells.com; for fitness videos, visit www.collagevideo.com.

When You're Flying

Flying is the most hectic, unpredictable method of travel. As a result of the increased stress, our rush-rush mentality, and poor planning, what we eat often ends up being the last thing we think about. How many times have you said, "I'll just eat something when I get there" or "I'll eat on the plane"?

It's that lack of planning that costs us when it comes to weight control. To make matters worse, airlines rarely provide meals these days, and because of tightened security, we're spending more time in airports, where most food choices aren't conducive to healthy eating.

So if we travel just five times a year and overeat by 2,800 calories each round trip (some pizza, a few sodas, a candy bar, or peanuts), that's more than 4 pounds gained every year. It adds up.

"Americans may think healthy and low calorie, but most of the time when they're traveling, it's a let's-splurge mentality," says Larry Meltzer, spokesperson for LSG Sky Chefs, one of the leading food service providers for most of the major airlines. If you want to make sure you're not the one overloading the plane, here are a few tips:

Bring Your Own

It seems like common sense to bring your own food so you don't get hungry. But people think they can make it without food, especially on short flights. Then when they end up getting hungry, they gobble the first doughnut or croissant they're offered. If you are carrying your own food, it's important to know that due to cabin pressure, the actual flavor of food changes, and your taste buds are dulled.

"That's why food has to be prepared differently for in-flight service," explains Meltzer.

If you add a bit more flavoring than normal, you should be fine. Food should be easy to carry, easy to reseal, hard to spill, and shouldn't require refrigeration.

Even if you ate before you left home, you are still going to get hungry. We often underestimate the amount of time a trip can take. A two-hour flight could mean four or five hours of travel.

"Travelers can take items from home, pick up food at a take-out restaurant, or avail themselves of the various options in airport terminals," advises Meltzer. Here are some ideas of what to bring:

- Water: Buy it after the security checkpoint to take on board. Dehydration can cause or exacerbate hunger, jet lag, and fatigue.
- Cereal: Kashi (a variety of healthy versions) and Cheerios are both portable, low-calorie choices.
- Beef jerky: Especially if you're a low-carb fan—but not if you're watching your sodium.
- Fruit: Apples, pears, and grapes are durable, and almost any fruit can be stored in a container.

- Rice cakes: Be selective, since calorie and fat content vary widely.
- Energy bars: Although they tend to be high in calories and fat, they often are better than a slice of pizza or a candy bar at the airport.
- Nonfat yogurt: Yogurt is a great portable snack, although it is perishable. You can pack a 3-ounce container or less in an insulated bag or take a small cooler, but understand that this can be counted against carry-on bag limitations.
- Sandwiches: Precut them into portion-controlled sections so you can pull them out at different times during the trip without making a mess. Chicken, turkey, cold cuts, and cheese (on 100 percent whole wheat bread) are all great options for sandwiches on the go.
- Soy chips: These are yet another portable, low-cal, high-fiber snack.
- Make sure to check with the Transportation Security Administration for the latest in-flight rules on bringing food and water: www.tsa.gov/travelers/airtravel/prohibited/permitted-prohibited-items.shtm#10.

The Best of the Worst

What happens when you get to the airport, you're hungry, and you have no food with you? Today most airport eateries have some healthy alternatives, including salads and burgers without buns or fattening condiments. Do your homework before you get to the terminal.

Most airports have websites that list the restaurants in each terminal so you can decide in advance where you'll eat. If you don't want to do the research, find a place with salads. Most are pretty healthy and low in calories, but beware of the dressing. With sandwiches, get in the habit of asking "Does this have mayo or any spread on it?" Mayo seems to sneak in everywhere these days, and at 100 calories per tablespoon, leaving it out is an easy way to save calories.

According to Susan Bush, concession stand manager at Kennedy International Airport in New York City, the airport requires all terminal food service operators to provide take-out service. Try a takeaway salad with dressing on the side, sushi, or a sandwich (with the unhealthy condiments on the side), all of which can be stored in your carry-on bag.

Just recently, I arrived at JFK Airport at six in the morning without breakfast. I went up to the food court and asked if they could make an egg white omelet using a cooking spray. I was shocked that the answer was yes. Ask for healthy food; you might be surprised.

Buy on Board

Many airlines have eliminated complimentary food service for coach flights under four hours and have started buy-onboard programs.

Generally speaking, there is some complimentary food service if your flight is longer than four hours, which means you might be stuck with no choice but to eat what is served. No matter how long your flight is, always ask the specific details of the food served when you make your reservation and keep these tips in mind:

Request a special low-calorie meal ahead of time. Request this at the time you purchase your ticket (even if it's an e-ticket) or call ahead. If not available, ask which meal comes with salad.

Learn to recognize the healthy (or least-unhealthy) option.

Eating after Dark

I'll confess: Snacking after dinner is one of my longtime eating behaviors. I kick back, watch a movie, and eat. Apparently, I'm not alone. According to Kelly C. Allison, PhD, a researcher in the Weight and Eating Disorders Program at the University of Pennsylvania School of Medicine, people generally eat about 10 percent of their daily intake (roughly 200 calories) after their evening meal. Those with Night Eating Syndrome consume 25 percent or more of their calories after dark. However, those who are overweight probably eat way more than 200 calories. Maybe there's something to the "don't eat after eight" diet.

The problem is that most people are able to restrict what they eat and resist their favorite high-calorie foods during the day, but "they allow themselves a treat at night, usually salty or sweet foods," says Allison.

Why Do We Eat after Dark?

"It's partly because we have time at night. We're not at work or busy taking care of the kids," explains Ruth Striegel-Moore, PhD, professor of psychology at Wesleyan University. Other primary causes: depression, sadness, anxiety, loneliness, or boredom. "Plus we're at home, in close proximity to food," says Allison, "whereas during the day, we may have to go through more trouble to obtain food."

Eat during the Day

Delayed eating is not helpful. All it does is create a desire to overeat later in the day. "Eating regularly is recommended because it helps maintain energy," says Dr. Striegel-Moore, adding that eating at night will only start a vicious cycle of shifting food intake toward the evening. Eat breakfast and at least two healthy snacks during the day.

Let It Pass

When you think you want a snack at night, ask yourself, "Am I really hungry, or is it something else?" Distract yourself for a few minutes, and the craving may pass. Try drinking a big glass of water or another low-cal liquid.

Break the Pattern

Are you tired, bored, lonely, or just snacking out of habit? If you're tired, go to bed. If you're lonely, call a friend. If you're bored, get busy. Learn to play an instrument, write letters, clean your house, paint your nails, surf the Internet, play with your kids, take a bath, or read a book. Or do something active after-dinner, such as going for a walk or a bike ride or taking tennis lessons.

."We can learn to feel hungry at set times or in set circumstances," says Striegel-Moore. Cravings can become a routine: Just as you might feel tired at night because you usually go to bed, you might feel hungry at night because you usually eat then. If you make a conscious effort to stop eating at that time and come up with alternatives, after awhile that hunger pattern could go away.

Be Prepared

Eating at night in moderation can be OK. In fact, an after-dinner snack is pretty normal. The problem arises when we overdo it and eat a pint of ice cream instead of the half-cup serving recommended on the package. So come up with five different low-calorie "replacement" snacks you enjoy and keep them readily available. For instance, if you normally choose nachos and cheese, replace them with baked pita chips and salsa for a similar snack that's lower in calories. Make sure these are substitutions you like and can live with in the long run.

Pre-Portion Your Snacks

Try premeasuring a reasonable, smaller serving of your favorite food and eating only that amount. Put away any leftovers before you start to eat, and never eat directly out of a bag or box.

Snack Consciously

According to the *British Medical Journal*, people tend to "forget" the snacks they eat that are high in calories, fat, and carbs. So pay attention to your snacks, especially if you're eating them in front of the TV or computer or at the movies.

Out of Sight

Don't keep food in the house that's hard to resist. Stock your fridge with healthy snacks, such as veggies and fruit, that won't leave you feeling guilty. Research from the University of Illinois shows that if a snack is within sight and easy to reach, you are going to eat it. When candy was six feet away from office workers, as opposed to right on their desks, they ate less of it. If you have a snack attack, and there is only good stuff around—well, that's probably what you'll eat.

Close the Kitchen

Once dinner is over, wash the dishes and turn off the lights. Come up with other techniques that signify the end of your meal, like having your favorite cup of coffee or a mint.

Brush Your Teeth

This doesn't work for everyone, but some people find that food is less tempting when they have minty-fresh breath. Plus, the thought of having to repeat the whole process may be enough to discourage you from eating.

Other Tips

- Eat only at the kitchen table. Consider all other areas of your home snack-free zones.
- No munching while on the phone, computer, or while watching TV!
- Serve all snacks on plates—make it formal. No picking while standing in front of the fridge or in the kitchen.

Acknowledgments

This book has been a long-time passion, and I have many people to thank for helping me finally bring it to fruition.

First, I would like to thank Amy Previato for her dedication, loyalty, and unyielding commitment to getting this book in working order. She is just amazing. Next, I would like to thank Kelly Frindell for her late-night manuscript and column reviews; Sarah Amer, M.S., R.D. for her diligent fact checking; and my literary agent, Farley Chase, for believing in the idea from the start and pushing to make this book a reality. Danielle Friedman, who was instrumental in producing, editing, and everything else that needed to get done—on this project as well as on *The Diet Detective's Count Down*. And last, but not least, Judy Kern, for her constant assistance and wise remarks that always managed to keep my writing in order, especially when it's out of order.

About the Author

Charles Stuart Platkin, J.D., M.P.H., is one of the country's leading public-health advocates, whose syndicated nutrition and fitness column, "The Diet Detective," appears in more than 165 daily newspapers across the country. Platkin is also the founder of the health and fitness network DietDetective .com, which offers thousands of original articles, bloggers, health tools, quizzes, interviews with leading health experts and celebrities, Calorie Bargains (food/beverage and health product/service reviews), a detailed food nutrient search engine with more than 10,000 foods, podcasts, a nutrition and weight-loss program, and a thriving online community.

He is the founder of the Institute for Nutrition & Behavioral Sciences, a nonprofit organization that conducts obesity-related research. He received his undergraduate degree from Cornell University, a Juris Doctorate from Fordham University, and a Masters in Public Health from Florida International University. He is also a certified personal trainer and is currently completing his Ph.D. in Public Health. He is an adjunct professor at the Robert Stempel School of Public Health at Florida International University in Miami.

Platkin is also the founder of Integrated Wellness Solutions, and the author of four books, including *Breaking the Pattern* (Plume, 2005) and *The Diet Detective's Count Down* (Fireside, 2007).

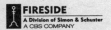